GOVERNING HEALTH AND CONSUMPTION

Sensible citizens, behaviour and the city

Clare Herrick

First published in Great Britain in 2011 by

The Policy Press
University of Bristol
Fourth Floor
Beacon House
Queen's Road
Bristol BS8 1QU, UK
t: +44 (0)117 331 4054
f: +44 (0)117 331 4093
tpp-info@bristol.ac.uk
www.policypress.co.uk

North American office:
The Policy Press
c/o The University of Chicago Press
1427 East 60th Street
Chicago, IL 60637, USA
t: +1 773 702 7700
f: +1 773-702-9756
e:sales@press.uchicago.edu
www.press.uchicago.edu

British Library Cataloguing in Publication Data
A catalogue record for this book is available from the British Library.

Library of Congress Cataloging-in-Publication Data
A catalog record for this book has been requested.

ISBN 978 1 84742 638 3 (hardcover)

Cover design by The Policy Press
Front cover: photograph kindly supplied by Clare Herrick
Printed and bound in Great Britain by TJ International, Padstow

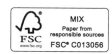

Contents

List of figures, tables and maps

Figures

Tables

Maps

Acronyms

AHRSE	Alcohol Harm Reduction Strategy for England
APS	Active People Survey
BBPA	British Beer and Pub Association
BMI	Body Mass Index
BRFSS	Behavioral Risk Factor Surveillance System (US)
CAMRA	Campaign for Real Ale
CDC	Centers for Disease Control (US)
CDZ	Controlled Drinking Zone
CGF	Clinical Governance Framework
CHD	coronary heart disease
CMO	chief medical officer (UK)
CSR	corporate social responsibility
CVD	cardiovascular disease
DAAT	Drug and Alcohol Action Team
DCMS	Department for Culture, Media and Sport (UK)
DEFRA	Department of the Environment, Farming and Rural Affairs (UK)
DfES	Department for Education and Skills (UK)
DCLG	Department of Communities and Local Government (UK)
DH	Department of Health (UK)
DHHS	Department of Health and Human Services (US)
DoT	United States Department of Transportation
DTLR	Department of Transport, Local Government and the Regions (UK)
DWP	Department for Work and Pensions (UK)
EFS	Expenditure and Food Survey (UK)
FDA	Federal Drug Agency (US)
FPH	Faculty of Public Health
FSA	Food Standards Agency (UK)
GHS	General Household Survey
GNR	Great North Run
HSE	Health Survey for England (UK)
LIDNS	Low Income Diet and Nutrition Survey (UK)
MF	*Men's Fitness* (magazine)
MPRE	mass participation running event
NAO	National Audit Office (UK)
NCC	National Consumer Council
NCD	non-communicable diseases
NDNS	National Diet and Nutrition Survey
NHANES	National Health and Nutrition Examination Survey
NHS	National Health Service (UK)

NICE	National Institute for Clinical Excellence (UK)
NPAOP	Nutrition and Physical Activity and Obesity Prevention Policy
NSF	National Service Framework (UK)
NSMC	National Social Marketing Centre
NTE	night-time economy
ODPM	Office of the Deputy Prime Minister (UK)
PCT	Primary Care Trust (UK)
PHO	Public Health Observatories (UK)
SHA	Strategic Health Authority
T2D	Type 2 Diabetes
PRD	Parks and Recreational Department (Austin, Texas)
PSA	public service agreement
RCP	Royal College of Physicians
TDHHS	Texas Department of Health and Human Services
TfL	Transport for London
WHO	World Health Organization
UNOSP	United Nations Office for Sport and Development
USDA	United States Department of Agriculture
VCS	Voluntary and Community Sector (UK)

About the author

Clare Herrick is Lecturer in Human Geography in the Cities Group, King's College London. She undertook her PhD at University College London and has held visiting scholar positions at the University of Texas, Austin, the National University of Singapore and, most recently, the University of Cape Town. Her research critically explores the intersections of risky health behaviours with urban space, political ecologies and contemporary governance strategies.

Acknowledgements

This book has been a pretty long time in the making. As is common among those having recently completed PhDs, the idea of translating a thesis into a book is enough to send chills rampaging through even the most diligent of graduates. Suffering from a bout of a similar illness, I set about delaying the inevitable and instead seeing if some of the bigger questions that have always fascinated me about the governance of health pertained to a series of other realms of unhealthy lifestyle choices. For this, I thank the Royal Geographical Society for supporting the research on alcohol in London and also the receipt of the Jasmin Leila Prize in 2008. The British Academy supported the work on physical activity and urban regeneration, and the Economic and Research Council funded my PhD research on obesity; I thank them both.

Writing a book has been harder than writing the original PhD thesis ever was and I am incredibly indebted to a number of people for helping me see it through. First, I would like to thank Professor Matthew Gandy for being a better PhD supervisor than even the UCL handbook ever imagined possible. His patience, support and intimidating intellect have always been a source of inspiration. Dr Nicola Shelton has consistently been of great intellectual and personal support and I thank her for her immense input into my PhD and continued friendship.

Throughout the multiple phases of fieldwork that have made this book possible, there have been many people that have made the process easier and better by always conveying an infectious enthusiasm for their work. In particular, I would like to tank Kim Bandalier at the Texas State Department of Health and Lyn Davis at Steps to a Healthier Austin. Kirsten Gray was my guide and mentor in Texas and my constant hankering after some decent bbq is all her fault. I also thank Richard Nerurkar at the Great Ethiopian Run for his time and insight into the ways and means of mass participation events. While I could not include any sustained commentary on his event in this book, the work that he has done in creating one of the most incredible races I have ever attended can never be praised highly enough.

Finally I would like to thank my colleagues, family and friends. In particular Mike Raco, Rob Imrie, Emma Street and Katie Jones as well as the rest of the Cities Group at King's, who have always provided enormous support for some of my more unusual research ideas. I am also grateful to the geography departments at UCL and QMUL for allowing me to come and talk about my fledgling book ideas at departmental seminars and for the helpful comments from attendees. Last but never least, my friends, brother and parents always listen patiently to me talking about my work, for which I thank them greatly. But, for his supreme patience, boundless enthusiasm, love and support, I cannot express my gratitude to my husband David deeply enough.

ONE

Introduction

In 2006, the UK's Health and Safety Executive carried out what it termed a 'sensible risk debate' as a direct response to growing public fears that government intervention in private decision making had reached excessive and, in many cases, simply untenable levels. Action had been catalysed by then-Prime Minister Tony Blair's 2005 speech to the Institute for Public Policy Research in which he set out the UK's commitment to placing the theme of better regulation at the heart of its 2005 European Union presidency term. Stating categorically that 'we cannot eliminate risk, we have to live with it, manage it', Blair also acknowledged that within public service, 'the idea that it is the job of government to eliminate risk can lead to the elimination of common sense'. In a language that seamlessly combined the work of liberal governmentality theorists (Valverde 1998: 7; Dean 2007) and the concern with 'self-efficacy' by cognitive psychologists of public health (Bandura 2004); the ensuing debate aimed to determine where the 'sensible balance' lay between ensuring public protection and guaranteeing personal freedom and autonomy (Nuffield Council on Bioethics 2007). When set against a backdrop of what has been branded an emergent 'risk culture' of a 'kind of perpetual uncertainty' (Dean 2007: 66), such keen government interest in the appropriate management of those 'fine-grained risks and the balance of probability' (Blair 2005) has opened up space for a consideration of what it might mean to be 'sensible' in the face of new and emergent risks, especially those linked to the contested and under-explored realms of consumption and behavioural choices expressly linked to (healthy) lifestyles. This is the chief concern of this book.

The demise of Blairite politics in 2010 and the ascension of the Conservative–Liberal Democrat coalition have done little to dampen this debate in the UK. The 2010 White Paper Healthy Lives, Healthy People reiterated this governance tension:

> The dilemma for government is this: it is simply not possible to promote healthier lifestyles through Whitehall diktat and nannying about the way people should live. Recent years have proved that one-size-fits-all solutions are no good when public health challenges vary from one neighbourhood to the next. But we cannot sit back while, in spite of all this, so many people are suffering such severe lifestyle-driven ill health and such acute health inequalities. (Department of Health 2010: 2)

While the UK debates the appropriate role of the state in crafting healthy outcomes, on the other side of the Atlantic, the passing of President Barack Obama's Healthcare Bill through Congress in early 2010 has ensured that personal health behaviours are now deeply political. While risk may be an inevitable and essentially unavoidable part of everyday life, *managing* individual risk behaviours raises important questions concerning the limits to free choice and where the duty and burden of care to protect individuals and wider society from harm must be placed, raising, in turn, ethical, political and policy contentions. This is particularly pertinent in the case of those behaviours identified as posing marked challenges to public health. Indeed, the recognition that 'many of the choices that affect our health . . . are choices we make as consumers' (Department of Health 2004a: 19) demonstrates that managing or governing risk is inextricable from the wider market context within which decision making is both made and given meaning. Moreover, and as geographers have expressly identified (Kearns 1991, 1993; Macintyre et al 1993, 2002; Kearns and Gesler 1998; Gesler and Kearns 2002; Kearns and Moon 2002; Cummins et al 2007), the enterprise of governing health risks is also inextricable from the broader socio-spatial contexts from which such risks emanate, are shaped, given meaning and, ultimately undertaken. Thus, this book also aims to contribute to the broadening canon of work within the subdiscipline of health geography, where the politics of health practices are figured as existing in complex recursive relationships with places. As such, in speaking and writing about health, geographical perspectives offer up valuable spatial insights that, in the examples explored in this book, aim to deepen our understanding of the contemporary urban condition.

As Offer (2007: 74) contends, societal prudence does not necessarily follow societal affluence, and, instead, 'novelty tends to produce a bias towards short-term rewards, towards individualism, hedonism, narcissism and disorientation'. The tension generated by the freedom and necessity to consume and the concomitant risks cultivated by doing so in ways cast as 'irresponsible' or 'uninformed' consequently mark out numerous behavioural domains – including eating, drinking, inactivity, smoking and sexual activity – as peculiarly and particularly problematic. These causes have been taken up with varying degrees of alacrity at a range of spatial scales, from the local to the global. At each of these levels, the multi-tiered and complex structures of governance in the multiple agencies and departments charged with public health improvement offer especially fertile ground for prescient empirical research on the management of the three 'risk behaviours' that have been chosen as the core focus of this book: eating, drinking and physical (in)activity.[1] In this way, this book follows Petersen and Lupton (1996: ix) in its foundational belief that 'in contemporary Western societies the health status and vulnerability of the body are central themes of existence'. Health is all-pervasive, however unhealthy we may or may not be, and it thus demands and commands our attention.

As rates of obesity and the multiple elements that constitute the category known as 'alcohol-related harm' climb year on year in the UK (Cabinet Office 2004; Department of Health 2004a), inculcating sensible eating, activity and drinking habits has become a key cross-governmental priority. However, while the empirics of such governmental programmes have been subject to consistent critical attention, relatively little weight has been given to how those 'risks that people face [that] are dealt with by individual choices and market interactions' (Select Committee on Economic Affairs 2006:7) are reworked through and by the construction, definition and deployment of what might be considered 'codes of sensibleness'. While part of the broad suite of governmental tools and techniques aiming to create a healthier populace, these codes of sensibleness present distinct points of contrast with those mechanisms of government that encourage the development and exercise of qualities such as 'informed choice' (Hunter 2005; Clarke et al 2006) and 'personal responsibility' (Minkler 1999; Guttman and Ressler 2001). These concepts have courted considerable attention in social science, especially in relation to what has been termed the 'new', prevention-oriented public health (Lupton and Peterson 1996) and New Labour's 'Choice Agenda'. However, this book argues that the admonitions and expectations placed on ordinary citizens to 'be sensible' underpin both the aspirations of informed choice and personal responsibility and should also, therefore, not be discounted. Indeed, to underplay the potency of the term 'sensible' is to miss a fundamental governmental aspiration at a time of proliferating risks: that it is possible to normalise 'sensible' approaches to risky behaviours without jeopardising the present and future health of the economy. Such assertions thus merit further exploration, not just for what behaving sensibly might reveal about the complexities and contestations contained in the wider regulation of unhealthy behaviours, but also for what it might say about how we might think in a better way about risks and risk taking in (neo) liberal economies in general.

Therefore, in contrast to the attention devoted to conceptualising and critiquing the governmental rhetoric and tools of 'informed choice' and 'personal responsibility', this book takes a step back to examine the fundamental assumption undergirding the conditions of the tools' existence. The first assumption is that people can and will apply common sense to act in reasonable, rational, wise and proportionate ways; the second is that these can be defined, measured and communicated. As a consequence, this book asks what it is to be sensible and, consequently, why such a thoroughly mundane character trait must not be discounted as simply 'unproblematic' and therefore unworthy of scrutiny. Instead, given the degree to which the belief that sensible behaviour can mitigate the risks of obesity, alcohol-related harm and sedentarism has now infiltrated policy discourse and practice, it would seem logical to explore the workings of this empirically. Asking what being sensible means in practice necessitates exploring how those stakeholders charged with mitigating the effects of certain behaviours go about trying to create revised social relationships to risk and, as a consequence, the unavoidable tensions, conflicts and negotiations that form part of these efforts. In so doing, and by focusing on a series of relevant examples from both the UK and the US, it is hoped that this book will offer a novel and comparative perspective on the governmental drive to create healthier, more productive, engaged citizens.

In order to achieve this, the book is structured around three key arguments that are woven throughout the chapters and revisited in the conclusion. The first asserts that personal responsibility and informed choice may be discursive bedrocks of neoliberal health policy, but the relative influence of people's circumstances or 'luck' has received far too little attention. Given that to be sensible, people need to be able to overcome the effects of their (bad) luck, how responsibility is ascribed is both a thoroughly moral as well as practical question. Geographical circumstance or fate present a direct challenge to this moralisation by both undermining the possibility of responsible action and assigning culpability for irresponsible lifestyle choices to the inanimate realm of the environment, charting the porous boundary between what is theoretically possible and what is practically plausible. Public health is perhaps at the fore of this debate as its complex web of political, economic, moral and medical exigencies means that optimal healthy outcomes are not always compatible with the demands of the neoliberal market economy that so often works directly against aspirations of sensibleness.

The second argument builds on the first and posits that the call for sensible behaviour emerges from the need to manage tensions internal to many neoliberal economies – balancing self-restraint and self-indulgence; coercion and freedom; supply and demand – in a manner that produces socially acceptable types and degrees of regulation. The need to tread a plausible middle ground between regulating risk and permitting the choice needed to optimise market functioning is contested particularly in the context of health. In short, eating, drinking and exercise represent distinct market opportunities. However, such opportunities (in the shape of innovative techniques for increasing volume sales) also present clear health risks (through increased calorific or alcohol consumption). The food and alcohol industries have thus been roundly criticised for their instrumental roles both in creating the kind of chronic poor health that this book critically explores as well as in offering up solutions to the negative externalities of their products and actions. At root, therefore, the realm of being sensible remains an under-theorised and empirically sparse field that offers great potential to shed light on the seeming inability (or unwillingness) of government to address a range of societal and political economic concerns that interlock with health.

Third, the book argues that, with personal lifestyle choices now accepted as having a complex array of negative externalities, encouraging sensible lifestyle choices has become a tool in a range of public policies that extend far beyond public health. As such, the drive to govern lifestyle has melded public health with an array of spatial governance agendas ranging from crime, disorder and social inclusion to urban planning. This conceptual assertion is most potently and effectively demonstrated through the three examples of eating (unhealthy, to the point of obesity), drinking (hazardous or harmful quantities of alcohol) and inactivity; all interlocked domains of behavioural choice that require the delicate management of supply and demand in order to produce optimal health outcomes. These risk behaviours must therefore be conceptualised as part of a wider system of governance 'in the name of health' that has distinct moral and ethical implications, rather than as discrete social, economic or health problems. Thus, in charting the drive to be sensible, this book will also chronicle the increasingly amorphous nature of health governance in late modern society.

To digress briefly, this book sprang from my own curiosity about how what we might call 'codes of sensibleness' have become an inescapable element of the ways in which not just our health but our lives are governed. I am a fairly sensible person by any account: I eat well, exercise regularly and drink in a quasi-moderate way on a pretty regular basis. I believe that, by and large and for the majority of the time, I sit comfortably in the realm that might be broadly defined as 'sensible'. Yet, somehow, I remain particularly averse to the term and all that it stands for. I just don't want to be seen as sensible even though my own self-interest welcomes the range of benefits that this prudence brings: lower insurance premiums, the trust of others, and infrequent visits to Accident and Emergency to name but a few. I don't think that I am alone in my lifestyle choices. I also believe that the majority of people either are sensible or genuinely consider that they are sensible. Yet, such faith in the public's intentions seems controversial when we are constantly confronted by hyperbolic media reports to the contrary and associated reactionary policy responses. Sensible behaviour is not far from the norm, but really *is* the norm for most people. Yet, because unremarkable behaviour is not a particularly enthralling spectacle, it is rarely the issue that concerns us. Rather it is those singular and collective deviations from the norm that have come to occupy the minds of the vast array of actors now concerned with the governance of health behaviours. It is therefore the process by which such deviations become deviances that interests me. When and why did eating, drinking and being inactive suddenly become so bad and in such a uniquely emotive and urgent way? Tudge's words are thus particularly emblematic of such emotive appeals:

> Over-nutrition, and all that follows from it, should be seen as a disaster . . . Death comes early and horribly, with amputated limbs and blindness brought on by diabetes. And what is it all supposed to be *for*? Drunks may die early, but some of them at least have some riotous times on the way. Before the days of antibiotics, syphilitics traditionally died early too, but they presumably had some fun. But to endure such morbidity for burgers and coke? It makes no sense at all. (Tudge 2004: 111)

While I am not necessarily in agreement with his forceful assertions, I do think that they serve to highlight why this work is significant and timely. In essence, the debate about sensible behaviour is one that, on a theoretical level, operates at a population scale. However, in reality, it is underpinned by stark judgements about personal behavioural choices based on a presumed correlation between demographic, socioeconomic, geographical or educational characteristics and decision making (including the *capacity* to make decisions). Being sensible is therefore not merely about being healthy, it is also about acting in predictable, rational and categorisable ways. It is thus a debate about people, their similarities and differences and must consequently be unpicked in order to avoid punitive moral judgements over personal choice. It is for the simple reason that the ability to exercise choice is unevenly distributed between people and places, and that these differences are often judged as evidence of personal failure rather than stemming from broader structural barriers, that this work is important.

Chapter overview

Chapter Two examines the conceptual significance of the term 'sensible' and explores it in relation to the irrevocable tension between freedom and coercion that characterises the government of liberal societies (Valverde 1998; Joyce 2003; Dean 2007). Being sensible, it is argued, sits at the precarious fulcrum of the need to invest in and engage with the market as consumers while at the same time identifying and managing the negative externalities of such consumption choices. As such, this fulcrum sits uneasily within theoretical and empirical ethical, political, ideological and policy concerns. The chapter argues that maintaining this delicate balance between self-indulgence and self-restraint require the creation and deployment of what this book terms 'codes of sensibleness' – or, in other words, expected, socially normative behaviours – and that these can be defined, measured, rationalised and communicated within policy and beyond. Furthermore, while these codes may be generated through an adherence to regularised definitions of acceptable levels of risk exposure, this is far from an exact science. Instead, the injunction to be sensible in relation to behavioural choices is filtered through distinct socio-spatial frames of reference that, in turn, redefine the parameters of sanctioned behaviours. Put another way, being sensible as a tool of governance is given relevance not just by *who* is acting, but *where* these actions are taking place. As a consequence, space itself should start to be considered as a means though which risky behaviours can be shaped and corralled and, in the process, as a vehicle to shape a particular form of sensible citizenry.

The third chapter explores the intensification of governmental attention on the realm of personal behavioural choices in the context of health in the UK over the last 20 years. It examines this in the context of the mounting tension between behaviouralist and environmentalist perceptions of risk. It asks how public perceptions of risk feed into techniques of behavioural governance that are fraught with tension and uncertainty about where attention and resources should be directed. The chapter therefore examines the increasingly hazardous nature of everyday life and the UK government's changing response and stance towards this. In essence, individual risk taking through lifestyle choices (for example smoking, unsafe sex, drug taking and drinking) is plagued by numerous contentions: of correlating cause and (definitive) effect; of the habitual nature of risk taking (and therefore its normalisation); of the inequitable distribution of its negative consequences; of the inability to compute the long-term and cumulative nature of certain health effects; of the perception that risk taking can be controlled adequately by individuals; of a persistent lack of trust in those assuming the burden of managing those risks; and of the role of poor-quality environments in imposing constraints on behavioural choices. As a result, exercising

–

common sense, or being sensible has emerged as a pragmatic attempt to try and neutralise the conflict between the public realms from which both market and environmentally/structurally generated risks emanate (for example alcohol supply within the broader temptations of the night-time economy) and the private realms within which behavioural decisions are fashioned and undertaken (for example the home). This need to balance the public with the private has raised inevitable questions about the degree to which the state should and can intervene to mitigate the health risks caused by, for the most part, behaviours that are otherwise socially sanctioned.

Chapter Four claims that the act and aspiration of sensible behaviour serves three strategic roles in the governance of what has been hyperbolically termed the 'obesity epidemic': first, as a collective and personal risk mitigation strategy; second, as a means by which to overcome individual and geographical luck; and third, as a driver of growth within the political economy of food and leisure. In order to ground and contextualise these assertions, the chapter first explores the contrasting rhetorical and policy stances towards obesity in the two case study countries, dwelling on the controversial new vision of public health set out in late 2010 by the UK's secretary of state for health, Andrew Lansley. Moving on from here, the chapter turns to an exploration of the contested aetiological explanations for the rise in population-scale obesity prevalence. Given that epidemiological studies concerning the individual risk factors for obesity underpin the logic and enterprise of prevention efforts, the profound uncertainties in obesity research need further consideration in order for us to think through how obesity is framed as a 'problem' and thus consider the potential social, cultural and moral ramifications of the solutions proffered. In so doing, the chapter also critically unpacks the very notion that we are in the midst of an obesity epidemic and instead argues that obesity represents multiple and situated "epidemics of signification" (Treichler 1988). Building from this, the chapter then turns to the three assertions in order to explore the strategic role that sensible behaviour places in both the politics of obesity and the political economic demands of the neoliberal state.

The fifth chapter explores the rapidly expanding canon of work examining the 'obesogenic' nature of urban environments and the ways in which this epistemology crosscuts efforts to create an incidentally sensible city. The turn from the behavioural to the ecological framings of health offer up very different readings of risk and responsibility and thus warrant further empirical and conceptual attention. As such, the chapter examines the conflicting body of evidence concerning the causal relationships between the environmental determinants of health, body mass index (BMI), physical activity and nutrition. It questions the consistencies, limitations and generalisability of such studies when transferred across into the pragmatic realm of obesity prevention policies and interventions. Given that concern with the environmental determinants of health cuts across a wealth of urban policy agendas, it is hardly surprising that health is now a measure of the 'good city'. The recent trend of ranking cities based on a host of factors such as liveability by publications such as Business Week and Human Resources company, Mercer, now extends to their citizens' relative fitness or fatness. Trite as this may seem, such league tables not only demonstrate the methodological complexities of measuring the environmental determinants of health, but they also serve as an impetus to actions that might improve collective 'city' fitness. The chapter then turns to two empirical examples from the US and UK to question the ways, means and effects of the endeavours to create an *incidentally sensible* populace by focusing on the environment, rather than behavioural change. To illustrate this, the Steps to a Healthier Austin (Texas, US) programme is considered before we turn to the example of active travel promotion in London. In so doing, the chapter not only teases out the practical limits to creating a sensible city, but also explores the ways in which spatial and social differences and features become elided in obesity prevention efforts.

With sport now being cast as a solution to a range of social, economic, health and urban-related ills, Chapter Six explores the contentious role played by mass participation running events (MPREs) in achieving these aims and fostering, in the process, a lucratively sensible city. MPREs blend commercial means with the ends of mass participation to achieve a unique mix of profit and healthy lifestyle promotion. However, within public health circles, opinion remains divided as to whether they are an appropriate vehicle for catalysing sports participation in any sustained way. In order to explore this, the chapter first examines the ways in which sports participation is measured, defined and delineated and, therefore, how it becomes the benchmark against which MPREs are judged. After detailing the nature and characteristics of MPREs, the discussion turns to the example of Austin's proliferation of events and Newcastle's major event – the Great North Run – in order to think through the discrepancies between the rhetoric and reality of MPRE participation in these two very different cities.

Chapter Seven explores the ways in which drinking epitomises the deeper paradoxes of consumption, especially in the UK. On one side, drinking alcohol has been a normal component of Northern European culture for hundreds of years; on the other, those drinking behaviours deemed excessive or irresponsible have long been subject to scrutiny and moral judgement with episodic variations in intensity. At present, drinking is being subjected to an exceptionally intense degree of governmental attention due to its chronic and acute health effects, its evident impact on the social (dis)order of town and city centres and its recent inclusion in the World Health Organization's (WHO) global health remit. After setting out the ways in which alcohol is now deemed to be problematic and why, the chapter moves onto a critical analysis of the ways in which individual consumption choices have been corralled by a flurry of experts, groups and organisations into a series of tightly defined, but uniquely contentious, risk parameters. These parameters lay down what it is to be sensible in relation to drinking and have, therefore, taken on powerful political salience in the ongoing struggle to curb the nation's drive to drink.

Moving on from the definition of sensible behaviour in relation to alcohol, Chapter Eight explores the rise and rise of London's night-time economy as a particular example of the potentially risky environments within which individuals are being asked to regulate and modify their own behaviour. Just as with the food economy, London's night-time economy – composed of the nation's largest selection of bars, pubs and nightclubs – is now an important element of the city's broader economic success (Hadfield 2006). Over the past two decades, the landscape of London's leisure industry has changed beyond all recognition and, with this, so have the consumption habits of those who frequent the city's diverse range of night-time entertainment venues. Beyond the issues raised by the commodification and commercialisation of the night-time experience, changing drinking environments also raise associated questions of how these may problematise existing codes of sanctioned behaviour. Indeed, with the conscious efforts to create the '24-hour city', or to encourage 'café culture' through licensing reform, the ways in which people drink and, therefore, the risks associated with these practices, have inevitably altered. London therefore provides an exemplary backdrop in discussions of recent machinations to invoke sensible drinking in the UK through spatially targeted strategies. These include legislation for controlled drinking zones (CDZ) and designated public place orders (DPPO) that effectively render certain behaviours (such as having an open alcohol container) in defined spaces subject to fixed-penalty fines or, for persistent offenders, prosecution.

The final and concluding chapter recapitulates the central theoretical contentions of the book and examines the contrasts and comparisons between its case studies. In so doing, it sets out five key findings of this work and, moreover, reflects on what might be learned from bringing into analytical conversation a series of risk behaviours that are usually considered in isolation. It is argued that the 'siloed' thinking so prevalent in government work around health is unsurprising given the disaggregation of health risks into discrete work bundles or strategies. Instead, there needs to be greater recognition of how risk behaviours interweave and their composite influence on wellbeing and urban quality of life. This compartmentalisation also often has the effect of undermining the ability to think through what problematisations of health may reveal about place and, therefore, the indications it can give as to how best to refashion space in order to mitigate risk. The research also demonstrates the overwhelming influence of a few motivated and empowered individuals. The question, however, remains as to whether this influence is being harnessed in the most productive way possible as, particularly in the case of MPREs, missed opportunities tended to be the norm rather than the exception. Two interrelated final points contend that there is a blurring of the line between public and private responsibilities for health and, thus, more attention should be paid to the interaction of political economy and health behaviours. To do this will mean interrogating the practices of industry by working *with* key players and, in so doing, developing a critical vantage point that sheds light on the geographically entrenched and embedded nature of health risks.

A brief methodological note

This book is the product of three conceptually interlinked, but nonetheless distinct, research projects exploring the current ubiquity of injunctions to be sensible and to act sensibly in the lifestyle domains of eating, drinking and exercising. It also aims to make these three projects speak to each other in both empirical and theoretical terms. As such, it is also representative of particular moments in time, with reflections on the data necessarily influenced by a period of great political change in the UK in the wake of the 2010 general election.

The first of these projects was my doctoral research on the comparative biopolitics of obesity in London and Austin, Texas. The rationale for the choice of these seemingly incongruous case study cities was the expositional value presented by *exceptional* 'thin' spaces in otherwise 'fat' environments. To clarify, both cities have lower rates of obesity than the national and regional average; a situation that raises the simple question 'why?'. The 2008 Behavioral Risk Factor Surveillance System (BRFSS) survey data suggest that the US has an average obesity rate of 26.7%, the state of Texas 28.9%, while Austin (Travis County) is a more modest 22.5%. The 2008 Health Survey for England (HSE) finds that the obesity rate in England is 24.5%, while the 2006 HSE data boost shows that London has an average rate of 16.5% (Coyle and Fitzpatrick 2009), with marked differences in rates between boroughs and between inner and outer London. The two cities are exceptionally useful examples in that they have been at the fore of developing and implementing local-scale obesity prevention strategies. They therefore provide a valuable resource for looking at what Evans (2006) calls 'anti-obesity policy' and, related to this, the wider questions of how the built environment and the social have become interwoven in questions of health improvement. The empirical material for Chapters Four and Five is drawn from this research, which was undertaken in 2005–7.

The second project came from a Royal Geographical Society small grant to explore the conceptual and substantive links between the governance of obesity and alcohol, this time using London alone as a case study. This research sought to map out qualitatively the parameters of the alcohol control debate at a national policy scale and at a local authority level, drawing on three central London boroughs (Islington, Camden and Westminster) and two outer London boroughs (Harrow and Croydon) as specific case studies. In addition and recognising the centrality of the alcohol industry to the alcohol control debate, interviews with key players in alcohol production, retail (for example, on-trade) and trade associations were also conducted. In so doing, the project critically explores the complex governance of alcohol as an issue of both public health and public order that necessitates regulating the intersections of personal behaviour, spaces of consumption, the legislative environment, retailing and social mores concerning drinking. This research forms the basis of Chapters Seven and Eight and is further elaborated later on.

The third project, funded by the British Academy from 2008 to 2009 and explored in Chapter Six, investigated the emergent relationships between physical activity and the city as seen through the lens of MPREs, with Newcastle and the Great North Run as the project's case study. Such events have seen a huge surge in popularity since the 1970s, when Fred Lebow reformulated the New York Marathon to take in all five boroughs (it had previously been laps of Central Park), attracted sponsorship, permitted women entrants and thus dramatically increased the inclusiveness of the event. Since that time, not only have marathons mushroomed across cities of the Global North and, in the past decade, the Global South, but they have been joined by a host of mass participation events of lengths ranging from one kilometre to ultra marathons. A host of commercial ventures and charitable organisations have become entwined with the enterprise and rhetoric of health improvement through sporting participation. These events, therefore, highlight points of intersection between the commercialisation of sport and public health and, as a result, serve as a useful vehicle to explore the conjoining of urban improvement objectives with a faith in the potential of sport to address social and societal problems (Sport England 2007, 2008a; UNOSDP 2008). Sport and physical activity are now at the heart of the will to induce a sensible population as an inducement to social and cultural capital accumulation, economic growth, social inclusion, active citizenry in order to make and shape 'better places' and thus they merit closer scrutiny than they have, thus far, enjoyed. The precise methods undertaken in these three projects are further explored next.

In the first instance, all three research projects draw on descriptive statistics from health survey, census and consumption survey data at a variety of spatial levels in order to contextualise and reinforce the book's conceptual arguments. In the UK, the HSE 2004 and 2007/8, the UK Census (2001), the National Diet and Nutrition Survey (NDNS) 2002, the Expenditure and Food Survey (EFS) and the General Household Survey (GHS) have been used to gauge fruit and vegetable intake (as a risk factor for obesity), body mass index and alcohol consumption habits. The Active People Survey (APS) (2005–10) administered by Sport England has also been drawn on to provide data on baseline activity levels in a variety of geographic places. In addition, the new Department for Communities and Local Government (DCLG) Place Survey has also been used to ascertain public attitudes towards local environments (for example crime and disorder, active engagement through volunteering and perceptions of drunk and rowdy behaviour). Where discussions turn to the US, the surveys chosen were the BRFSS, the National Health and Nutrition Examination Survey (NHANES) and the US Census (2000). These open-access data sets together provide a basis for understanding the demographic and socioeconomic composition of the case study area (and how this compares to the rest of the country) and lifestyle habits (such as physical activity, nutritional intake and alcohol intake) as well as more general data about self-reported health status, insurance coverage and increasingly important measures of attitudes towards place of residence.

Second, the three projects share a common grounding in a thorough critical discourse analysis of key national, regional and local policy documents pertaining to obesity reduction and prevention, alcohol control and physical activity promotion strategies. Policy discourse analysis has been recognised as an effective method for critically approaching the role of language in politics and political constructs through tropes such as narratives, framing and metaphors (Hajer 1995; Kearns 1997; Lawrence 2004; Hajer and Versteeg 2005). Moreover, in thinking through the text and its situation in multiple sociospatial contexts, an analysis of the discourse provides a potent constituent of any methodological armoury designed to investigate the governance of health, wellbeing and behavioural decision making. It therefore provides a conceptual framework from which to tease out the rhetorical foundations of political language. This insight is central to the arguments presented here as the will to create a sensible populace operates across numerous registers and domains within and beyond government. Thus, in practical terms, at each of the three stages of the research, the policy landscape was first mapped (for example, in the key institutional actors, networks and domains of responsibility) before a detailed policy document search was undertaken. This had the twin aims of ascertaining the temporal development of policy rationale and the conceptual shifts in the delineation of obesity, alcohol and physical activity, respectively, as a problem and, related to this, the techniques proposed to ameliorate emergent or existing situations of individual, community and societal risk. This discourse analysis helps to constitute the core arguments presented in this book and is consequently interwoven throughout the chapters which follow.

In order to augment the quantitative data and discourse analyses, and to make them speak to the sociopolitical realms within which this work is situated, semi-structured stakeholder interviews were conducted across all three research projects with a variety of stakeholders. For the doctoral research, a total of 80 interviews were conducted in London and Austin with those involved in the governance of obesity. In order for the research to be comparable, stakeholders were chosen from five key groups of actors: the departments of health/public health bodies, other central government departments with an identified role in obesity prevention, local government, non-profit organisations/charities/activist organisations and the 'consciousness industries' (advertising, marketing, PR agencies and think tanks). These groups reflect the diversity of stakeholders engaged in the enterprise of preventing further rises in obesity in the two countries and also, interestingly, underlie the reason why the joined-up thinking and governance that many deem essential to really tackling obesity as a public health issue remains an optimistic thought. The second project, on alcohol control, involved interviewing 30 stakeholders from primary care trusts (PCTs), drug and alcohol action teams (DAATs), local authority licensing committees, the police, trade associations, the on-trade (for example PubCos) and alcohol producers. The third project, on physical activity, drew from a smaller pool of 15 interviews with a similar array of local stakeholders from local authority leisure services, PCTs, regional development authorities, local MPs, tourist offices and the race organisers. In each case, interviewees are identified by their domain of employment in the text, rather than their name. This allows the reader to get a sense of the context of the interviewees' words without compromising their identity.

In all three cases, interviewees were recruited through various methods, with pre-selection guiding the initial choices and sequential sampling later being used (Curtis et al 2002). Potential interviewees were initially identified from policy document authors, local authority key contacts, investigative work to identify corporate contacts, working group members or relevant non-profit groups, and they were contacted via email explaining the research and asking for their input. As is common practice when recruiting interviewees, initial contacts proved to be an invaluable resource in helping to find informative stakeholders for later interviews. Such sequential sampling methods, as Curtis et al (2002) point out, are an effective way of allowing the choice of interviewee to evolve alongside the development of theory induced from the data as they are collected and analysed. It should also be highlighted that such sequential methods bring rewards, but also frustrations, as a point inevitably emerges when all contacts start to lead to the same person, whose door remains stubbornly shut, blocking off potentially illuminating interview material. A point also arises when new opportunities for interview contacts become harder and harder to come by as interviewees suggest people that have already been contacted. This process happened at a disarmingly fast pace in London and demonstrates that although the stakeholders charged with governing obesity, drinking and physical activity are, in theory, many and varied, in reality they remain a relatively small and insular group of experts.

This work uses a variety of sources to examine the governance of obesity, alcohol and physical activity, of which interview material is a substantial component. However, the choice of interviewees deliberately reflects only one side of an incredibly multifaceted debate. This research draws on the opinions and expertise of those endeavouring to govern and/or have a role in a governance debate that is defined by its propensity to use sensible behaviour as a point of practical and conceptual navigation. This inevitably means that, across all three projects, the voices of those subject to these techniques and rationales of governing health behaviours have been consciously omitted. The research therefore deliberately sought the opinions of those governing at the expense of those they are rendering governable for two reasons. First, to incorporate the individual voices of those citizens marked out as obese, harmful/binge drinkers or physically inactive and therefore subject to the wide array of interventions identified and discussed in this work would stray from the path laid down by the book's concern with the governmentalities reflected in the drive to create a sensible population. The voices of, for example, obese bodies are often silenced or marginalised by those claiming to be acting in their 'best interests' and there is an existing wealth of literature critiquing this tendency from social science, activist and feminist perspectives (Orbach 1978; Klein 1997; Gilman 2004). Given that obesity, drinking and physical inactivity are deeply entwined with health inequalities, there is also a substantial body of literature from a rights-based perspective that examines the effects of poverty, race and marginalisation on health (Farmer 1993, 1997, 1999; Pickett et al 2005; Wilkinson 2005). The second reason for the omission of 'the governed' as interview subjects was due to the author's own subject position; an issue that crosscuts other methodological critiques and therefore warrants further attention.

Researchers do not and cannot always research subjects that have a personal relevance or linkages to them. For example, while feminist studies of gender roles and positions are overwhelmingly conducted by women, not all studies of racial identity are conducted by those from the same ethnic background as the researched. Such distance between the position of the researcher and the researched inevitably raises questions concerning the ability and right to speak for and about others. Just as with many types of identity politics, fat activists tend to decry the overwhelming number of 'underweight', white public health officials deciding what policies are in their best interests (Wann 1999). They criticise the ability of the non-obese to understand the challenges faced by those who are overweight or obese and also suggest that this lack of understanding is accompanied by a lack of real empathy, often reflected in overly paternalistic policy decisions. While this is not such an issue in alcohol research and, even less so in physical activity research, there is still a remaining question of empathy and the ability to speak for others. As an example, the highest rates of obesity in Austin and London are found among minority ethnic communities and those on low incomes. Therefore, questions of racial and class differences confound the ability to speak about and for others. This was an issue repeatedly encountered in the process of research, although more frequently during periods of reflection than during interviews themselves. With the exception of four interviewees, none was obese and the overwhelming majority were white. This was not a conscious sampling method (indeed it would have been impossible to deduce the physical appearance of an interviewee from their name alone), but rather reflects the demographic and class profile of those in the position of making, reacting to or implementing public health policies. For example, in Texas, there is a clear divide between the non-Hispanic whites working in public health and their large 'high-risk' Hispanic target population. The divide is less marked in London as, despite the fact that ethnic monitory groups such as Bangladeshis are identified as particularly 'at risk' for obesity, their numbers do not begin to approach those of Hispanics in Austin.

Drinking and physical activity pose fewer issues. However, there remains a significant disparity between those charged with addressing alcohol-related harm and the nature of the high-risk groups (for example those delineated and popularly understood to be young 'binge drinkers' and those dependent on alcohol). In most cases, though, there was a shared understanding between the author and interviewees that drinking has both positive and negative effects; that drinking habits change throughout the life course, but that the risk of alcohol-related harm was greatest among those already rendered vulnerable by poverty. Discussions of physical activity were perhaps the least contentious, but interviewees were keen to stress that the middle-class concern with exercise as a route to moral and physical self-improvement highlighted by a number of authors (Gillick 1984; Glassner

1989) was not a belief shared, understood or relevant to all. While being able to identify with those about whom you are writing can help provide a unique insight and depth of analysis, it is also interesting to note the manifold ways that other outsiders negotiate and reconcile their own differences with those they are charged with governing in order to find the most efficient and equitable solutions to current public health challenges. This outsider status and navigation is acknowledged throughout this book.

On a final critical note, this research raises questions concerning personal biases, experiences and general perspectives on the issues of personal autonomy, rights and health. Obesity and alcohol have been subject to such media attention in recent years, not just because of their potential cost to the state in terms of healthcare and lost productivity, but also because evidence of rising rates of overweight, obesity and binge/hazardous drinking among certain groups raises ethical questions about who has the right to good health, about education, the duty of a host of actors towards children, ongoing class divides, about how and what we consume, cultural and ethnic differences and about the right of the state to intervene in individual lifestyle choices and realms of personal freedoms. Naturally, with such an array of ethical concerns in the background, this research has uncovered and required the negotiation of my own personal biases, experiences and opinions in relation to rights, autonomy and health. The starting point for this research was that obesity, drinking and physical inactivity represent distinct biomedical risks that need to be mitigated. The questions of how and why such risks have become bound up within a broader governmental project of creating sensible citizens need to be subject to greater critical interrogation.

Note

[1] The core empirical focus of this book is on eating, drinking and physical activity. This is not to disregard or underplay the significance of sexual health and smoking to the broader debates explored here. There can be little doubt that sexual health and smoking are at the very core of governmental agendas for behavioural change as well as exemplifying the persistent tension between moderation and excess that characterise the 'citizen–consumer'. There is a wealth of literature on sexual health and smoking and, rather than adding to this, this book instead aims to elide discussions of those behavioural realms that have, in isolation, tended to dominate the public debate. Eating, drinking and physical activity are contentious domains alone, but when considered together as part of a broader drive to engender a sensible citizenry, they are exceptionally useful in conceptual terms.

TWO

Being sensible

Introduction

Health is essential to individual, social and economic wellbeing. For this reason, it is central to political wellbeing or, put another way, political viability. Political success is increasingly being judged against public health parameters; the intensely divided reaction to the Obama administration's passing of the Health Bill or the emotive debate over ringfencing the NHS budget in the UK's 2010 general election are clear cases in point. As such, any examination of health goes straight to the heart of the rationalities, modes, tools and techniques of liberal governance that have been so ably explored by governmentality theorists in sociology, law, anthropology, accountancy and, most recently, geography, across a range of empirical contexts (see in particular Osborne 1997; Crampton and Elden 2007). This chapter therefore starts from the assertion that health is vital for what it tells us about the governance of individuals and society and, as a consequence, what the enterprises of governance reveal about those individuals and societies. In exploring how and why we are governed by and through health, we also uncover the ways in which space and place have become instrumental to these endeavours – a critical conceptual undertaking in the health geography perspective that underpins this book (Kearns 1993). Space and place are increasingly part of the weaponry called on to achieve the kind of sensible citizenry needed to undertake the inherently intricate task of ensuring the optimal functioning of the neoliberal project, while also managing the well-documented negative externalities. In order to explore these assertions, this chapter and that one that follows present and examine the book's core conceptual thesis and its central objectives. In so doing, they make a case for why an exploration of the overlooked realm of sensible behaviour offers a novel perspective from which to analyse health, its governance, the settings within which this takes place and the subjects who are made by these interlocked discourses and practices.

To this end, this book is grounded in three contentions:

1. Personal responsibility and informed choice are the discursive bedrocks of neoliberal health policy, but the relative influence of people's circumstances or 'luck' has received far too little attention. Given that, in order to be sensible, people need to be able to overcome the effects of their (bad) luck, the ascription of responsibility is both a 'moral enterprise' and a practical problem. Geographical circumstance or fate present a direct challenge to this moralisation by both undermining the possibility of responsible action and

assigning culpability for irresponsible lifestyle choices to the inanimate realm of the environment.

2. The call for sensible behaviour emerges from the need to manage tensions internal to neoliberal economies – balancing supply and demand, self-restraint and self-indulgence, coercion and freedom – in a manner that produces socially acceptable types and degrees of governance. Ensuring health thus requires risk management in the name of optimal market functioning. In other words, being sensible involves the application of a personalised risk calculation in pursuit of risk minimisation. This process also creates new market opportunities. Thus, sensible behaviour becomes a field of mediation between these neoliberal tensions, sparking a host of innovative market and policy fixes to optimise health outcomes without alienating consumers and avoiding the need to intervene in the supply of risky goods and services.

3. With personal lifestyle choices now accepted as having a complex array of negative externalities, encouraging *sensible* lifestyle choices has become a tool of a range of public policies that extend far beyond public health. As such, the drive to govern lifestyle has melded public health with an array of spatial agendas ranging from crime, disorder and social inclusion to urban planning, which in turn have recast the value and utility of health in distinctly spatialised terms. In so doing and through invoking the language, logic and practices of behavioural and cultural change, it has also fundamentally reworked the popular image of those living in places deemed at 'high risk' of obesity, irresponsible drinking and physical inactivity.

This chapter will focus on the theoretical underpinning of the first two contentions, while Chapter Three will introduce the empirical focus of this book before expanding on the third contention. Here 'governance' is understood as 'the institutionalized political compromises through which capitalist societies are negotiated' (Heynen and Robbins 2005: 6). Nettleton further elaborates that these compromises function at the 'levels of political rhetoric, institutional practice and individual conscience' (1997: 213). Contemporary public health challenges thus offer remarkable insights into the conceptual and practical tensions at the heart of these institutionalised compromises and their negotiation across a range of scales, domains and geographic settings. An exploration of these tensions also brings their contextual constitution into sharp relief. In other words, in examining why it consistently proves so difficult to produce sensible citizens predisposed to healthy lifestyle choices, much is also said about the interrelation between specific spatial, social and political economic settings.

This book thus aims to meld two theoretical standpoints. The first is health geographers' concern with 'the processes of putting health into place' (Gesler and Kearns 2002: 1), where place is understood as having both materiality and meaning. This expansive notion of health goes beyond the biomedical (Parr 2004) to undertake what (Brown and Duncan 2002) have termed a 'critical geography of public health'. The second viewpoint is the perspectives and frameworks offered up by Foucault's governmentality thesis and its later adherents (Rose 1996; Rose et al 2006; Miller and Rose 2008; Dean 2010) as a route by which to start to unpick, bit by bit, the practices involved in creating a sensible citizenry. This body of work, which geographers Kearns and Reid-Henry have usefully termed a 'sociology of possibility' (2009: 554), focuses on analysing the 'rationalities, techniques, goals and identities formed in the practices that seek to guide the conduct of oneself or others' (Dean 2007: 83) in particular 'zone[s] or space[s] of governmental intervention' (Osborne 1997: 176). Yet, as Dean further argues, it is essential to examine the points of disjuncture between the rationalities of government and their effects (or the 'logic of practices'); as Kearns and Reid-Henry assert, 'possibilities are not everywhere and for all people the same' (2009: 555). It is thus the messiness of the sites where ideology, aspiration and everyday realities clash that this book seeks to explore. In so doing, it also hopes to speak to a burgeoning interest among a diverse array of social scientists about governance *of* and *through* health.

This chapter proceeds in two stages. First, it approaches contention one through a critical exploration of the twin concepts of personal responsibility and informed choice in the context of risky lifestyle choices. Neoliberal economies require both the exercise of personal responsibility and a shared belief in its potential in order to function effectively. Related to this, there is a large volume of work charting the entwined development of neoliberal ideologies and the politicisation of responsibility in the context of health (Clarke 2005). Informed choice is inextricable from personal responsibility, given that individuals are rendered responsible for seeking the information necessary to make choices and for understanding the consequences of their choices. As such, the contractual role of government becomes one where choice is offered *on condition* of the exercise of responsibility. This has been particularly marked in the UK with the ascendency of New Labour's much-criticised 'Choice Agenda' (see Jordan 2005, 2006), but has also been a central feature of other neoliberal economies such as the US, where 'workfare' policies have consistently and often painfully highlighted the very partial nature of 'choice'.

Contention two expands on this theorisation of sensibility – or the ideology and state in which being sensible is possible, practicable and desirable – by exploring the ways in which these injunctions highlight some of the core tensions inherent in neoliberal economies and societies. In turn, these tensions then help illuminate why obesity, drinking and physical activity have obtained such political currency. Reducing the risk of chronic disease effectively means leading our lives in a continual state of balance between the need and desire to consume induced by affluence and the necessity to mitigate the negative externalities of such consumption through the exercise of self-restraint or what Offer (2007) has termed 'commitment'. In theory, self-restraint seems antithetical to the optimal functioning of the economy (given that it should involve a rejection of consumption). Yet, the market in self-restraint has proved to be exceptionally lucrative, with a raft of products and services catering to the consumption of self-denial. While much has been written about the diet, exercise and self-help industry, especially in the context of rising rates of obesity, there has been little attention paid to the broader 'enterprise of sensibleness'. This is expressly concerned with managing risks while permitting the coexistence of choice and, as a result, now delineates the parameters of the present debates over the plausibility of behaviour and cultural change in relation to obesity, alcohol and exercise. The second section of this chapter will therefore examine how health risks are increasingly choreographed in the context of market economies with a keen eye for profit.

This provides the bedrock for the detailed discussion in the next chapter of the empirical examples that form the substantive core of this book, setting out why they are of key significance in any discussion of the governance of health, people and places. Obesity, drinking and physical activity have emerged as national policy priorities for almost all developed countries and are increasingly afflicting countries of the Global South (Yach and Beaglehole 2004; Yach et al 2005a, 2005b, 2006) as they face a punitive 'epidemiological transition' from an infectious to a chronic burden of disease (Omran 1971). As examples, they hold huge conceptual power for their ability to shed light on the three contentions at the heart of this work. The third contention is key in this respect, for these lifestyle diseases and the politics that encircle them have fundamentally shifted the ways in which spaces and places are now conceptualised. The rash of work stemming from Egger and Swinburn's (1997) notion of the 'obesogenic environment' has been crucial in this respect. However, there has also been a great deal of interest in the spatial governance of the night-time economy (see in particular Jayne et al 2006) and the ways in which measures to encourage physical activity are also now thoroughly entwined with the refashioning of space (Sport England 2008b; Herrick 2009a). This interweaving of the physical and behavioural realms will be discussed in depth in Chapter Three. Health is inextricably geographical, not just in the uneven spatial patterning of wellbeing and illness, but for what health 'maps' onto geographical settings. In short, it is through examining health that we can shed new light on the nature, meaning and significance of places and place making, and this book aims to do that.

Responsible, sensible citizens

> Because of the centrality of lifestyles, risk taking and other individual choices in determining health outcomes, health policy cannot avoid the need to give careful and critical attention to personal responsibility for health. This is, however, a minefield in which we must proceed with caution . . . the appeal of the notion of personal responsibility masks an ideological vulnerability that is ripe for exploitation. (Wikler 2002: 55)

Tracing responsibilisation

The 2009 NHS Constitution asks Britons to recognise that they 'can make a significant contribution to [their] own, and [their] family's good health and well-being, and take some personal responsibility for it' (NHS 2009: 9). Health and responsibility rarely venture out unaccompanied by each other because individual lifestyle choices condition the risk of chronic disease. Wikler highlights this: 'at the population level, it is increasingly clear that individual choices – "healthy lifestyles" – are at least as significant in achieving good health outcomes as costly medical interventions' (2002: 47). As he also avers in the earlier quotation, health policy is now thoroughly embroiled in philosophical debates concerning the limits and expectations of responsibility, not least as the very concept of responsibility is ideologically malleable and thus vulnerable to appropriation. This vulnerability has courted academic interest, but there remains huge scope to extend and deepen these discussions to a comparative study of lifestyle diseases and behaviours. To do this requires attention to the genesis of such thinking.

This is not the place to rehearse a brief history of neoliberal epistemology, which has been amply covered elsewhere (see Harvey 2007 for an excellent treatise), but it is important to consider the development of what might be termed 'responsibility in choice narratives' in the context of health. The politicisation of lifestyle represents a relatively recent shift in health and social policy, and one that can be traced back to the 1974 report *A New Perspective on the Health of Canadians* by the Canadian minister of national health and welfare at the time, Marc Lalonde. In it, he explicitly outlined the role of 'adverse environmental factors and behavioural risks' that meant that the health care system was acting as a 'little more than a catchment net for the victims' (Lalonde 1974: 4, 5). The paper outlined the Canadian government's commitment to addressing the four broad and interrelated 'health field' concerns of human biology, environment, lifestyle and a well-financed health care system in order to 'add life to our years' and ensure 'economic and social justice' within the dictates of neoliberal welfare state deregulation. From this point, not only was the complex volitional and situational aetiology of chronic diseases outlined, but so was an ideological framework for mitigating and managing the risks associated with individual and collective lifestyles.

Notably, the paper recognised that 'there are national health problems which know no provincial boundaries and which arise from causes embedded in the social fabric of the nation as a whole' (Lalonde 1974: 6). In order to address these problems the government proposed to offer the necessary 'protection, information and services' by which Canadians could become 'partners with health professionals in the preservation and enhancement of their vitality' (ibid: 6). This working paper was viewed by some as seminal in that it proposed that attaining 'vitality' was not just a task for health care professionals, but rather required multi-agency collaboration, reflecting the complex multifactoral aetiologies of so-called chronic 'lifestyle diseases' (such as type 2 diabetes, certain cancers and liver disease). The

---

conclusion that 'future improvements in the level of health of Canadians lie in improving the environment, moderating self-imposed risks and adding to our knowledge of human biology' (ibid: 18) reflects the idea that health is governed by a complex interaction of active choices and factors over which individuals have no control. This, in turn, marks a significant change from an essentially passive biomedical model where disease risk was seen as lying extraneous to the body, to the active (and therefore theoretically controllable) risks of lifestyle choices.

This early turn to 'responsibilisation' in health also signalled the elision of moral judgement with hopes for autonomous decision making. While health and morality have long been entwined, the application of the neoliberal logic of financialisation means that immorality in decision making now comes with a quantifiable cost, thus layering personal responsibility with marked political and economic significance. As Osborne writes, 'a neo-liberal government acts directly on health by giving the ideal of health a series of surrogate values, entailing a sort of constructivism of goals and targets intended to bring about strategically limited objectives'(1997: 181). As such, when morality – as judged through health outcomes – is given a surrogate value, human life itself is reconfigured and rationalised along these surrogate-defined lines. In short, in response to the 'indeterminacy of health policy' (as evidenced by this discussion of the limitations of ascribing responsibility), neoliberalism 'constructs the possibility of its strictly de-limited determination' through 'surrogate variables that will stand measure for otherwise abstract ideas of health' (Osborne 1997: 185). Sensible behaviour in relation to eating, drinking and physical activity is a clear example of such determination and in this way opens up questions about the worth of surrogate values (for example BMI, binge drinking and physical activity uptake rates). These questions will be revisited in Chapters Four to Eight.

This book is concerned with how the aspirational politics of a responsible, informed citizenry (Raco 2009) is often exercised through the language and practices of sensible behaviour, reinforced by a move towards theories and techniques of behavioural and cultural change (see Cabinet Office 2004, 2010) in order to effect changes in health outcomes. However, before critically approaching this policy realm, it is first necessary to question how responsibility is theorised, before asking how it is applied to the behavioural realms explored in later chapters. From Lalonde's early vision of a prevention-oriented health care system aligned to the individual and personalised nature of chronic disease aetiology, we have now moved to a situation where health outcomes require careful moral ascriptions of social and individual responsibility and, with this, culpability. In this circumstance, people are figured as 'monads of conduct' rather than 'agents passive before power' (Osborne 1997: 175) with distinct ramifications for how their actions are rationalised. However, it is also essential to think through how personal responsibility itself is theorised, especially when the expectation of an 'active society' (Etzioni 1968; Gass 1988; Dean 1995) where individuals are called on to be 'entrepreneurs of their health' (Osborne, 1997: 181) is now so normalised in policy. This logic is embedded, for example in the Wanless Report (Department of Health, 2001), in its calculation that by 2022 it would cost £30 billion more to manage the 'unengaged' than a more cost-effective 'engaged' population.

Personal responsibility is conceptually inescapable, but is still not entirely comfortable among social determinants of health theories as both sides hold wildly disparate philosophies. As Schmidt rightly argues, 'appeals to individual responsibility generally do not sit easily with a social determinants perspective, for it is all too easy to "victim blame" people in disadvantaged positions by holding them responsible for factors that are beyond their control' (2009a: 137). This raises the question of the degree to which actions are voluntary and, therefore, the extent to which people have the kind of choices that neoliberal economies have been so forthcoming in promising (Department of Health 2004a). Kearns and Reid-Henry's recent (2009) exploration of 'vital geographies' is instrumental here. In taking neo-Foucauldian accounts of government to task for focusing too much on the ways in which the *capacities* of life are being maximised by the application of novel technologies, they open up a more fruitful discussion of the role of 'geographical luck' in *limiting* life. The theory of 'luck egalitarianism' has received little attention from geographers, despite its centrality to ascribing and delineating the boundaries of personal responsibility of interest to health geography. This omission must therefore be addressed before returning to Kearns and Reid-Henry's interpellation of the geographic and asking where this leaves a health policy torn between recognising the social determinants of health and the unwelcome minimisation of responsibility that this stance promotes.

Luck egalitarianism, responsibility and lifestyle diseases

Philosophical analyses of responsibility make a distinction between forward-looking (prospective or consequentialist) and backward-looking (retrospective or causal) views. In the first, individuals are held responsible for choices they *will make* or their obligations. In the second, they are held accountable for choices *already made* or their accountability. The contention consequently centres on the degree to which individuals have the capacity to choose or whether this is constrained by their circumstances. Offer suggests that neoliberal rhetoric may push notions of freedom and choice, but in reality such societies do not represent anything like a 'paradise of personal discretion' (2007: 357). This is particularly salient to the preventative turn in public health, where people are expected to act of their own volition to avert or at least reduce the risk of future poor health. In turn, this is premised on a particular view of the role of the health care system itself. The liberal contractual view of society asks that we consider what obligation the state has to its citizens and, therefore, what reciprocal duty they have to the state. However, it also considers that this obligation is mediated by responsibilities to both oneself and others. To luck egalitarians, those voluntarily causing their own or others' ill health should be held accountable for the consequences of such decisions. In contrast, those whose 'luck' or circumstances cause them to become ill should benefit from a policy of redistributive justice. Luck egalitarianism is thus a choice-orientated view of responsibility and is of particular salience to any empirical examination of the neoliberal health experience.

As Feiring contends, 'theoretically there has been a shift in the general idea of equality of opportunity from the traditional ideal of equality of condition to an ideal of equality that incorporates responsibility by compensating individuals for unequal circumstances while holding them responsible for their choices' (2008: 33). Yet, luck egalitarianism, for all its laudable redistributive aspirations, is often criticised for being too harsh a stance, for being unclear about the plausible extent of personal responsibility and the clear difficulties in disentangling choice from luck (Vincent 2009). To this I would add that the difficulties inherent in identifying clear patterns of causality for chronic health outcomes means that delineating where responsibility lies is endlessly problematic. As Vincent contends, 'we face epistemic barriers in trying to ascertain the degree of . . . responsibility' (2009: 42). The examples of obesity, drinking and physical activity highlight these epistemic barriers in action by bringing to the fore the conceptual and pragmatic limitations of ascribing responsibility to behavioural realms where circumstance so often impedes choice. For, even where people are deemed to have made irresponsible choices, this does little to mitigate their effects. If personal responsibility is 'the cost of freedom' (Roemer 1993) or the cost of exercising our free will, then this cost is also borne out in ascriptions of culpability for freedom's more negative outcomes. These play out in markedly different ways for obesity, alcohol and physical activity and these examples serve as a potent vehicle for a critical return to the concepts of equality, luck, responsibility, risk, choice and culpability.

From the personal to the social to the geographical

It is fair to say that 'not all choices leading to illness are counted alike'. Moreover, 'those that are targeted tend to be sins (sloth, gluttony, lust to use their old-fashioned names) or to be behaviour (such as drug addiction) of the marginalised' (Wikler 2002: 52). It is unsurprising therefore that academic consideration of personal responsibility in the context of health has often been very much focused on an empirical consideration of the culpability of particular actions – whether it is substantively the same to take responsibility for your body weight as it is for your alcohol intake. This is further complicated by the political context:

> In political debates, the argument on the left is typically that individuals cannot be held responsible as external constraints (socio-economic status, access to healthcare etc) thwart responsibility ascriptions, whereas the right generally takes a 'get real' view according to which the environment matters, but ultimately people are seen as free agents, aware and hence accountable for the consequences of their actions. Consequently, the argument about holding people accountable seems to turn mainly on proving, in an either-or fashion, that individuals are responsible (or not) for particular actions. (Schmidt 2009b: 23)

The adjunct to the debate on personal responsibility asks where *social* responsibilities lie, a notion that clearly invokes questions about the role of consequences and context. This version of 'luck' goes beyond biological predisposition or fate and centres on the relationship between structural inequality, political economic disparities and environmental justice and health. As Schmidt argues:

> Since health is affected by both personal behaviour and factors generally beyond immediate individual control (socio-economic status, access to healthcare, infrastructural arrangements etc) it is neither an exclusive matter of personal nor of social responsibility. As the element of personal control admits of degree, conceptually, personal responsibility also needs to admit of degrees. By necessity, health responsibilities are therefore *co-responsibilities*. (Schmidt 2009a: 24)

This co-responsibility between individuals and the multiple parties that represent the governance field cannot be considered without thinking through what locational fate or 'geographical luck' (Kearns and Reid-Henry 2009) might contribute to the personal responsibility/choice debate and, therefore, what it also says about the admonition to be sensible. Geographical luck challenges the philosophical foundations of the personal responsibility agenda, principally because it demeans freedom of choice and provides an antidote to moralisations of behaviour. In this case, the question becomes one of proportionality and, thus, where choice might reasonably be considered to exist within a broad constellation of responsibilities. Vincent perhaps sums up this complexity best in that 'responsibility is more of a "syndrome" than it is a single concept, or, put another way, there is not just one single concept which answers to the name "responsibility"' (2009: 44). Moreover, this syndrome is inescapably bound to the question of how well circumstances – including the attributes of place – permit the 'correct' choices. Places or circumstances sit in recursive and varied relationships with everyday life in that 'possibilities are not everywhere and for all people the same' (Kearns and Reid-Henry 2009: 555). The next chapter will expand on this spatial embedding of choice and responsibility in order to think through the consequences of such a 'spatialisation of virtue' (Osborne and Rose 1999) and its significance for the plausibility of current health policies.

The consumption of self-control

> How are freedom and constraint balanced in the right/duty of individual control over individual bodies? (Bauman 2005: 91)

Bauman's question lies at the very heart of endeavours to maximise individual and collective health within neoliberal economies; balancing the twin poles of freedom to consume and the exercise of restraint as a form of risk mitigation. Health lies at the heart of a series of ideologically, politically and economically conflicting behavioural realms, including: self-restraint and self-indulgence, coercion and freedom, supply and demand. It therefore demonstrates Osborne's assertion that:

> Such issues [of health] are always the product of particular problematisations. Problematisations are not modes of constructing problems but active ways of positing and experiencing them. It is not that there is nothing 'out there' but constructions, but that policy cannot get to work without first problematising its territory . . . the function of problematisations is to reduce complexity, to provide a field of delimitation regulating what can and cannot be said. (Osborne 1997: 175)

In this case, problematisation acts over a 'field of delimitation' that, at root, is concerned with mediating and managing the internal and palpable tensions between these clashing ideological poles and their associated health risks. The second contention at the core of this book suggests that being sensible functions as the bridge between these two poles, in the sense that moderation and prudence choreograph the interplay between indulgence and denial. Furthermore, the admonition to be sensible and the delineation of what this means and requires also identifies it as a 'tool of social change' (Hackley et al 2008: 63). Optimal economic functioning requires constant demand, freedom to choose and a weakness for self-indulgence, all of which can ideally be augmented in order to ensure the continued cycle of consumption. That this results in clear negative health outcomes is obvious and well-documented. How policies premised on the science and rationale of behaviour and culture change fit within this dichotomous system is less clear in spite of its evident centrality to contemporary public health debates. There is a glaring omission in current discussions of public health: little attention has thus far been paid to the ways in which sensible behaviour serves as an intermediary between the dictates and negative externalities of neoliberal societies and economies. By examining this, the genesis of behavioural and cultural change policies with respect to lifestyle diseases will also be explored. This will then form the conceptual foundations for later empirical discussions.

Being sensible and the management of neoliberal tensions

Being healthy should involve self-denial, but increasingly it 'involves the consumption of a range of goods and services which are increasingly marketed for their health-giving properties, such as food, exercise machines and health clubs' (Nettleton 1997: 208). The mediation of the tension between supply and demand, indulgence and restraint is a clear market opportunity, and this commercialisation pervades contemporary health discourses and practices. Moreover, such marketisation also legitimates and renders possible certain ideologies of health governance and the interventions that they require. It is evident that, as Nettleton suggests, 'healthy profits can indeed be made from health' (ibid: 209) or from the selling of the 'reflexive resources' that make up the entrepreneurial, reflexive self (Giddens 1992). But the question must be: what does the existence of such a market say about the inherent philosophical and pragmatic tensions with neoliberal ideology and practice? Then, in turn, what do such tensions say about the role and value of health in contemporary society? The marketisation and commodification of health has a distinct relationship to the constitution of the self and the body, an assertion already ably discussed by sociologists of health and illness (Turner 1984, 1995, 2004). Moreover, it is the act of being sensible and the aspiration to achieve this that have most clearly been transposed into market opportunities. The market for the tools, techniques and expertise that aim to facilitate sensible behaviour and, therefore, minimise future risks to health is infinite, principally because health can always be further optimised. More than this, such a market is underpinned by the expectation that sensible behaviour can be clearly defined, delineated, quantified and communicated and translated into action. Very little in the long history of regulating eating, drinking and exercise habits suggests that this is the case, but still the expectation persists. In order to clarify this, the three tensions highlighted as central to the will to create sensible citizens need to be explored, before we turn to the policy expectations that accompany them.

Supply and demand

Health is clearly a political economic question. Yet, because lifestyle diseases encompass such a cornucopia of behavioural risk factors, the category of 'health' itself is rarely subject to any holistic form of political economic analysis. Instead, the relationship between political economy and health is usually figured as one in which economic growth or success has the twin capacity to improve health and to generate health risks *at a population scale* (Brenner 1995). Political economy is therefore factored at a macroeconomic scale in which aggregate consumption and production are reconfigured as risk factors. However, and as Wilkinson's work (1996, 2005; Wilkinson and Pickett 2009) has persuasively argued, the impacts of economic growth are invariably cyclical and its effects (both negative and positive) are unevenly distributed among people and places, thus producing marked inequalities. Such inequalities have profound effects on health, with clear epidemiological and economic evidence to suggest that *relative* poverty *within countries* has a greater effect on health than *absolute* poverty both *within* and *between countries*. This is not just the case for life expectancy rates, but also for a broader host of social problems and health risks that are closely correlated to inequality.

Obesity, stress, anxiety, drinking practices, drug taking, crime, educational attainment and social capital filtered through the processes of social mobility and the forces of anxiety, self-esteem, social status, shame and pride are all adversely affected by income inequality (Wilkinson and Pickett 2009). The health inequalities that result have profound effects on wellbeing and have have had severe repercussions for policy development. Health and social inequalities are mutually constitutive and are socio-spatially conditioned. Such an argument, which is firmly rooted in the social determinants of the health field (Marmot

1998, 2001, 2005; Commission on Social Determinants of Health 2008), suggests that economic growth does not infinitely improve quality of life in the Global North. This is principally because 'the diseases which used to be called the "diseases of affluence" [for example degenerative cardiovascular disease and cancer] [have become] the diseases of the poor in affluent societies' (Wilkinson and Pickett 2009: 44); a situation that is increasingly being replicated in the Global South, with even more punitive consequences for longevity and quality of life.

In this context, the political economic systems of supply and demand are overlaid with complex social, demographic, cultural and geographic topographies that condition their characteristics and the possibilities for the management of their associated risks. In reality, therefore, the effects of political economic structures and systems are far more individualised than is accounted for by macroeconomic analyses. So it is no surprise that there has been such intense academic and public interest in supply-side explanations for our poor eating, drinking and, more recently, exercise habits (Guthman and DuPuis 2006). Political economic systems are not monolithic structures that mediate between supply and demand in identical ways across all market sectors. Rather, supply (in terms of quantity, product type, quality and so on) is actively predicated on active calculations and estimations of demand. Consumption relies on generating demand which, in turn, involves eliding need and desire. Health promotion policies, however, often require *need* to be divorced from *desire* in consumer demands for goods and services, even if this is not expressly communicated. Supply, on the other hand, enjoys minimal regulation, except on health and safety grounds. For example, food safety is regulated and, in recent years in the UK and the US, the sugar, salt and transfat contents of packaged foods have come under close scrutiny after concerted consumer group campaigns, especially by the (now threatened) UK Food Standards Agency (FSA). Yet, there is little suggestion that food manufacturers should fundamentally alter the nature and properties of the products, nor their retail prices. The debate is slightly different in the case of alcohol, where current concern in the UK is centred on the need to regulate supply through the imposition of minimum pricing (per litre of pure alcohol) such that the cost then reflects the relative risk of the drink (Thomson et al 2010).

In the case of both food and alcohol, however, the neoliberal logic of industry self-regulation through voluntary codes of conduct means that the interplay between supply and demand in the name of health is strongly skewed towards demand-side solutions. Supply, by contrast, is often left relatively untouched. As a result, the onus thus falls on consumers to ensure their own health through the exercise of informed choice. Food manufacturers and alcohol producers argue that all their products can be enjoyed as part of a healthy lifestyle when consumed 'in moderation'. Therefore, 'moderation' becomes the language and technique by which healthy outcomes and continued profits can coexist. Moderation is now increasingly being encouraged and enacted by the application of a range of corporate social responsibility (CSR) techniques, which have seen the seemingly improbable entry of companies such as British American Tobacco into fields such as the cessation of smoking for young people. It is therefore possible to argue that CSR has become an important mediator between supply and demand by minimising individual risk exposure by providing information and hoping that knowledge is converted into action, while legitimating the continued existence of such risky products through an assertion that CSR facilitates the exercise of informed choice. CSR thus ensures that supply remains free of regulation and that demand is effectively responsibilised, with any failure to exercise this responsibility being the fault of the individual's information-seeking capacity, willpower or logic (Herrick 2009b). Supply and demand exist in extreme tension in the context of health outcomes, with corporate innovation continually seeking to remedy these tensions by making demand malleable. The end result is rarely more regulation of those industries selling products that increase risk, but rather an increased expectation that consumers will exercise appropriate and needs-based demand. The market for desire has not, however, been eradicated; rather it now serves a definite purpose, mediating the tension between self-restraint and self-indulgence.

Self-restraint and self-indulgence

Self-restraint and self-indulgence, while apparently diametrically opposed, are, in reality, two sides of the same coin. Good citizen–consumers both indulge and exercise restraint. While they may undertake the former in the pursuit of pleasure and the continued health of the economy, they may undertake the latter either because they are forced to by circumstance or because they actively choose to. A restrained lifestyle might well thus be considered an indulgent lifestyle, given the effort, willpower and determination that self-denial requires. As Petersen and Lupton contend, this reading of restraint 'is not based on the asceticism of self-denial or an obedience to an authoritative imperative, but rather is supported by a narcissistic approach of "caring for and about oneself"' (1996: 70). Restraint is therefore as self-interested as it can be self-sacrificing and, even where it might require sacrifice, this can be discursively reworked as a facet of self-interest. For this reason, to think of these behaviours as two poles is to miss the tension inherent in their interactions: being a healthy citizen requires the ability to exercise restraint and indulgence, and judge *when* and *where* these might be *appropriate*. However, it is increasingly obvious that defining and communicating where the borders of appropriateness (personalised risk gradients across all consumption possibilities) lie is a far from exact science. The uncertainties and gaps in knowledge that accumulate in this vacuum have again created a distinctive market opportunity. Healthy lifestyles require a balance between restraint and indulgence, such that pleasure is permitted, but is also redirected and recoded under conditions of self-control and self-denial. Thus, making self-control both pleasurable and possible is now an industry in and of itself.

Being sensible is another way of balancing indulgence and restraint in that it calls on the individual to exercise an informed judgement about which behaviours might optimise health outcomes or at least minimise possible risks. However, as Offer asserts, 'choice is fallible because psychic arousal, which is desirable in itself, can mask out some of the larger opportunities for wellbeing' (2007: 367). The pursuit of such 'psychic arousal' or pleasure is an inextricable part of a contemporary society founded on the belief and expectation of immediate gratification and the endemic impatience that this breeds. Pleasure, however, comes at a cost – lung cancer from smoking, weight gain, hangovers and poor fitness through the pleasures of sloth. The irresponsible quest for pleasure, underpinned by the insatiable exercise of 'impulse and instinct' (Offer 2007: 372) acts (despite the best intentions of health promotion) as a causal explanation for continued poor health outcomes. Discourses of pleasure (such as the gluttony or sloth explanations for obesity discussed in Chapters Four and Five) also act to refocus attention on demand rather than supply, again absolving big business from blame. However, in response to the potentially punitive application of pleasure as an explanatory discourse of culpability, there has been a call for greater attention to its role in health (Coveney and Bunton 2003). Pleasure has been ably explored with respect to drinking and drug taking (Measham 2004; O'Malley and Valverde 2004; Hadfield 2007; Moore 2008; McGuire and Hallsworth 2010); the visceral pleasures of eating (Berry 1999; Coveney 1999; Petrini 2003) and a recent rash of popular books extolling the multiple virtues of running (McDougall 2004; Murakami 2008). Pleasure is not theorised in any universal way in these accounts, with perhaps the most marked difference being the delineation of the boundary between self-restraint and indulgence. As such, it might be possible to think of sensible behaviour as marking the parameters of this boundary. Furthermore, it also demonstrates that being sensible with respect to health is difficult precisely as the lines between restraint and indulgence are redrawn according to the particular behaviour in question, who is undertaking it, where, why and to what end. These ideas will be further explored in later chapters.

Coercion and freedom

The role of freedom in neoliberal market functioning has been hotly debated since Milton and Rose Friedman's (1980) treatise *Free to Choose*. The Friedmans' anti-interventionist, anti-welfare, anti-centralisation stance called for Adam Smith's 'invisible hand' of the market, propped up by the associated freedoms of consumers to choose. In their words, 'economic freedom is an essential pre-requisite for political freedom' (Friedman and Friedman 1980: 22). This 'fecundity of freedom' (ibid) comes only when political control is curtailed and its concentration is actively resisted. However, it is clear that the freedoms guaranteed in the name of legitimating the neoliberal project have come at a dramatic health cost, especially in the case of ever-widening health inequalities (Davey Smith et al 2002; Shaw et al 2005). At the same time, addressing the adverse effects created by the workings of neoliberal economies actively challenges the very logic on which the processes of what Peck calls 'neoliberalisation' (Peck and Tickell 2002; Peck et al 2010) are founded. Thus, ensuring healthy lifestyles may well mean curbing freedoms through a kind of 'disciplinary work on the self' or an imposed system of disciplinary measures and sanctions, rather than a disciplining of the neoliberal system per se. This aversion to addressing the system has found particularly contentious expression in the UK, where the coalition government's public health 'Responsibility Deals' seamlessly inculcate corporate interests. With Unilever chairing a committee charged with improving the nation's health it would seem that any coercion of the system looks unlikely.

Liberal governmentality theorists have explored how the creation and governance of the city was made possible *through* freedom (Joyce 2003). In this reading, freedom is actively deployed as a means of governing people, but to do so often involves the application of certain forms of coercion. Freedom is, ambiguously, not an absence of coercion, but may well be produced through its application. In the Foucauldian lexicon, freedom is a technology of government. Nik Rose (1999) builds on this to argue that an 'ethics of freedom' pervades contemporary understandings of how this technology should be deployed. Rose further contends that we must understand freedom 'not simply as an abstract ideal, but as material, technical, practical, governmental' (1999: 63). Thus, freedom is not something unfathomable; it works in ways that can be subjected to empirical analysis and has material outcomes. Valverde's sociopolitical history of the governance of alcohol regulation is a case in point here for its analysis of the limits to free will and the 'dialectic between freedom and necessity' (1998: 15). In the case of drinking, Valverde suggests that freedom is 'defined largely as self-control, as the will's power to manage desires' (ibid: 17) and this gives some indication of the constant proximity of coercion. As she further explains, 'individual freedom is not a utopian force threatening the status quo . . . but is rather the means through which the status quo perpetuates itself in our very souls' (ibid). As such, self-control is necessary in order to ensure the freedom of self and society from the ties of medical or state dependency; poor health foists such a relationship on even the most well-intentioned person.

Being sensible might therefore be understood as the process of acknowledging and accepting personal limits to freedom in return for escaping direct coercion. However, the ways in which this coercion is applied vary in accordance with the specificities of the risk calculation appended to the particular freedoms in question. For example, smoking in public was deemed sufficiently risky for passive smokers to legitimate a ban across a vast and diverse list of cities, states and countries including: Bahrain, Australia, the US, Colombia, Hong Kong, India and Nigeria. In all, over 90 countries now have full or partial bans on smoking in public (indoor and/or outdoor) places. However, there is far less agreement around the individual risk thresholds associated with alcohol as well as the acceptable costs that society is prepared to tolerate. This means that alcohol control policies vary from Sweden's supply-side control policies exercised through a state monopoly on alcohol retailing to the far more liberal, laissez-faire stance found in the UK.

Coercion is not equally applied and, moreover, is rarely applied in any logical or consistent way in relation to risks. This says much about the contested, constructed and complex nature of risks in society. It also says a great deal about the faith being placed in individuals' sensible behaviour to mediate between freedom and coercion – to assign certain limits to freedom in exchange for the promise of minimal coercion. From a geographical perspective, the situated nature of sensibleness is clear and this also starts to expose why freedoms are unequally granted and coercion unequally applied. For example, New Labour discourses on youth characterised by such ill-fated policies as the Respect Agenda demarcate a disproportionate application of a deeply moralised form of coercion to young people (for example through anti-social behaviour orders) and a heavy handed limitation of freedoms through technologies such as curfews (Cobb 2007; Minton 2009), however sensibly they may be acting in reality. The discontinuities in such a 'governance of shame' (Cobb 2007: 360) are clear and it will be through empirical exploration that the three tensions explored above are more thoroughly unpacked and reassembled in the name of being sensible.

Conclusion

This chapter introduced the first two contentions that sit at the heart of this book, to pave the way for the discussion of the third in the next chapter. In so doing, it has highlighted the extent to which and manifold means by which, as Rose (1999: 267) has suggested, 'citizenship [has become] conditional upon conduct'. If the 'art' of (neo)liberal government can be figured as the 'conduct of conduct', then conduct is inextricable from the projects of citizenship that are so thoroughly embroiled in health practices, policies, debates, experiences and outcomes. As Norris and Williams (2008) have suggested, this has been especially marked in New labour's version of citizenship, where choice has been so readily linked to public service provision. As such, 'there is now a strong accent on the idea of a welfare contract between the state and citizens: benefits should be offered only in exchange for disciplined and orderly lives and can be withdrawn as a lever to effect behavioural change' (Rodger 2008: 18). In this case, health forms part of this bundle of benefits. Since Lalonde's 1974 report, the delineation of responsibility – and therefore the configuration of citizenship – with respect to health has been fundamentally reworked. The report laid the foundations for a retheorisation of the duties and obligations of state and citizens vis-à-vis each other to address rising rates of chronic disease. In addition, it also made a clear case for the importance and role of citizens' active choice making – a significant shift from the biomedical model's figure of the passive patient. This has been further politicised by the neoliberal passion for financialising life through a series of 'surrogate values' such as BMI or binge drinking rates (Osborne 1997). Not only does this ascribe responsibility a clear value, it also places a clear financial worth on sensible behaviour. Being sensible is therefore important as it saves state money and can improve individual quality of life. However, such an aspiration relies on the individual capacity to exercise free choice, which is rarely a given and is conditional on far more than individual will.

The first contention argues that while personal responsibility and informed choice are two of the central pillars of policies of the 'new public health', the effects of circumstance or 'luck' have remained relatively under-theorised in the sociology of health and illness and within health geography. This is surprising given that the effects of luck problematise the moralisation of responsibility, in that luck marks a domain of blamelessness. Furthermore, when the effects of what Kearns and Reid-Henry (2009) have called 'geographical luck' are considered, then ascriptions of responsibility become even more morally contentious. Advocates of the theories of social determinants of health argue that poor health results from a wide and socio-spatially differentiated range of structural determinants including: poverty, the unequal distribution of resources and power, unemployment, poor environments, a lack of human rights and insufficient access to health care. This is the case across the Global North and South. A framework with a social determinant of health sits very uneasily with a personal responsibility framework, not least because most factors listed above are frequently far beyond the reach of individual control. Ascribing and expecting the exercise of personal responsibility is further problematised by the difficulty of delineating the relative riskiness of certain lifestyles, even without the added complication of individual circumstances. The responsibilisation agenda may, therefore, set expectation levels with respect to individual comportment improbably high. The call to be sensible, with an appreciation that the possibilities of its undertaking are contingent circumstance, might thus provide a more realistic framework for encouraging healthy lifestyles.

The second contention builds on the first in that it explores some key tensions and incongruencies in the neoliberal enterprise. Sensible behaviour, in this reading, is thus a vehicle through and by which these tensions might be managed and their effects mitigated, without impinging on optimal market functioning. If being sensible does not entail the fundamental restructuring of political economic systems – as social determinants of health advocates would demand – then it also creates novel market opportunity. In short, the secrets to sensible behaviour sell and, in turn, are saleable. Clear examples of these tensions include the dichotomy of supply and demand, self-restraint and self-indulgence and freedom and coercion. In all cases, but in markedly different ways, sensible behaviour shifts the dichotomous into the recursive, by acting to moderate those tensions that mark out neoliberalism as continually at odds with its own ends and means. However, because the sensible choice is not always the most pleasurable choice (who wouldn't want to eat chocolate, after all?), such behaviours are understandably not immediately popular. As such, they are thus clear targets of market innovation and development that shift the focus onto demand-side solutions, while leaving the supply-side creation of risk relatively untouched. This is reinforced by the ubiquity of CSR strategies that aim to displace responsibility onto consumers by the industry assuming responsibility only in so far as it *provides* choice (a full product range, for example) and information (such as sensible drinking or healthy eating advice), while sticking to the logic that, when consumed in moderation, all products can be part of a healthy lifestyle. Again, supply is rarely targeted in the same way as demand, which is thoroughly responsibilised.

Being sensible is a technique that also mediates between restraint and indulgence, especially where 'sensible choices' are materialised in such a way that restraint can become reworked as indulgence. Food is perhaps the clear example of this where light, low-fat or no added sugar versions of indulgent foods permit an illusion of sensibleness without the inconvenience of restraint. Humans are coded to seek pleasure in indulgence. Pleasure seeking is both dangerous to health and often called on as evidence of culpability. Yet, pleasure is not alone in being blamed for poor health outcomes; too much freedom and too little coercion are also cast as culprits. There is a fine line between freedom and coercion, as liberal governmentality theorists have shown (Valverde 1998; Rose 1999; Joyce 2003; O'Malley and Valverde 2004). Such authors see freedom as a 'technology' of government or a state that renders governance possible. In this case, we can think of being sensible as a form of limited freedom in return for the promise of minimal coercion. The 'responsible majority' argument made ubiquitous in the UK's alcohol control debate is the intended target of this promise. However, and as geographers are deeply cognisant, freedom and coercion are never equally given or applied, once again rendering the hope of a sensible populace particularly troubled. The ability to choose freely or, in other words, to be and act in sensible ways straddles the divide between *de jure* and de facto rights. In other words, the right to free choice is not always congruent with the duty to act in ways requiring the exercise of free choice. Moreover, de facto rights are constrained by complex mediating structures and contexts (Bauman 2005) that make *du jure* hypothetical rights a dangerous norm. Treading the line between the tensions at the heart of neoliberalism is a task tailormade for each sensible citizen. However, being sensible is a charge of self-management that is always undertaken in situated contexts. Abstraction is of little use in understanding health and the workings of health policy. Instead, these conceptual assertions must be territorialised to be meaningful. The next chapter will undertake this task.

THREE

Governing behaviour change in risky environments

Introduction

Sensible, healthy citizens require an environment conducive to the exercise of appropriately sensible and healthy behavioural choices. However, the interplay between individual behaviour, environmental/structural attributes and health outcomes is extraordinarily intricate. As a result, identifying *causal* relationships between these factors is fraught with methodological difficulties. This is further complicated by the current trend within social policy of conflating the health costs and long-term effects of chronic diseases induced by lifestyle choices with a broader critique of an 'urban condition' characterised by decline, inequality and congenital irresponsibility (Peterson and Lupton 1996). Yet, despite recognition of the distinctive relationships between the urban form and health outcomes, public health and urban planning have been remarkably slow to amalgamate their means and ends in order to address these social and structural determinants of health (Corburn 2004). This is particularly curious given the well-documented historical co-emergence of public health and urban planning through a shared dream of sanitising the city to eradicate infectious disease (Hamlin and Sheard 1998). Despite this entwined history, we have recently been told of an 'emerging field' of the built environment in health (Jackson 2005: 218). In this iteration, the built environment is being cast as a tool for meeting specific public health goals (Curtis et al 2002; Cummins 2003; Foster and Hillsdon 2004) as part of a wider range of urban policies and objectives. Therefore, it is increasingly the case that to explore the problematisations of public health is also to explore the problematisations of the urban environment and, by extension, the urban condition in far broader terms. In other words, constituting sensible behaviour in relation to acceptable levels of risk opens up new sites of urban governance in order to flip the built environment from a *cause* of poor health to the *solution* for optimal health.

The emergence of what have been described as 'epidemics' of chronic, lifestyle diseases has been instrumental in refashioning attitudes towards the value and utility of the built environment in health. It is for this reason that this chapter turns first to an extended discussion of the three empirical examples that drive this book – obesity, drinking and physical (in)activity – in order to highlight why, how and where they have become such a significant component of everyday, lived experiences and the political machinery. Later chapters expand on these discussions, but there is a clear need to justify the choice of these examples not just for what they show in and of themselves, but for what their comparison reveals about the limits to our ability to generalise about a unitary 'new public health' and how it might best be conceptually interrogated. In this vein, attention is given to the striking discord between constructivist accounts of these public health 'epidemics' and biomedical/epidemiological assertions of their unbridled severity. This book charts a productive middle ground between the two stances and this is further explicated in this chapter.

Turning to the third contention of this book, the second part of this chapter asks how the enterprise of encouraging sensible lifestyle choices has become a tool of a range of public policies that extend far beyond public health. Governing lifestyles has brought public health into close conversation with an array of associated spatial agendas ranging from crime, disorder, social inclusion, citizenship and participation to urban planning. As a result, health is increasingly being figured in spatial terms: as an outcome of certain environments and, in turn, a route by which environments might be improved by the strategic actions of responsible or sensible citizens. This has recast the value and utility of health in distinctly spatialised terms, with defined implications for the depiction of risk taking and risky environments as well as for the conceptualisation of the urban within public health discourses. This trend is further reinforced through invocations of the language, logic and practices of the kind of behavioural and cultural change policies that have attained such popularity in places such as the UK. As such, there is a need to reconsider how these now-ubiquitous policy frameworks and expectations sit within the context of a respatialised public health. These geographical approaches to health draw attention to the possibility that invoking spatial strategies for health improvement goals may seem morally innocuous when set against explanations that focus on the fallibility of individual will, but, in practice, may shift responsibility back onto individuals when such goals fail to be realised. Spatial strategies to govern health move the boundaries of responsibility, but this book will explore how accusations of individual culpability are rarely far away.

The 'problems' of obesity, drinking and inactivity

Health, space and governance

This book empirically examines the ways and means through which the drive to be sensible has been normalised in and through the current concern with three interlocked health domains: addressing mounting obesity rates; the rising health and social costs of drinking; and the impacts of sedentary lifestyles. From a conceptual and methodological standpoint, the three examples are comparable in that all represent significant contemporary health 'challenges' across a variety of spatial and governmental scales, from the global to the local. Furthermore, they are 'challenges' that demonstrate, in exceptionally clear ways, not only the marked social, economic and environmental changes that have occurred since the Second World War, but also the profound limits to the effective governance of their negative externalities.

These limitations arise precisely because obesity, drinking alcohol and physical activity sit so uneasily at the fulcrum of the tensions endemic to late capitalist societies explored in Chapter Two. As we have seen, the active pursuit of healthy lifestyles highlights the irrecoverable tension between the desire to consume and the self-control needed to mitigate the risks of such consumption practices. This tension is most strongly marked in urban environments, where the city not only ensures its own continued viability by providing consumption opportunities but is also, increasingly, being called on to offer solutions to the effects of its own success. For this reason, exploring the enterprises of governing health through the examples of obesity, drinking and physical (in)activity directly and indirectly sheds light on the contestations *within* and *for* urban spaces and environments. As such, while this is a book about the contemporary governance of health, it is also an exploration of how those governance conundrums are entwined with urban political aspirations and set within particular problematisations of the urban environment. As Petersen and Lupton have highlighted, there needs to be greater critical reflection by the new public health 'on the concept of the city and on the political strategies deployed in advancing the ideals of the "healthy city"' (1996: xv). Therefore, in recognition of this call, the book empirically explores the ways in which we are now governed 'in the name of health' by asking how health is being governed 'in the name' of urban liveability and quality of life, social cohesion, social justice and economic growth. In so doing, it aims to offer a vantage point from which to shed new light on what some urban theorists have termed the 'urban condition' (see for example Brenner and Theodore 2005)

Given the current furore around our unhealthy lifestyles and their far-reaching adverse effects, it is unsurprising that a plethora of authors have sought answers by tracing the changing political economic landscapes of consumption and the shifts in the built form that have necessarily accompanied these (Schlosser 2001; Critser 2004; Gard and Wright 2005). This work has been most developed with reference to the genesis of the current 'obesity epidemic' (see Campos 2004 for a critique of this), however the story of how we have become increasingly sedentary is always entwined with accounts of how our eating habits have changed and how, as a result, our weight has climbed. Such accounts have been overwhelmingly situated in the US, where post-war suburbanisation, environmental concern, an inescapable nostalgia for simpler ways of life and an optimism that change is possible have combined to produce a rash of work chronicling the loss of American community (Ehrenhalt 1995; Putnam 2000, 2002; Putnam and Feldstein 2003), the loss of authenticity and the rise of 'defensive living' in gated communities (Davis 1990; Blakely and Snyder 1999; Minton 2009; Oduku and Bageen 2009) and the manifold societal and aesthetic horrors of suburban 'sprawl' (Kunstler 1993, 1998; Marshall 2000; Duany et al 2001). These topological shifts have been replicated, although to a slightly lesser extent, in other countries, and a large canon of work is now devoted to finding solutions for an urban condition indelibly marked by neoliberal political economic processes and their associated profound inequalities (Navarro 2004, 2007; Navarro et al 2006). Obesity draws attention to the built form by shifting causal explanations from individual behaviour alone to behavioural drivers or triggers that emanate from what have been termed 'obesogenic environments' (Swinburn et al 1999; Lake and Townshend 2006; Jones et al 2007). In this reading, obesity is cast as a logical result of a flawed environment, producing what Swinburn and Egger (2004) have termed a 'runaway weight gain train' in which unhealthy behaviours and an obesogenic environment mutually reinforce an inexorable march towards obesity.

While narratives about the changing landscapes of alcohol consumption point to more complex cyclical shifts in production, retailing, consumption and, therefore, regulation, they are also interlaced (at least in the UK) with a sense that we are currently enduring the adverse health and societal effects of too much drink and an urban environment hardwired to encourage the profligate consumption of alcohol (Hadfield 2006; Hall and Winlow 2006; Plant and Plant 2006), leading to violence, drunkenness and anti-social behaviour. New Labour's liberalisation of the licensing laws in 2003 to encourage a café culture style of drinking in the regenerated 24-hour city is said to have fuelled a dramatic shift in the political economy and retail environment of alcohol (Loveday 2005; Talbot 2006; Norris and Williams 2008). Through this, the temptations posed by the growth in the night-time economy have increased in line with the ease of satisfying them. The affordability of alcohol has increased markedly over the past few decades; drinking spaces and places have become more welcoming to women and it is now possible for young people to buy alcohol in a far greater range of outlets over an extended number of hours (for example in supermarkets). This policy of liberalisation has had a profound effect not just on urban drinking spaces and people's drinking behaviours, but also the general public and politicians' perception of alcohol as a problem. In this reading, drink is a problem not just because of how much people consume, but also because of where, when and how they consume. Drinking places and their occupants are thus indelibly marked as loci of risk and subjected to an ever-increasing degree of indirect and direct forms of control as a way of mitigating this (for example the Best Bar None scheme in the UK and controlled drinking zones). Drinking, physical activity and obesity thus hold a clear potential to illuminate varying aspects of the neoliberal 'urban condition' (Brenner and Theodore 2005) – that is, the experiential and material realms of everyday life in cities and the ways in which these are both problematised and governed. When urban liveability is governed in the name of health, then the debates that underpin the enterprise of being healthy serve to illuminate the limits to achieving optimal, liveable environments.

Why are obesity, drinking and physical (in)activity important?

Obesity, drinking and physical activity represent key 'modifiable risk factors' for what have been aptly termed 'diseases of comfort' (Choi et al 2005: 1031). This

—

'global chronic disease epidemic of heart diseases, cancers, respiratory disease, mental disorders, diabetes, musculoskeletal disorders etc' (ibid), the authors suggest, have four causal layers. Obesity is an 'immediate' cause (along with high blood pressure, high cholesterol and stress). Physical inactivity and excessive alcohol are 'underlying causes', along with an imbalanced diet and smoking. Underpinning these causal factors are 'technological advances', which include: mechanisation (for example cars and domestic technological advances), the advent of energy-dense foods, poor urban planning, modern life and the global economy. More than this, though, Choi et al describe the root of the problem as the inexorable 'human progress towards "perfection"' in the shape of 'comfort, convenience and pleasure' (2005: 1031). This drive for perfection through comfort, convenience and pleasure is at the heart of the debates around the governance of obesity and also crosscuts the associated concern with the risk presented by urban environments physically and psychologically conditioned to pose a risk to health.

Diseases of comfort have long been considered a phenomenon of the Global North, but this is no longer the case. As countries of the Global South work their way along the epidemiological transition model, they are likely to endure a devastating 'double burden' (Boutayeb 2006) of mounting rates of chronic disease coexisting with high rates of infectious disease. Indeed and as Table 1 shows, at a global scale, alcohol accounts for 9.2% of the disease burden, a figure which puts it in third place behind tobacco (12.2%) and hypertension (10.9%). Overweight (which includes obesity) accounts for 7.4% of the global disease burden and physical inactivity a relatively small 3.3%. While there are clear limitations to the ability to calculate and disentangle the precise causal influence of each of these risk factors at a global scale (and thus any calculation of the global disease burden must not be accepted uncritically), the global line-up of major health risks nonetheless demonstrates that all are *modifiable*. As such, they are politically potent in that they are deemed to represent risks that can be alleviated by individual

Table 1: Leading 10 risk factors as a percentage of causes of disease burden

Risk factor	% Cause of disease burden
Tobacco	12.2
Blood pressure (hypertension)	10.9
Alcohol	9.2
Cholesterol	7.6
Overweight	7.4
Low fruit and vegetable intake	3.9
Physical inactivity	3.3
Illicit drugs	1.8
Unsafe sex	0.8
Iron deficiency	0.7

Source: WHO 2002; cited in Cappelen and Norheim (2005: 47)

behaviour change. At the root of this change is therefore a vision of what such risk-averse behaviour might be. However, the question of how to make the shift from a risk-taking to a risk-avoidance culture in a market context that saturates the consumption landscape with potential health risks remains at the core of the governmental conundrum.

As significant negative externalities of economic growth and urbanisation and their resultant impact on lifestyle habits, 'diseases of comfort' represent a dramatic economic burden to both the state and individuals. Importantly, this is a burden set to climb relentlessly in both developed and developing countries unless there is definitive prevention-orientated action. At a global scale, obesity and physical (in)activity appear as World Health Organization (WHO) concerns in its *Global Strategy on Diet, Physical Activity and Health* (2004). Alcohol is a more recent global health concern and the members of the WHO reached a resolution on the *Global Strategy to Reduce Harmful Use of Alcohol* in 2010 (WHO 2010a). At the national level, obesity, alcohol and physical activity are key public health policy priorities across a broad range of countries. However, within Anglo-Saxon academic circles, it is unsurprising that the bastions of neoliberalism – the US, New Zealand, Australia and the UK – have been subject to the greatest degree of conceptual and empirical scrutiny by social scientists. While this book charts the same geographical course, it does so in full acknowledgement of the spatial partiality of the arguments presented here. It should not be taken as read that 'governing in the name of health' (Rose 1996; Osborne 1997; Osborne and Rose 1999) has become a de facto feature of all late modern societies. To do so risks reinforcing the 'Western imperial vision of good health' identified by Brown and Bell (2008: 1571) and, in the process, understates the vast political, cultural, structural and geographical complexities that condition the governance of health at all scales (see Gesler and Kearns 2002).

Paying the price(s) for neoliberal success

Managing obesity, alcohol consumption and physical inactivity are national public health priorities both for the chronic health risks they pose and the economic burden these present to the state, the private sector, society and individuals in terms of lost productivity and treatment costs. The UK government has been prolific in its quantification of costs associated with these diseases of comfort and such estimates serve as a direct legitimation of a host of governmental interventions to render behaviour more malleable. Drinking alcohol poses a complex array of negative consequences, for the individual drinker, their immediate environment and society more broadly. This is in addition to the costs that the management of alcohol-related harm poses to the NHS, the police and local authorities. Alcohol is estimated to cost the NHS over £2.7 billion a year, of which £167 million is directly attributable to alcohol misuse and £1 billion indirectly attributable (Health Improvement Analytical Team 2008). When the cost of addressing the crime and disorder that stems from alcohol abuse and use are added into the calculation, drinking represents a cost of between £18 billion and £20 billion to the British state (HM Treasury 2009: 3). In terms of the burden of cost, drinking is a societal issue rather than one of individual dependence. While this is not to claim that dependent drinkers do not pose a significant cost in terms of treatment, that cost is far smaller than the broader costs of managing the negative, anti-social consequences of the UK's night-time economy and penchant for home drinking. By contrast, in the US, the debate about alcohol has tended to concentrate around underage binge drinking, especially by college students (Wechsler et al 1994, 2003; Hingson et al 2005). While this problematisation is a reflection of the legal drinking age of 21 in the US, it is also a marked response to a nation in which abstinence rates are far higher than in the UK and the conservative right holds strong sway over the moral delineations of 'problem' drinking.

Obesity also places a significant cost on the NHS. In 2008, this direct cost was estimated at £4.5 billion (Department of Health 2008). The 2007 Foresight Report (Government Office for Science 2007) from the Parliamentary Office of Science and Technology (POST) estimated the broader costs of obesity to the UK economy to be in the region of £16 billion, with the potential to reach £50 billion by 2050 if no effective preventative measures were in place. While the UK is facing definitive challenges in dealing with the costs of obesity, drinking and sedentary lifestyles, the US remains the heartland of chronic disease. The US is an iconic and perspicuous site for any examination of obesity, given the assumed synonymity between the American built form and a lifestyle response that encourages sedentarism, excessive consumption and weight gain. It is, therefore, a useful counterpoint to the UK, especially in explorations of behavioural responses to the built form. Obesity directly contributes to an estimated 112,000 deaths a year in the US (Flegal et al 2005), although the accuracy of this calculation has itself been subjected to vehement critique (see Herrick 2007). The national obesity rate – defined as those adults with a BMI greater than 30.0 – has climbed from 13.4% in 1980 to 34.3% in 2008, while the rate of 'extreme' or 'morbid' obesity (BMI greater than 40.0) now stands at 6%. Rates of children classified as having a BMI in the 95th percentile or above for their age has undergone an equally sizeable leap, from 5% to 17% over the same time period (United States Surgeon General 2010). In terms of absolute percentages, obesity hardly seems to pose the threat that its 'epidemic' label suggests. However, it is the growth in prevalence rates over the past three decades that signals the more significant concern – what obesity says about the pathogenic nature of late modern society, lifestyles and environments. It is here that the public and political anxiety is situated.

In 2000, shortly before the surgeon general's 2001 *Call to Action to Prevent and Decrease Overweight and Obesity* was published, the economic cost of obesity was set at $117 billion. More recent estimations of the economic cost posed by obesity are hard to obtain, but a recent report prepared for the Centers for Disease Control (CDC) suggests that obesity now accounts for 10% of all medical expenditure in the US, or $147 billion (Finkelstein et al 2009). The same report also calculated that per capita annual medical spending was $1,429 higher for an obese person than for someone of normal weight. The health care costs attributed to obesity are generated from treating not obesity itself, but rather the conditions that obesity causes and perpetuates. Type 2 diabetes (T2D) is one example, given that excess body weight is its single most significant predicting factor. Diabetes is a chronic condition that requires a lifetime of management and, with a prevalence rate of almost 8% across all ages in 2007, current direct and indirect costs of T2D are now $174 billion (Centers for Disease Control 2007). More worrying in the US is the increasing incidence of T2D (or 'adult onset diabetes' as it is more commonly known) among children, and the disproportionate affliction of African Americans and some Hispanic groups (for example Puerto Ricans).

The cost of physical inactivity is far harder to quantify exclusively given that sedentarism is itself a risk factor for obesity. Regular physical activity is linked to the reduced risk of cardiovascular disease, some cancers, T2D and also has marked psychological benefits. Physical inactivity and obesity are inextricably linked: sedentary lifestyles increase the risk of obesity; obesity increases the chance of being sedentary. It is unsurprising, therefore, that the 2004 report of the UK chief medical officer (CMO) suggested that the costs of physical inactivity were as high as £8.2 billion (Chief Medical Officer 2004: iii), with the direct contribution of physical inactivity to obesity costing an extra £2.5 billion. With only 37% of adult men and 24% of adult women in the UK meeting recommended levels of 30 minutes of 'moderate activity' (for example brisk walking, cycling, swimming) five days a week (Department of Health 2005b), the target of 50% participation by 2020 laid down by Derek Wanless in his 2004 report, means that uptake rates among adults need to climb by 1% a year across the UK. However, concern over low rates masks the fact that recent studies suggest that uptake is actually climbing, albeit slowly.

This is also the case in the US, where physical activity rates seem to be on the rise. In 1988, data from the BRFSS showed that 30.5% of all adults were inactive. However, by 2008 this had fallen to 25.1%, marking a clear upwards swing in the uptake of leisure-time activity. This change of heart is not necessarily replicated evenly across the country, and social and geographic disparities in uptake rates remain as significant in the US as they are in the UK. Figures from Sport England's APS shows a range in uptake rates (here defined as 30 minutes on three days a week and not five days a week as suggested by the CMO) from 29.8% in Richmond-upon-Thames to 14% in Boston, Lincolnshire. As in the US, there is evidence to suggest that the appeal of physical activity is growing. Between 1999 and 2004, those meeting the CMO's recommended levels of physical activity actually rose by 1.7% among all age groups, with the percentage of those in the 35–49-year age band meeting these levels increasing by over 6% (Stamatakis et al 2007). While overall participation increased in the period 1997–2006, it is important to note that this increase 'did not occur equally across socioeconomic, demographic and ethnic groups' (Stamatakis and Chaudhury 2008: 6) and so clear socio-spatial divides in the uptake of healthy lifestyles remain. This has distinct ramifications for interventions to address this imbalance as well as an obvious impact on the way in which low uptake rates are figured as problematic. Such contentions will be further explored in Chapter Six.

Constructed 'epidemics'?

This book starts from the assumption that obesity, drinking alcohol and being inactive have discernable and significant negative effects on health when taken to excess. It therefore also starts from the premise that they represent *real* problems, rather than the completely constructed fictions that have been suggested in some poststructuralist accounts of health (Campos 2004). To say that these health behaviours and lifestyles are real in the sense that they can be understood as objective biomedical *fact* is far from true. In this reading, they are real only to the extent that it is acknowledged that they have negative consequences for individuals, society and the state, and that action needs to be taken to mitigate these. The *scale* and *extent* of this problematisation must be treated with more cautious scepticism given its repeated subjection to the multiple constitutive processes that 'make up' lifestyle as a governance concern. There has been an impressive volume of work critiquing the ways in which biomedical concerns are constructed as societal imperatives and, therefore, how diseases (whether chronic or infectious) become what Paula Treichler (1988) has so notably called an 'epidemic of signification'. The perspective adopted here aims to respond to Brown and Duncan's (2002) call for critical approaches to public health understood as 'a socio-cultural practice and a set of contingent knowledges' (Peterson and Lupton 1996: x), which filter conceptualisations of disease, illness and health behaviours. Thus, as both practice and knowledge, any study of the 'contingency' of public health must always be critically attuned to its politicisation and its multiple 'significations' to ensure that it remains sufficiently grounded to read its material effects.

There has been sustained debate in social science studies of health concerning the extent of the 'crisis' or 'epidemic' nature of public health challenges, with the growing canon of work in critical obesity studies perhaps the most notable example (see for example Monaghan 2005; Campos et al 2006; Evans and Colls 2009). There has also been significant attention to the criminalisation and demonisation of (particularly youth) drinking practices as part of a broader moral panic around drinking cultures, especially in the UK (Measham and Brain 2005; Hayward and Hobbs 2007; Szmigin et al 2008). In both cases, the object of concern is the *social interpretation* of disease, thus operationalising the idea that such interpretations are based not simply on 'the facts' or reality, but rather 'what we are told' about such reality (Treichler 1988: 35) through the multiple outlets that now communicate health (newspapers, web forums, internet search engines and so on). Approaching health concerns thus means studying 'a nexus where multiple meanings, stories and discourses intersect and overlap, reinforce and subvert one another' (ibid: 42). These nexuses are frequently the cause of the kind of 'hysteria' that Campos contends undermines the possibility of any sane discussion of 'what constitutes a healthy lifestyle and a desirable body' (Campos

2004: xvii), reinforcing the current 'phony war' on fat. He further argues that the causal relationship between body weight and health is far from assured and that, therefore, America's 'anti-fat warriors' ensure that "overweight" is a 'cultural construct, not a scientific fact' (ibid: xxiii).

Similar lines of logic are drawn by those concerned with tracing the deep uncertainties and discontinuities in risk calculations in relation to (binge) drinking (Herring et al 2008b). This work is further complemented by those arguing that public health and biomedical accounts of drinking rarely inculcate the potency of pleasure and, therefore, the role of individual decisions to take risks in full knowledge of the possible consequences of their actions (Moore 2008). Sociological and anthropological examinations of drinking have yet to align themselves with Campos's vehement disavowal of obesity as a health concern *tout court*, but have instead expressly critiqued the validity and accuracy of risk calculations attached to drinking practices. Binge drinking has been a clear target in this respect, especially given that public health advice on 'sensible drinking' limits is at odds with normative codes of acceptability in relation to social drinking. This points to a middle ground where, as Gard and Wright argue, we might think of the central health concerns of this book as 'a complex pot-pourri of science, morality and ideological assumptions about people and their lives which have ethically questionable effects' (2005: 3). In this mix, social concerns and health aspirations are conflated to produce a reading of illness as something more than merely poor health. It is not just the metaphor that Susan Sontag's (1979) admirable work suggests, but rather an expression of the multiple disequilibria between self/society/environment that characterise late modern society across the Global North and South. Health, therefore, has distinctive metonymical value in that it holds huge explanatory potential when employed to examine the aspirational politics of creating a sensible populace. In turn, admonitions to be sensible act as a lens through which to interrogate contemporary health challenges and how they unfold in diverse urban settings.

Spatialising health agendas

The third contention at the heart of this book asks how encouraging sensible lifestyle choices have become a tool of a range of public policies that extend far beyond public health into an array of spatial agendas ranging from crime, disorder and social inclusion to urban planning. This expansion has reworked the value and utility of health in distinctly spatial terms, producing reworked geographical imaginations of risk, risk taking and at-risk groups. In this logic, spatial and social explanations of health are frequently conflated in order to sanction public health interventions. However, adherence to the language, logic and practices of behavioural and culture change policy in the broader pursuits of sensibleness means that the ('choice') environment (see Cabinet Office 2010) is often reduced to a simple classification of 'barrier' or 'facilitator'. Such reductionism is at odds with the forceful arguments being made in health/ medical geography for the inclusion of explicit theorisations of the dialectical and relational relationships between people and places in conditioning health (Cummins et al 2007). This core tenet of geographical reasoning is now appearing as innovation in government policy agendas increasingly concerned with 'place-focused principles' (Department of Communities and Local Government 2007). Explorations of being sensible with respect to healthy lifestyles are no exception in this regard and it is clear that a blind faith in the ability of behavioural/cultural change policies to induce improved health outcomes undermines the possibility of public health once again being a vehicle for urban improvement goals. The two policy stances are therefore highly conflicting in that behaviour change presents solutions as individual modification to adverse environmental settings, whereas an entwined public health–urban planning agenda would view space as instrumental to optimal behaviour. In order to explore this contention thoroughly, the call to re-inject space into health (research and policy) agendas is briefly explored, before a discussion of the rise and rise of behavioural and cultural change perspectives in public health.

This book is situated squarely within a health geography framework in that it recognises that the new diseases of comfort are directly influenced by the interplay between people and places, both in the generation of risk and in techniques to mitigate risk (Kearns 1991, 1993; Kearns and Moon 2002; Macintyre et al 2002; Cummins et al 2007). As a consequence, this has endowed places with huge political significance. The new public health as 'an area of expert knowledge and action' (Peterson and Lupton 1996: ix) has also been instrumental in this respect by aiming 'to redirect the attention of public health theorists and practitioners back towards structural and environmental influences on health and health behaviours' (Macintyre et al 2002: 126). The 'new public health' takes the environment as an express focus and, moreover, one that functions by casting health as 'an antidote to all kinds of problems linked to modern life, particularly problems of the urban milieu' (Peterson and Lupton 1996: x). Shifting the focus to the more holistic, environmental understandings of health advocated by health geographers (Gesler and Kearns 2002) reveals that governing obesity, physical activity and drinking is now an enterprise that takes place inside, outside and in between the state and a plethora of non-governmental stakeholders amid a wider concern with identifying and addressing these 'problems of the urban milieu'.

In this rationale, places are now both the *cause of* and possible *solution to* poor health, and it is logical that their management and strategic re-engineering would thus come to occupy the minds of an ever-expanding and diverse array of actors (Herrick 2009a). Such attention to place in the context of chronic disease is inextricable from the vast resources devoted to the collection of baseline epidemiological, demographic and consumer data for alcohol consumption, inactivity and activity levels and BMI that do not delineate problems at an individual level, but rather aggregate collective risk taking, constructing spaces of risk and deviance. Therefore 'high-risk' places containing 'at-risk' groups have now become loci of intervention through measures to change and modify behaviour. However there remains a clear conceptual and empirical divide between those calling for this to be undertaken through the provision of an 'enabling' built environment that is conducive to healthy lifestyles and sensible behaviour (Srinivasan et al 2003) and those favouring the individual or community-scale behavioural change techniques that have risen to such prominence in government circles.

Over the past decade, the UK's policy strategy towards obesity, drinking and physical activity has been firmly orientated towards a profound faith in the power of and need for behavioural and/or cultural change (Department of Health 2004a; 2005a; 2005b). Behavioural/cultural change policies are underpinned, in the first instance, by the assertion that individuals are personally responsible for some aspects of their health and that health improvements will only be met in a sustained fashion when people live up to these responsibilities. Second, behaviour change occurs 'not only through a focus on individual persuasion, but through an ecological approach' (Cabinet Office 2004: 7). In this case, however, the ecology in question refers to the *social* context – individual, interpersonal and community – that constitutes an individual's 'choice environment'. The uptake of social and behavioural psychology within public policy has been reinforced through the profound and concomitant political influence of behavioural economics, where *Nudge* author Cass Sunstein now heads the White House's Office of Information as Barack Obama's 'regulatory czar'. Moreover, it has also been reinforced by an epistemology of public engagement in which government suggests that it 'can't go it alone' (nor can it rightfully be expected to do so) and works only when citizens are active and engaged with respect to their own health.

Behavioural economists argue that the state should adopt a stance of 'libertarian paternalism' towards its citizens, allowing some freedoms in return for engineering expected norms of behaviour. In reality, this is enacted through setting default norms as the desired behaviour and working with assumptions of apathy by creating systems that ensure that individuals have to opt out of this norm. This is in direct recognition of the failure of the traditional tools and techniques of behaviour change usually leveraged by government (such as legislation, taxation, information and so on) to address the UK's perceived drinking 'problem', mounting rates of obesity and low rates of physical activity uptake. As such, governments have increasingly turned to the commercial realm (for example using behavioural psychology as applied to management science) for innovative ways of influencing individual behaviour at an ecological scale of decision making. However, the mismatch between the 'place-based' governance expounded by departments such as the Department for Communities and Local Government (DCLG) in recent years and the largely aspatial behavioural psychology now holding sway in a range of social and health policy agendas seems stark.

If public health policy is increasingly orientated towards generating sensible (conducive) attitudes towards healthy lifestyles, then the barriers to these behaviours are a particular topic of concern. As such, the '(un)healthy city' as the locus of such refusals, has necessarily become an 'object of a particular kind of understanding and action' (Peterson and Lupton 1996: 137). However, while

—

the city is subject to the deployment of particular kinds of knowledge, 'it is not urbanisation *per se* that is the problem, but rather the processes of managing the city environment' (ibid: 136). These limits to management effectively point to the multiple pressure points in the 'dynamic and symbiotic, rather than linear, relationship between people, their "internal" environment (or psyche/spirit) and their "external" environment (or social and material milieux)' (ibid: 109) that produce the risks of obesity, drinking and physical activity. This assertion also highlights a profound gap in the ability to ease these pressure points effectively, often reinforced through perceptions of a more generalised lack of 'self-efficacy' in society or a paucity of self-confidence in one's own ability to take a particular course of action (Bandura 1982, 1995).

The need to reinforce and cultivate self-efficacy has been noted by the UK government as a way of converting individual behaviour change into the more pervasive culture change that they suggest is really needed to address the societal ills of obesity, drinking and sedentarism. In other words, there needs to be a clear shift in societal norms so that risk-taking behaviour becomes the exception rather than the rule. In so doing, however, not only have the contested realms of risk in relation to health behaviours been comprehensively glossed over, but the health agenda has become subject to the same general concern with correcting a flawed culture that now underpins causes as diverse as pension reform, the Respect Agenda and congestion charging (see Figure 1). In this reading, risk is recast as a generalised feature of (poor) urban environments, where the existence of social problems also points to a high probability of low self-efficacy or, in Raco's (2009) reading, a poverty of 'aspiration' and, therefore, a high likelihood of poor health. As self-efficacy pertains to the individual, but is moderated by levels of cultural capital which derive from the more complex interplay of geographic and social scales, a focus on behaviour change to elicit culture change invariably ascribes certain pathogenic attributes to particular 'ecologies'. Under the rubric of self-efficacy, however, the onus ultimately falls on the individual to address their attitudes and actions as this is seen as a more effective level of 'investment' (Cabinet Office 2008: 31) than widespread restructuring of, for example, the political economy of food or drink. In devolving responsibility for culture change to individuals and communities, governmental responsibility for addressing the very features of geographical 'luck' (Kearns and Reid-Henry 2009) that code for some health outcomes is skirted. An appreciation that geographical fate is only rarely undone is thus undermined by an adherence to a behavioural psychology that codes fate only as an impetus for self-betterment.

The drive to govern the risks surrounding obesity, phyiscal activity and drinking in order to improve health outcomes could never be a universal enterprise, despite a generalised adherence to the tenets of behaviour and culture change policy rationales (Cabinet Office 2010). Indeed, the explorations that make up the rest of this book show that conflating all three realms of lifestyle within one general category of 'healthy living' as circled in Figure 1 risks downplaying the clear distinctions between them. In essence, individual risk taking through lifestyle

---

Figure 1: Examples of UK culture change interventions

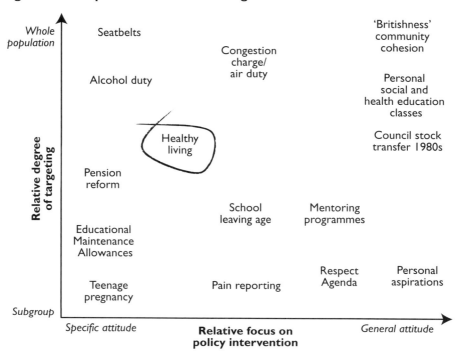

Source: Cabinet Office, 2008: 28

choices (for example smoking, unsafe sex, drug taking, drinking and so on) is plagued by numerous contentions: of correlating cause and (definitive) effect; the habitual and normalised nature of risk taking; the inequitable distribution of the negative health consequences; the short-termist nature of risk-taking behaviour; an inability to compute the long-term, cumulative nature of certain health effects; the perception that risk taking can be controlled adequately by individuals; a persistent lack of trust in those assuming the burden of managing those risks; and the role of poor-quality environments in imposing constraints on (sensible) behavioural choices. As a result, encouraging the exercise of common sense, or being sensible is also a politicised and pragmatic strategy to neutralise the conflict between the public realms from which both market and environmentally/structurally generated risks emanate (for example alcohol supply within the broader temptations of the night-time economy) with the private realms within which behavioural decisions are fashioned and undertaken (for example the home, family or community).

This need to balance the public with the private again raises some familiar questions about the degree to which the state should and can intervene to mitigate the health risks caused by, for the most part, behaviours that are not only socially sanctioned and exceptionally commercially desirable, but also conditioned by environments that are usually beyond individual control. Therefore, it also means questioning the ecological influences on rationality (Cabinet Office 2010: 71), deeply problematising the current UK government's hope of 'nudging' citizens into 'acting by going with the grain of [their] automatic brain' (Cabinet Office 2010: 73). Behavioural psychology tells us that the automatic brain needs to be nudged for optimal functioning, whereas an environmental reading of health would argue that an automatic brain can only ever be a fallacy. This opposition constitutes the third contention of this book and will be explicitly explored in Chapters Five, Six and Eight.

Conclusion

This chapter has set out why and how obesity, drinking and physical activity are valuable examples in explorations of the governance of health in urban environments. To do so, it has discussed how these 'diseases of comfort' have become recognised as significant contributors to global burdens of disease, expressly included within WHO *Global Strategies* (2004) and also come to compose significant national public health challenges. In the US and UK, obesity is an explicit target of public health policy, where health survey figures show rising prevalence rates and econometric analyses show that excess body weight poses significant costs to the state in terms of elevated health care costs, absenteeism, lost productivity and the extra cost associated with modifying environments to cater to larger body sizes (such as modified hospital equipment). The direct causal influence of physical activity on both body weight and health is far harder to calculate with any accuracy. While studies demonstrate that exercise has a beneficial effect on health, they have struggled to ascertain a causal relationship between physical inactivity, weight and poor health. As such, obesity and physical inactivity are often (falsely) elided in calculations of their relative cost. The cost of drinking is also exceptionally high on governmental agendas, particularly in the UK, where the 'binge drinking' culture seems to have plagued efforts to address both anti-social behaviour and public health. Alcohol poses a complex array of costs to the UK economy (for example policing, Accident and Emergency, lost productivity, street cleaning, security and surveillance) that spread across the crime and disorder and health agendas. Drinking also presents an excellent counterpoint to obesity and physical activity agendas in discussions of both the urban condition and its governance. While there are clear areas of conceptual overlap between all three areas of risk, their governance plays out in markedly different ways, thus constituting them as distinct urban governance conundrums.

Addressing and redressing obesity, alcohol-related harm and sedentary lifestyles means trying to cultivate a sensible citizenry predisposed to sensible behaviour. It also means creating the kind of places where sensible behaviour is an easy and desirable choice, and exercising personal responsibility is the norm. Does this necessarily mean creating sensible places? This chapter has examined the continued disjuncture between the individual-scale focus of behavioural change programmes concerned with promoting and increasing self-efficacy to produce a more widespread culture change and an emergent concern with 'place-focused principles' (Department of Communities and Local Government 2007: 11) that aim to engender behaviour change through changes in the built form. In so doing, it has also highlighted that while public health theorists have become more cognisant of the complex mechanisms through which urban environments can present health risks as well as opportunities, public health policies and practices are not as overtly attuned to the spatial as might be expected. This is curious given that, in reality, public health practices operate according to a highly spatialised logic, where a reliance on epidemiological data derived at an individual level (but aggregated to formulate and delineate risk groups by socioeconomic status, race, age and so on) means that interventions are targeted over high-risk people and, by extension, high-risk places. Behavioural and environmentalist readings of health are thus not as conceptually distinct as their false separation in policy might suggest. As health geographers have long argued, health outcomes result from the interplay between people and places, and these in turn refashion both individuals and their geographical contexts. Neither can therefore be meaningfully considered in isolation. Moreover, in recognising that the central behavioural tenets of neoliberal policy – choice, personal responsibility, rationality – are shaped, enabled and also constrained by the dictates of certain spatial settings, it is clear why the governance of health speaks to a far broader set of political, cultural and economic agendas than public health alone. It is also apparent that questioning the governance of health facilitates the kind of critical interrogation of urban liveability that can only aid in meeting public health improvement objectives.

FOUR

Obesity and strategies of rule

More than any other phenomenon, fat encapsulates, condenses and blends the fears emanating from the poorly-mapped 'frontier land' stretching between the body of the consumer and the outside world, crowded with incapacitating dangers while simultaneously filled to the brim with irresistible temptations. Because of its unique status . . . the 'fat phenomenon' may offer a useful insight into the ambivalence intrinsic to the consumer's condition. (Bauman 2005: 96)

Introduction

This chapter argues that being sensible has three strategic roles in the context of governing the purported 'obesity epidemic' (Flegal 2006; Mitchell and McTigue 2007; Chiolero and Paccaud 2009; Wright and Harwood 2009): as a personal and collective risk mitigation strategy; as a way of overcoming both individual and geographical luck; and as a core driver of growth within the food and beverage market. Being sensible thus does not necessarily entail self-denial and the avoidance of consumption, but rather the creation of new market opportunities for the instrumental deployment of purposeful and informed consumption choices. As Bauman's quote above suggests, obesity thus renders consumption a political battleground with inevitable and definitive tensions within the multiple enterprises that, as is explored throughout this book, constitute the governance of health. Moreover, the governance of obesity is inherently contingent and contextual, with strategies developed, mediated, legitimated and gaining meaning in situ. For this reason, this chapter will draw on examples from both the US and the UK. The active comparison of national-level policy discourses and stances is important in order to situate obesity as a public health 'crisis' (Ebbeling et al 2002; Carmona 2003; Campos et al 2006; Lobstein 2006; Orbach 2006) relative to 'crises' unfolding in other places. This also offers a means by which the condition can be excised from a situation of moral panic and, instead, held up as a societal concern representative of broader structural failings and limitations. Kwan's suggestion that 'obesity is not an unambiguous medical fact. It is a social fact that various cultural producers vie to define' (2009: 45) is thus useful here. This is not to suggest, as the growing band of obesity sceptics do (Gaesser 2002; Campos 2004; Campos et al 2006; Oliver 2006), that obesity is simply a medical fiction and constructed category that acts to discipline, control and coerce. Instead, while this book accepts that obesity is a constructed 'epidemic', it also concurs that a generalised rise in weight represents a significant public health concern for which viable solutions have been predictably slow to materialise.

This chapter is squarely situated within the growing canon of a poststructural and interdisciplinary critical obesity studies, which 'question[s] particular medical, moral and political obesity truths' (Colls and Evans 2009: 1012). More than this, and as the authors further argue, there is 'an imperative for geographers to question the content and the practices of such politics through critically interrogating the drivers for, and implications of, the increasingly stringent, often knee-jerk policies which unilaterally define certain bodies and places as fat and problematic' (ibid; see also Longhurst 2005). Such 'critical geographies of obesity' are small in number, but are invaluable in their recognition that 'space and place are becoming increasingly important to the conception and deployment of obesity politics' (Colls and Evans 2009: 1012), and their associated governmentalities (Guthman 2009). In exploring examples from the US and UK, this chapter and the one that follows discuss how obesity is never a universal or unitary problem, but rather a series of qualitatively distinct 'problematisations' and 'fields of delineation' (Osborne 1997) that change through time and space. Thus to talk or write of a singular obesity epidemic is conceptually and empirically misguided (Ross 2005), especially given the degree to which the accuracy of obesity being described as an 'epidemic' has been critiqued by social scientists (see for example Gard 2009). Instead of rehearsing this comprehensive debate, this chapter starts from the position that obesity is as much an 'epidemic of signification' (Treichler 1988) as it is a biomedical challenge and significant commercial opportunity. This offers a valuable conceptual lens through which to consider how admonitions to be sensible (often justified in the language and logic of biomedicine) in the name of reducing current weight and preventing future weight gain cut across and mark out specific social, spatial and temporal zones of signification and, in so doing, may also point to new commercial opportunities and realms of moralisation.

To this end, the chapter first explores the current obesity debate and sets out how and why obesity has risen to the lofty status of 'public health problem', the rationales underpinning this moniker and thus the strategies of governance that are sanctioned in the US and the UK. In so doing, it highlights the core differences between the UK and the US's current ideological stance towards rising rates of obesity. In particular, the controversial vision of the UK's secretary of state for health is outlined and set in contrast to that of the Obama administration. Building from this, the chapter then sets out the contested aetiological explanations for a generalised rise in obesity rates which serve as the basis for governance and risk communication strategies that aim to prevent further rises in obesity. The idea that obesity is a function of 'energy in' exceeding 'energy out' as represented by the now-ubiquitous 'energy-balance equation' has become commonplace, but explanations have tended to fall on the side of either gluttony or sloth (Prentice and Jebb 1995), often corresponding to the way in which obesity is framed as a problem and, therefore, the kinds of solutions that are suggested.

—

The discussion then turns to the three assertions. First, it asks how sensible behaviour is delineated with reference to these aetiological explanations such that it becomes an active strategy of risk mitigation and management. This mitigation takes place in the present and in the future, for both the self and, given research detailing obesity as socially and culturally contagious (see for example Cohen-Cole and Fletcher 2008), anyone an obese person might unwittingly 'pollute'. More than this, it also represents a strategy of intergenerational risk minimisation, extending as far as a mother's unborn child (Wardle et al 2002; Davey Smith et al 2007). Second, it argues that being sensible is cast as a tool to overcome the effects of 'luck' as well as 'geographical luck'. In this reading, being sensible offers lifestyle strategies that skim over deep structural inequalities and avoid the need for the kind of redistributive policies that luck egalitarians might call for. The choice of whether or not to take this path is then left up to the individual, with the choice to remain disengaged often cast as evidence of the entrenched negative externalities of luck, thus reinforcing the perception of a fundamental divide between those taking charge of their health and those, in effect, letting the side down. The third assertion is that sensible behaviour is a fundamental engine of market growth in that the 'right kind' of consumption serves to mediate between discipline and pleasure (Smith Maguire 2008). It is this active mediation of the tension between discipline (self-denial) and pleasure (self-indulgence) that serves as a key motor of market activity and opportunity. This is in stark contrast to the suggestion that a healthy lifestyle is about consuming less. Instead, recent areas of growth in the leisure and food industries are testament to the marketability of sensible lifestyle choices. In exploring these assertions in both conceptual and empirical terms, this chapter hopes to think through the entanglements of neoliberal political economies and the governance of health. Being sensible is thus about far more than simply behaving in a responsible way and making the correct choices to do so. It is also about ensuring that these choices perpetuate continued growth.

The 'obesity debate'

Obesity is cast as an 'epidemic' in the biomedical sense (see also United States Surgeon General 2001) due to its global prevalence and increasing occurence (World Health Organization 2003b , 2004). However, this appellation has been subject to recent and numerous critiques (Chopra and Darnton-Hill 2004; Ross 2005; Flegal 2006; Oliver 2006; Mitchell and McTigue 2007; Saguy and Almeling 2008; Chiolero and Paccaud 2009; Wright and Harwood 2009). The question of how obesity has simultaneously risen to the status of twin epidemic – biomedical and of meaning – is one that critical health geography is in a methodologically and epistemologically fortuitous position to address. The World Health Organization (WHO) defines obesity as 'a condition of abnormal or excessive fat accumulation in adipose tissue, to the extent that health may be impaired' (World Health Organization 2005: 6). The biomedical definition of obesity is based on a simple standardised ratio or anthropometric reference value of weight to height (weight in kg/height in m^2). Since 1995, the WHO has differentiated body mass index (BMI) between underweight (below 18.0), normal (18.0–25.0), overweight (25.0–29.9), obese (30.0–39.9) and morbidly obese (over 40.0). This classification system is underpinned by the assumption that there is a statistically significant correlation between increased BMI and mortality and morbidity risk from a range of non-communicable diseases (NCD) (Kuczmarski and Flegal 2000). Weight-responsive co-morbidities include type 2 diabetes, coronary heart disease (CHD), cardiovascular disease (CVD), hypertension, sleep apnoea and certain cancers (Hubbard 2000) and, most recently, the risk of preterm birth for overweight pregnant women (McDonald et al 2010). In addition, being obese also increases the severity and complications associated with a broad range of conditions, as well as making treatment and surgery more complex and more costly. Using BMI to define obesity is not without its conceptual problems and there is a substantial debate around the validity of a universal index of weight/health (see Evans and Colls 2009). Indeed, the WHO acknowledged that 'public health action' cut-off points should be lower among Asian and Pacific populations as such groups have an increased risk of type 2 diabetes and cardiovascular disease at lower body weights. There has also been substantial debate over whether BMI or waist–hip ratio (central obesity) is a better measure of health risk for such populations, with central obesity now the favoured measurement for British Asians. Despite its contested hegemony, BMI still has a useful function as a tool for international comparison of population risk and has thus permitted a quantitative exposition of the scale of obesity's global and national spread, catalysing current calls for public health action.

The BMI's 'probabilistic notion of risk' (Chiolero and Paccaud 2009) underpins the current ubiquity of the 'epidemic' label when describing the global and national prevalence of obesity and its rapid rate of increase over the past two decades. The WHO (2003b) estimate that there are over one billion people worldwide who fall within the overweight category, and of these, 300 million are classified as obese. Indeed, with 46% of the global burden of disease currently apportioned to non-communicable diseases (WHO 2003b: 4), and the prevalence of obesity rising annually, there is little surprise that the WHO has classified overweight as a 'chronic' NCD (2003: 2). At the national level, concern has been mounting over evidence of a marked increase in adult and childhood obesity rates. For example, HSE data from 2003 show that 22% of men and 23% of women in England were obese. This represents a marked increase on figures from 1993 of 16.4% and 13.2% respectively. In addition, by 2003, 43% of men and 33% of women were classified as overweight (see Figure 2). There has been a similar rise in the percentage of men and women classified as having a 'raised waist circumference' of greater than 102 cm in men and 88 cm in women (see Figure 3) from 20% of men in 1993 to 34% in 2008 and from 26% to 44% of women over the same time period. Using waist circumference as a measure of risk also demonstrates the elevated risks faced by women. By 2010, the proportion of obese men is predicted to climb to 33% and 28% for women. However, by contrast, predictions for overweight are

Figure 2: Changing proportions of overweight and obese among men and women 1993–2008 in England

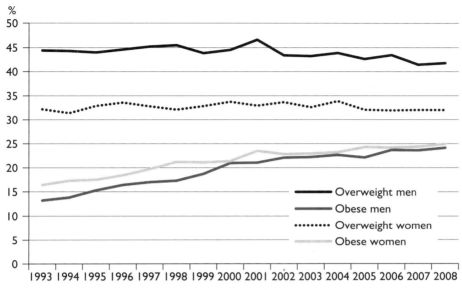

Source: NHS Information Centre (2009)

Figure 3: Changing proportions of men and women with an increased waist circumference 1993–2008 in England

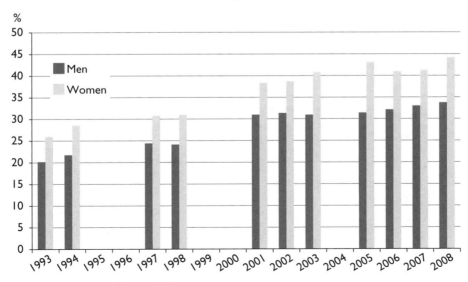

Source: NHS Information Centre (2009)

slightly more optimistic, with men expected to see a fall to 42% and women a fall to 30% (Zaninotto et al 2006). However, while these calculations are based on extrapolations of historical trends (and only the upcoming HSE will be able to demonstrate their veracity), the figures are nonetheless significant in that they highlight that any cause for optimism based on projected rates of overweight are undone by significant projected climbs in obesity.

In the US, national median obesity rates stood at 15.9% in 1995. By 2009, these were 26.9%, with little evidence of any reversal of this upwards trend. As Figure 4 shows, what is perhaps as notable as the continual upward climb in national obesity rates is the denormalisation of 'normal' weight as, in 2009, being overweight became the norm. National rates also mask significant variations between the states (see Map 1). Mississippi, for example, has an obesity rate of 35.3%, while Colorado bucks the trend at 18.9%. In a similar vein, there is a distinctive geography to overweight and obesity in the UK with 'the balance of evidence [suggesting] that obesity prevalence tends to be higher in the Midlands and Northern England' (Moon et al 2007: 23). However, Moon, Quarendon et al are careful to conclude that the geographies of obesity are complex and should be subject to multiple caveats given that their conclusions are based on synthetic estimations of prevalence, which, in effect, describe 'geographic variations in the socio-demographic profile that is associated with obesity/ overweight' (ibid: 29). In effect, while the quantitative and geographical exposition of obesity prevalence is a clearly biopolitical exigency, it also serves to communicate a particular vision

Figure 4: Percentage of US citizens of normal weight, overweight and obese, 1995–2009

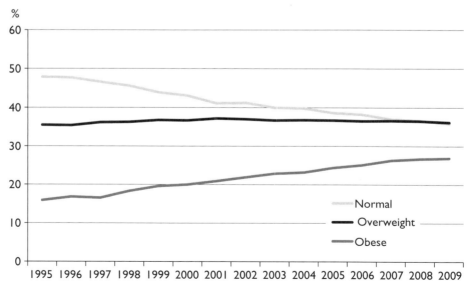

Source: Centers for Disease Control (2009)

Map 1: Geographical variations in obesity rates across the US in 2008

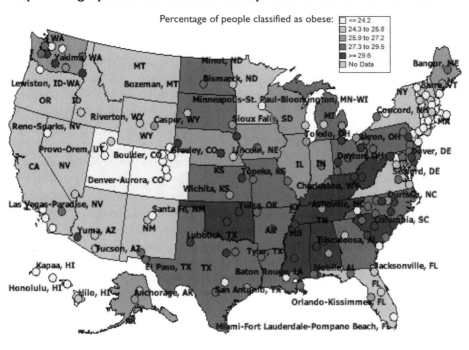

Percentage of people classified as obese:

□ <= 24.2
■ 24.3 to 25.8
■ 25.9 to 27.2
■ 27.3 to 29.5
■ >= 29.6
□ No Data

Source: BRFSS GIS Maps 2008, http://apps.nccd.cdc.gov/gisbrfss/

of risk situated within normative discourses of culpability and responsibility which, in turn, sanction and necessitate particular strategies of governance.

Taming obesity: governing health and lifestyles in the US and UK

The WHO's reclassification of body weight as a disease has raised public and political interest in personal dietary and lifestyle choices and the ways in which these might be managed to produce better health outcomes. In the UK this has taken the form of funding for local obesity strategies attached to the 2004 Choosing Health White Paper (Department of Health 2004a) and an associated public service agreement (PSA) to 'halt, by 2010, the year-on-year increase in obesity among children under 11 in the context of a broader strategy to tackle obesity in the population as a whole'. The more recent White Paper Healthy Weight, Healthy Lives (Department of Health 2008) then sets out a further strategy to address the key issues raised by the Government Office of Science's Foresight Report on obesity (Government Office for Science 2007). However, with the Foresight Report indicating no sign of any movement towards meeting the PSA target, the Labour government quietly set this back to 2020, where it has remained ever since (Boseley 2007; House of Commons Committee of Public

Accounts 2007; Kmietowicz 2007). In the US, *Healthy People 2010* set a goal for 60% of adults to be at a 'healthy weight' by 2010 and to reduce the proportion of those classified as obese to 15% (United States Department of Health and Human Services 2000). A target was also set to reduce the proportion of children who are overweight and obese from 11% (1994) to 5% by 2010. Federal targets also include increasing those eating five servings of fruit and vegetables a day, consumption levels of wholegrains and lower fat and salt intake. The latest 'Healthy People 2020' document is still in the planning stages, but looks likely to have the additional (and slightly vague) objective of preventing 'inappropriate weight gain in youths and adults'.

In the US, overweight and obesity officially became 'leading health indicators' in the *Healthy People 2010* report (United States Department of Health and Human Services 2000) and the surgeon general commissioned a consultation on the issue. The resultant *Call to Action* aimed to 'promote the recognition of overweight and obesity as major public health problems', 'identify effective and culturally appropriate interventions to prevent and treat' and impose 'environmental changes that would help prevent overweight and obesity' (United States Surgeon General 2001: iii, see earlier). In 2001, the CDC also announced that it would fund state-based Nutrition and Physical Activity Programs to Prevent and Decrease Obesity. Most recently, under the 2009 American Recovery and Reinvestment Act, $650 million has been made available for community-scale 'prevention and wellness initiatives'. While both the UK and US have declared their intentions to address childhood and adult obesity, the deployment of these goals has involved contrasting ends and means. However, at a very basic level, it is underpinned by a common discourse of what it is to be sensible with respect to obesity (for example eat healthily, move more). Yet, this discourse of sensibleness is further marked by differing recognitions of *how* people might be sensible, *who* might hold responsibility for facilitating this, the *barriers* that might hinder such efforts and the behavioural/cultural *transformations* required. In short, while information about healthy lifestyles has generally been stripped back to commonsense labels (for example targets such as five fruit and vegetables a day), the governmentalities underpinning their realisation have remained moving targets.

In this vein, the shift to a new Conservative–Liberal Democrat coalition government in the UK in 2010 has brought in ideological shifts with regard to health which merit further consideration. In July 2010, the Faculty of Public Health's (FPH) annual conference hosted Andrew Lansley, the newly appointed secretary of state for health, as its keynote speaker. The speech was Lansley's first since the formation of the coalition government and garnered huge media attention as he reiterated the UK's ongoing struggle to curb 'the highest obesity rates in Europe', 'among the worst rates of sexually transmitted infections' and 'rising rates of alcohol and drug problems' (Lansley 2010). The Conservative Party's general election campaign had clearly stated the will to transform the Department of Health (DH) into a Department of Public Health, an objective welcomed by the incoming president of the FPH in a preconference interview with *The Guardian*

(Campbell 2010a). Initial optimism over the transformation of the DH had been high, but alarm bells had started to sound when the coalition ignored its own National Institute for Clinical Excellence's (NICE) advice to impose legislation and regulations to limit saturated fats, transfats, sugar and salt in food sold in the UK and impose a junk food advertising watershed in order to reduce deaths from cardiovascular disease (National Institute for Clinical Excellence 2010).

When Lansley finally took the stage at the FPH conference, he outlined a vision of poor health rooted in 'factors like dysfunctional families, poverty, worklessness, weak family and community structures, lack of good parenting, or mental illness', all underpinned by a 'lack of self-esteem' (Lansley 2010). Yet, as he suggested, 'you can't legislate for self-esteem from Westminster'. Instead of legislative change, therefore, the nation must recognise the value and influence of social norms in driving behaviour change at a time when 'social and individual responsibility' in Britain is in 'decline'. Thus people need 'nudging . . . in the right direction, encouraging positive choices. Not lecturing or nannying, but making people feel empowered'. Casting aside the predictable castigation of the outgoing Labour Party's 'nanny statist' approach to health, the social vision expounded in Lansley's speech is not only one of a terminal decline in responsibility, but a clear statement that responsibility is necessarily personal and, in contrast to Labour's vision, not always 'shared' with government. Instead, it is government and business that are expressly given the task of promoting 'innovation in thinking and practice'. The speech closed with the suggestion that the government's flagship healthy lifestyle campaign, Change4Life, inaugurated in 2009 with £75 million in government funding over three years, should be handed over to the food and drinks industry in a new 'Responsibility Deal'. This was, understandably, greeted with disbelief; *The Guardian*'s Felicity Lawrence summed up the sentiment as follows:

> What's not so much risible but truly frightening about Lansley's speech is that it lays bare the underlying Tory philosophy. In their 'Big Society' – which casts everything as personal responsibility – social injustice, like obesity, is indeed a moral failure, but only on the part of those who suffer it. (Lawrence 2010)

Lansley's controversial words thus offer up a vision of the ways and means of public health that contrast starkly with that of a medical and research fraternity staunchly and outspokenly opposed to the involvement and practices of big industry. Freudenberg sums up this tension between state, industry and individual health outcomes as follows:

> The primary obstacle to comprehensive and effective policies to control obesity is not our lack of understanding of its biology, but rather opposition from the global food industry. Like the tobacco and alcohol industries, most food and beverage companies emphasise that individual responsibility rather than public protection is the best route to reduce obesity, a strategy that conveniently preserves their right to

transfer the health-related costs of their products to consumers and tax-payers . . . To date, the industry has successfully framed the policy debate as a conflict between proponents of individual responsibility and those who want to impose an overbearing nanny state that deprives us of sweet, salty, and fatty pleasures. (Freudenberg 2010: 365)

Shortly after Lansley's contentious speech, the coalition announced its intention to close the Food Standards Agency (FSA), despite the significance of its work on nutrition and food labelling to the obesity agenda. Instead, the closure more likely reflects the FSA's antagonistic relationship with the food industry over proposals for its traffic-light food labelling scheme which, after significant industry lobbying at an estimated cost of €1 billion (Ecologist 2010), were rejected by the European Union. Despite their unpalatable nature, Andrew Lansley's words do resonate with the conceptual arguments made in this book concerning the enterprise of delineating, encouraging and facilitating sensible behaviour and the relative role of the state and individual within this undertaking. His speech therefore marks a fitting starting point for this discussion of obesity, as it sets the UK in stark contrast to the current stance of the US administration.

On the other side of the Atlantic, Michelle Obama is actively working to 'end the plague of childhood obesity in a generation', linking the efforts of the Food and Drug Administration (FDA) and manufacturers to impose mandatory front of pack nutritional labelling and a Healthy Food Financing Initiative to improve access to healthy foods for low-income communities. The contrast between the UK and US ideologies seems clear. The UK is backing corporate interests at the expense of the kind of regulation and legislation repeatedly called for by expert advisers (see Campbell 2010b). By contrast, the US is productively aligning state involvement with industry accountability, recognising that a call for personal responsibility alone cannot overcome the effects of structural and social inequalities. As such, the delicate interplay (intended and actual) between the state, industry and the individual (or community) forms the basis of the *geographies* of governmentality, that are, in turn, underpinned by a far more generalised hope that people have the capacity and desire to be sensible with respect to their health and body weight.

The contested aetiologies of obesity

The aetiology of obesity is complex and contested, with Jebb arguing that:

At its simplest, obesity will only develop when energy intake exceeds energy expenditure over a prolonged period, but this overview conceals the multiple influences on energy intake and expenditure and ignores the potential for a genetic predisposition. Accordingly, there is unlikely to be a single unifying theory to explain the aetiological basis of obesity. (Jebbs 1997: 281)

The lack of a 'single unifying theory' stems from the fact that obesity is not a single disorder but:

> A heterogeneous group of conditions with multiple causes each of which are ultimately expressed as an obese phenotype . . . body weight is ultimately determined by the interaction of genetic, environmental and psychosocial factors acting through the physiological mediators of energy intake and expenditure. (Jebb 1997: 264).

Therefore, at the root of virtually all explanations of the sudden and dramatic rise in obesity rates in the US and UK, lies the simple energy balance equation:

Energy consumed – energy expended = net weight change

As Jebb further contends:

> The second law of thermodynamics is one of the few incontrovertible facts in this field. Obesity will only develop if energy intake exceeds energy expenditure over a prolonged period of time, but the mechanisms underpinning increases in energy intake or decreases in energy expenditure remain elusive. (Jebb 1999: 2)

The idea that obesity is rising because we are all eating more of the wrong types of food and exercising less (whether willingly or unwillingly) has produced two main schools of thought: gluttony or sloth (Prentice and Jebb 1995). However, this bifurcation may mask additional complexities. For example, Lang and Rayner (2005) identify no fewer than eight theories for obesity's rise, ranging from genetics to technological changes in agriculture and food manufacturing. Yet, even these numerous theories fall back on either the assumption that energy consumption has increased, or that energy expenditure has fallen over the past two decades. In so doing, they highlight the ongoing and deeply politicised tensions between the array of stakeholders trying to unravel the complex linkages between diet, exercise, body weight and health to develop workable and legitimate interventions on the contentious terrain of individual lifestyle.

Common sense dictates that if a person eats too much, they will gain weight. Of course, not all individuals who overeat become obese and, conversely, not all obese individuals overeat. Obesity often pushes common sense to its limit as generalised statements hold little sway against the diversity of empirical reality. Proponents of the gluttony camp contend that there is statistical evidence suggesting that per capita calorific intake has been rising steadily since the early 1980s. This change has occurred against a backdrop of (assumed) static or declining energy expenditure due to a 'Western lifestyle' characterised by sedentarism, car usage, service sector jobs and domestic technological advances. The gluttony argument has found a particularly powerful voice with those authors falling into the category termed 'science for the people' (Gard and Wright 2005). The cultural histories of consumption in the US, set against a backdrop of technological changes in agriculture and food production that made disposing of surplus fat and sugar a national imperative (Schlosser 2001; Nestle 2002; Critser 2004; Spurlock 2005a, 2005b), suggest that fast food consumption has been increasing year on year since its inception in the 1960s. Indeed, Young and Nestle (2002) calculate that from 1978 to 1995, Americans started eating an extra 200 Kcal a day per person. The authors also compared portion sizes with United States Department of Agriculture (USDA) guidelines and noted that in 2002, muffins were on average 300% larger and soda servings 35–100% larger than recommended by federal guidelines. Their suggestions chime well with an anti-corporate discourse linking the increased availability, desirability and marketing of fast food to the emergence of the obesity 'epidemic'. This argument has spurred a vociferous political and media critique in both countries of the ways and means of the food industry that has been especially potent in the context of evidence of food marketing to children, where questions of health and morality unhappily collide (Kraak and Pelletier 1998a, 1998b, 2009).

One of the main barriers to developing the unequivocal evidence base needed for obesity prevention policy is the fact that NHANES and the UK's National Diet and Nutrition Survey (NDNS) are self-reported. This means that those using the data set to ascertain temporal changes in calorific intake or composition have to be aware of complex reporting biases. Not only do people tend to underreport what they have eaten, but this underreporting is more marked among those classified as obese, women, low income, smokers and those known as 'restrained eaters' (Jebb 1999). Often this gives the paradoxical and misleading impression that obese people eat far less than their non-obese counterparts, undermining the gluttony argument. In addition to this, reporting methods, cohort sizes and questions asked have not been consistent since the 1980s, making temporal trends difficult to ascertain due to the incompatibility of data sets – a criticism that is also levelled at alcohol consumption data and will be further discussed in Chapter Six. For example, the National Food Survey in the UK underwent methodological changes when it became the NDNS in 2001. Furthermore, data sets are based on different methodologies in the UK and US and so are not immediately comparable for researchers seeking explanations for the similarities in the rise of obesity in the two countries. These problems have led some biomedical researchers to contend instead that the energy density of foods may be one potential explanation (Prentice and Jebb 2003), and that gluttony per se must only be considered a causal factor at an individual scale, rather than at a population level.

In 1995 Prentice and Jebb grappled with the idea that obesity could be caused by either gluttony or sloth, and reported that, in contrast to Ruppel Shell's (2003) figures, the proportion of fat in the diet has climbed 50% from 0.6 kJ for each kJ of carbohydrate in 1940, to 0.9 kJ by the 1990s (Prentice and Jebb 1995). They further suggested that, not only has the fat content (or energy density) of diets in the UK been rising (principally due to a generalised shift from food cooked at home using raw ingredients to processed foods), but that high-fat diets could themselves undermine the natural hypothalamic regulation of energy balance and have a neurological effect on appetite. High-fat diets, it was found, not only increased calorie intake (fat has more calories per gram than any other type of food) but also the fat itself could undermine feelings of satiety, leading to what Prentice and Jebb (1995) termed 'passive overconsumption' due to 'high fat hyperphagia'. This initial suggestion as to a potential aetiological basis of obesity was followed up in their later work. This 'passive overconsumption' is reinforced by the disjuncture between food's bulk and its energy content (Prentice 2001). Since people judge portion sizes based on their absolute bulk, overconsumption inevitably occurs when energy density is raised but portion sizes remain constant in volume terms. Prentice and Jebb term this passive overconsumption a 'mechanism of dysregulation' (2003: 192). This was an understandably popular assertion with a global media seeking biomedical proof to back up the popular suspicion that obesity could be blamed on multinational food manufacturers and retailers. Their conclusion that 'fast food retailers have a global impact and one that targets the most vulnerable members of society in terms of obesity' (2003: 193) was one repeated in newspapers and TV news bulletins on either side of the Atlantic. Most notably, it was the catalyst for some food companies to shift from the defensive to an aggressive reinvention of their corporate social responsibility (CSR) strategies, a revision of product lines to reduce their fat, sugar and calorie content and to take up new voluntary codes of conduct for advertising and marketing (Herrick 2007; Kraak et al 2009).

However, both Prentice and Jebb acknowledge that while the composition of diets is partly to blame for rising obesity, this would have had a benign effect at a population scale if energy expenditure had risen in tandem. As Jebb concedes, 'the paradox of increasing obesity at a time of decreasing food consumption can be reconciled only by an even sharper decline in energy requirements' (1999: 9). The sloth school of thought thus crystallises around the belief that rising rates of obesity can best be explained by a population-scale fall in physical activity, in the absence of any genotype change in such a short timeframe. The reasons for this assumption are largely the same as those underpinning the argument for increased energy intake, namely that technological innovation has permitted and involuntarily resulted in more sedentary lifestyles, perpetuated by the lure of activities such as TV viewing and videogames. No longer does work require energy expenditure, and increases in car usage mean that trips made on foot or by bicycle have fallen year on year, despite confounders such as a rise in the rate of cycle ownership in the UK from 14% to 32% between 1975 and 1996 (Lawlor et al 2003) and a doubling of cycle use in London since 2000 (Transport for London 2007).

The assumption of falling activity levels has become common in both the scientific and popular imaginations. As a result, obesity is most often viewed through the lens of nostalgia such that being sensible would require a return to more 'traditional' ways of living – home-cooked food, children being able to play outdoors and walking to local shops. Yet this received wisdom means that 'there is a recurring refrain in the overweight and obesity literature in which the relationship between food, physical activity and body weight is described as "obvious" despite a scarcity of evidence to that effect' (Gard and Wright 2005: 43). The relationship between physical activity and body weight is particularly fraught, with the added complication that not only must the link between weight and exercise be uncovered, but also the way in which these then interact with health. Indeed, measuring physical activity changes accurately across populations over time has consistently proved an obstacle to determining a definitive aetiology of obesity. Physical activity measures are included in the HSE and the BRFSS, and in both cases report the percentage of people claiming to have engaged in no, moderate or intense physical activity in the past week or month; among those that have exercised, the duration of time is taken into account. However, as Robinson and Sicard note:

> One of the challenges facing obesity research is the difficulty in feasibly, reliably and validly measuring many of the key exposure variables of interest . . . as a result, many associations identified are subject to measurement error that, at best, weakens relationships that truly exist or, worse still, introduces bias that leads to spurious conclusions. (Robinson and Sicard 2005: 198)

Just as energy intakes tend to be underreported by exactly those groups of people who have the highest rates of obesity, energy expenditure is overreported most frequently by men and those who are overweight (Wareham et al 2005). The notion that Britons and Americans have become irrecoverably sedentary, slovenly and slothful under 'modernity's scourge' (Waters and Baur 2003: 422) is one that has been transformed into received wisdom as well as forming the basis of London's successful Olympic bid (see Chapter Six). Yet, blaming 'modernity' and 'modern life' really just shifts blame away from individuals and onto wider forces beyond their control. However, the simultaneous adherence to the energy balance equation conveys the need actively to monitor and manage this delicate equilibrium. The coexistence of these two explanatory framings appear, therefore, to deliver the message that:

> The pro-obesity forces are unimaginably powerful, our defences against them are notoriously weak and unreliable and, worst of all, it is our own individual, imprudent inattention to energy-in and energy-out that has landed us in this situation. (Gard and Wright 2005: 84)

It is thus such imprudence in the face of a 'runaway weight gain train' (Swinburn and Eggar 2004) that has become a policy target in the US and the UK, underpinned by a shared belief in the need for personal responsibility, but differing in the extent to which individuals are deemed accountable for choices and their outcomes.

Being sensible

Risk mitigation and management

Aetiological explanations of obesity communicate the condition's causes as well as the consequences of certain lifestyle choices. They thus form the basis of risk communication strategies and, as a consequence, risk mitigation and management techniques. The relationship between being sensible and risk is of both an intrinsic and an instrumental nature. Being sensible is thus a means and an ends – to a longer happier, healthier, more fulfilled and vibrant life – realised through *active* strategies of risk mitigation and management applied to oneself and in relation to one's surroundings. However, communicating the behavioural risk factors for obesity requires some degree of aetiological consensus to produce a common risk narrative. Yet, the delineation of risk needed to inform categorisations of sensible behaviour has long been characterised by disagreement, conflicting evidence, swayed by social and cultural trends and, most recently, been subjected to sharp critical analysis. Furthermore, aetiological explanations for obesity are as political as they are physiological and psychological. Narratives of risk are thus reflective of a broad set of sociologies, rather than simply the state of biomedical research. As such, they often represent particular iterations of received wisdom and common sense in the absence of conclusive scientific evidence.

For example, while there is evidence to suggest that the increasing calorific density of food is one of the causes of obesity, on the other side of the energy balance equation, studies struggle to provide any definitive evidence for a generalised fall in activity rates over the past 30 years. Instead they rely on proxy measures of reduced activity such as car journeys, undermining suggestions that individuals need to be more active to prevent obesity. The behavioural and biological (for example genetic predisposition or obese parents) risk factors for obesity squarely overlap, which further complicates both the identification of objective risk measurements and their communication. As a consequence, without any clearly defined idea of the genesis of risk, proposed strategies to mitigate and manage risk often tread a precautionary line through these spaces of uncertainty. Being sensible is thus a cue to moderation that weaves a delicate path between both sides of the energy balance equation. Sensible behaviour needs to be defined to be worked and shaped into policy guidelines, but as the discussion here has shown, this process of definition strikes at the political heart of designating not just where the duty and responsibility to act lie, but also the limits to governing the risks of obesity given the lack of 'incontrovertible facts' within the aetiological evidence base.

As a further example, cohort studies show that increasing physical activity can aid weight loss, but it is far more problematic to prove that decreasing activity causes weight gain. In the absence of a clear population-scale correlation between weight and activity rates, research has instead focused on the link between health and activity rates. There is much clearer evidence suggesting that physical inactivity is correlated with a higher risk of cancer, heart disease, respiratory disease, hypertension (Department of Health 2004b) and that activity can reduce the symptoms of diabetes (Di Loreto et al 2005) as well as helping ensure mental health and dementia among older people (Rovio et al 2005). Since the evidence base correlating health and physical activity is relatively strong; health has been used as a proxy for body weight when arguing for the importance of physical activity as a strategy of risk mitigation, despite the fact that the two variables have very different mechanistic relationships with physical activity. Such arguments have also been used to great effect by the 'health at every size' movement, which states that it is possible to be fit and fat and that trying to attain a 'normal' BMI is not necessarily accompanied by better health (Provencher et al 2007).

However, such messages about the necessity of maintaining a healthy weight conflict with efforts to instil sensible behaviours to mitigate the risk of present and future obesity. Indeed, as discussions of 'sensible drinking' in Chapter Six will show, communicating risk in a way that is meaningful when set against socially normative practices and contexts (an upward rise in average body weights) that may favour risk taking is a challenge both in conceptual terms and in how it relates to the practices, policies and promises of the food and leisure industries. Information on how to eat sensibly to reduce the risk of weight gain or how to exercise for weight management now comes from a plethora of sources: government, non-profit organisations, the internet, magazines and newspapers, TV and word of mouth. Yet, to be effective, these 'sensible planners' (Sunstein and Thaler 2003: 178) must distil a thoroughly conflicting field of evidence into a series of universally applicable, communicable sound bites that are credible and workable. It is in this need to find workable advice (that is, advice that will be translated into action) that risk communication becomes embedded in the discourses of self-efficacy discussed in Chapter Two.

Communicating sensible behaviour as a strategy of risk mitigation is a means to overcome the 'intention–behaviour gap' (Sheeran 2002) that plagues the lifestyle choices discussed in this book. The route from good intentions to the uptake of healthy behaviours is determined by a multitude of factors, but it is the development and deployment of self-efficacy – or the belief that one is capable of behaving in a certain way to achieve a desired end – that is key. At the motivational stage of behaviour change, 'risk perception in itself is insufficient to enable a person to form an intention' (Schwarzer 2008: 6); rather an awareness of risk enables the individual to contemplate consequences and competencies (ability to enact change). Thus, being aware that obesity carries health risks is a necessary precursor to behaviour change. When a person's intentions are formed they need 'detailed instructions on how to perform the desired action' (Schwarzer 2008: 7) as well as support to maintain it. As an example, the NHS pamphlet *Your Weight, Your Health*, which is shared with patients demonstrating or expressing concerns about their weight as set out in the obesity 'care pathway', highlights that it is not concerned with 'miracle diets' but rather 'looking at your life and building up gradually to the changes that will make a difference' (NHS 2006: 9). The

—

ideas of getting beyond a compartmentalised focus on (unattainable) diets is also echoed in the CDC's Healthy Weight information website, which highlights the importance of holism in its declaration that: 'it's not a diet, it's a healthy lifestyle!' (Centers for Disease Control 2010). Both the NHS and the CDC's materials highlight that obesity poses clear health risks, with the NHS asking 'what's weight got to do with health?' and listing co-morbidities that are, in order of severity: life threatening, could be life threatening, cause pain and unhappiness and are disruptive and irritating. In pointing out the order of relative severity of these risks, it also ensures that individuals can identify with at least some aspects of the table and, therefore, the idea that obesity has got a *lot* to do with health.

Both the NHS and the CDC's materials iterate the importance of 'control' in the quest for healthy lifestyles. In this reading, control (the kind of self-efficacy also evident in Lansley's speech) is both cause and consequence of weight management and, therefore, better health. To take control, patients on both sides of the Atlantic are first asked to know their weight and BMI through using a chart or online calculator before being provided with an abridged version of the 'detailed instructions' needed to change their lifestyles. This process of knowing through measurement is necessary for individuals to personalise calls for behaviour change by identifying with the risk categories being presented. This notion of self-identification is also suggested in the NHS care pathway, where patients are asked if they are ready to change. If the answer is 'yes', the doctor will proceed through stages of information, advice and, as a last resort, treatment. If the answer is 'no', they are offered literature and reassured that appropriate advice and support will be there when they decide that they need it. Both the CDC and NHS are also quick to stress the importance of moderation and of learning new habits that are simple, manageable and achievable. This non-threatening language of attainability is a crucial motivator to inspiring the active choice to undertake risk mitigation strategies through a series of pro-forma, commonsense behavioural changes.

This view of risk mitigation is curious for being such an unsatisfactory variation on the libertarian paternalism (Sunstein and Thaler 2003; Thaler and Sunstein 2003, 2008) or asymmetric paternalism (Loewenstein et al 2007; Downs et al 2009) thinking now so favoured by both the US and UK administrations. Libertarian paternalistic thinking aims to bring about policies that have the 'goal of influencing the choices of affected parties in a way that will make those parties better off' (Thaler and Sunstein 2003: 175). Important for the conundrum of delineating sensible behaviour, the authors suggest that being better off should be an *objective* measure (for example changes in population or individual BMI). Libertarian paternalism differs from classic economic theory in that it assumes that people are irrational. For example, the existence of high obesity rates in the US serves as clear evidence that 'it is hard to claim that Americans are eating optimal diets' (ibid). The problem with such arguments in the context of obesity is that the default option that might be agreed on to counter the effects of the inevitable irrationality that produces obesity may be unattractive to citizen-consumers, politicians and industry. The default of a ban on junk food advertising and sponsorship and agreements to curb (and label) fat, sugar and salt content in foods is enormously popular among the health lobby (National Institute for Clinical Excellence 2010). However, making sensible behaviour inevitable runs counter to the rhetoric of consumer choice taken up by the food industry and, in the UK, government. To return to Andrew Lansley's speech, this notion of choice (through moderation) was reiterated in his statement that:

> It is perfectly possible to eat a Mars Bar, or a bag of crisps or have a carbonated drink if you do it in moderation, understanding your overall diet and lifestyle. Then you can begin to take responsibility for it and the companies who are selling you those things can be part of that responsibility too. It is not about good foods and bad foods it is about good diet and bad diet. (Smith 2010)

When set against his earlier assertion that 'no government campaign or programme can force people to make healthy choices', the unwillingness to reduce or offer alternative choices in order to facilitate risk mitigation seems to be directly lacking in paternalism, and overwhelmingly dominated by libertarianism. As set out in the Responsibility Deal document, this 'Conservative response to societal challenges which we know can't be solved by regulation and legislation alone' represents a partnership that 'balances proportionate regulation with corporate responsibility' (Public Health Commission 2010, n.p.). This ideology, however, runs counter to recent calls for transfats to be 'virtually eliminated' in the UK (Mozaffarian and Stampfer 2010) and 2010 NICE guidance echoing this. The tension between the freedom of choice promised by the market and research suggesting that unrestrained choice rarely results in optimal outcomes (Schwartz 2004; Salecl 2010) sits uneasily with an obesity policy that fails to address fully either the market or choice. Instead, there is an assertion that policy must focus on 'nudging individuals in the right direction'. Yet, with little suggestion of how these nudges might combine to produce sensible behaviour rooted in improved self-efficacy, obesity policy remains toothless in its aversion to challenging the machinations of industry actively. This weakness is further reinforced when individuals' situational and contextual vulnerabilities to obesity (luck) are considered.

Overcoming luck

Acknowledging that choice is neither universally granted nor universally taken up is at the heart of socioecological explanations of obesity. The effects of 'brute luck' – the social, economic, geographic or genetic situations over which people have no control – can, it is argued by luck egalitarians, be overcome by making responsible choices (Feiring 2008). The extent to which people can be held accountable for conditions outside their immediate control (for example having obese parents doubles the chances of a child becoming obese in adulthood (Whitaker et al 1997; Zaninotto et al 2006)) or that may have resulted from suboptimal choices or the 'voluntary assumption' of risk factors (Wikler 2002: 48) is a particularly fraught moral debate when applied to obesity. Because of the paucity of comparable longitudinal data, a definitive and generalisable aetiology of obesity has been slow to materialise. As a result, epidemiologists and public health specialists are increasingly pointing to changes in the food, physical activity, political and social 'environments' as explanatory variables (Smith and Cummins 2009). However, with the exception of Kearns and Reid-Henry's (2009) paper, there has been little to link the brute luck of these structural inequalities to conceptualisations of responsibility, especially in a geographical sense. This is curious given the expectations of self-control and self-transformation that accompany many policy discourses of obesity. Thus, running counter to the assumption of the 'active citizen' and the 'entrepreneurial self' (Rose 1991) set out by neoliberal governmentality theorists, attention to 'luck' highlights the importance of proscription in the absence of free choice. In this reading, sensible eating advice becomes central to endeavours to prevent obesity, as well as being a yardstick against which to judge individual and collective progress towards citizenship ideals measured quantitatively through key indicators. Thus, being sensible is often extricated from the realm of what Valverde has called 'common knowledge' (Levi and Valverde 2001) and instead coerced into a series of defined parameters and categories, often markedly out of step with a prevailing political economy of food premised on unbounded choice.

The idea of a 'lifestyle disease' sits at odds with the idea of luck, given that lifestyle, by its very nature, is assumed to be a product of active choices. Since luck is seen to exist outside the spectrum of control, it consequently suffers an uneasy relationship with obesity. However, it nonetheless adheres to the idea that 'human vitality is structured by geographically mediated inequalities: patterns of life chances that, although they might be locally articulated, are connected to events elsewhere' (Kearns and Reid-Henry 2009: 556). For example, the *Healthy People 2010* report (United States Department of Health and Human Services 2000) states that the proportion of adolescents from poor households who are overweight or obese is twice that of adolescents from middle- and high-income households. In addition, obesity is especially prevalent among those on lower incomes, African American and Mexican American women compared to white women. Furthermore, the proportion of African American women who are obese is 80% higher than the proportion of men. This gender difference also exists among Mexican American women and men, but among white, non-Hispanics, both men and women have the same prevalence rates (United States Department of Health and Human Services 2000: 57). Since vulnerability to obesity is not evenly distributed by race, income or gender, this reinforces the marked health disparities that prevail in both the US and UK. Yet this local articulation of life chances is also inextricably linked to events and contexts that exist beyond individuals' reach, including the global political economy of food production, retailing and marketing. Thus, there is a certain 'pathogenic challenge' (Kearns and Reid-Henry 2009: 562) in preventing obesity, given the prevailing, 'pathological environment' in which Egger and Swinburn (1997: 480) suggest we live. In order to overcome this challenge, sensible eating guidelines are used as a proxy for and tool to elicit sensible behaviour from individuals. As complex ciphers of risk communication, sensible eating guidelines aim to discipline the population while leaving the political economy of food untouched and undisciplined.

In the US, the 'Dietary guidelines for Americans' which have been issued by the USDA, DHHS and the Center for Nutrition Policy and Promotion every five years since 1980 are a key weapon in realising obesity prevention targets. This document is the definitive statement on the current state of knowledge pertaining to dietary advice and is thus used to underpin the messages and logic of health promotion messaging. At the centre of the dietary guidelines toolkit is the Food Pyramid, which is a representation of the proportion of each type of food that should make up a healthy diet (see Figure 5). From early advice in 1958 aiming to help reduce the effects of post-war nutritional deficiencies, the first 'Dietary guidelines' in 1980 emphasised the consumption of fruit, vegetables and grains. The first pictorial representation of this advice came with the USDA Food Wheel in 1984 and the development of recommended daily allowances (RDA) for each food group. The pyramid was developed between 1988 and 1990, but its launch was set back by calls for further testing of its applicability to low-income adults and school children. As Nestle and Dixon (2004) discuss, there was essentially a conflict between the USDA's mandate to protect US agricultural productivity and viability and the need to maintain and improve public health through achievable

Figure 5: USDA's 2005 MyPyramid

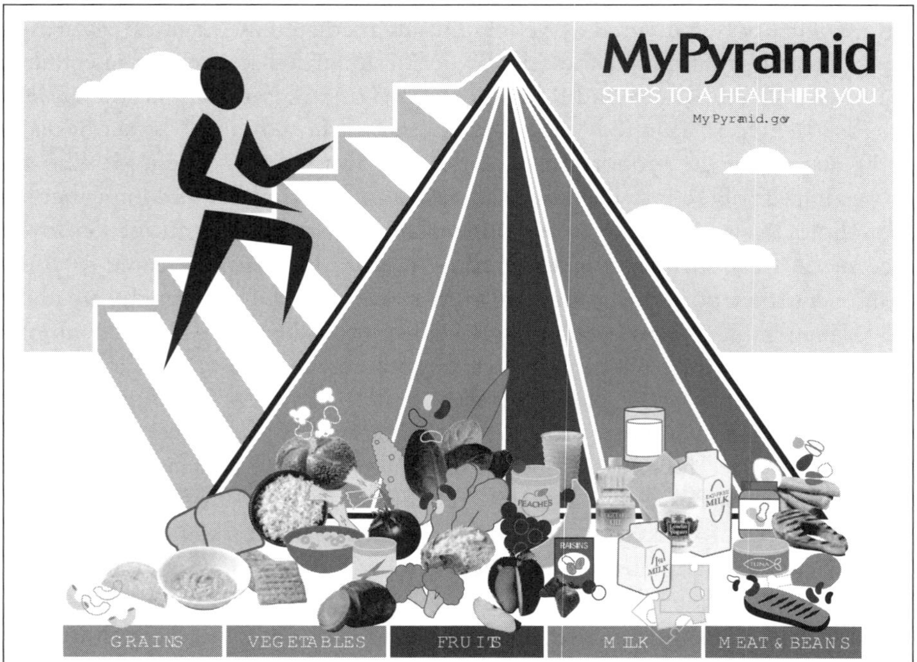

Source: www.mypyramid.gov/downloads/MiniPoster.pdf

and sound dietary advice. When the pyramid was eventually released in 1992, it was subject to criticism due to the lack of any guidance on exercise, salt, sugar or fat consumption. The powerful influence of the National Dairy Council and the Sugar Association ensured the favourable positioning of their products in the pyramid, with the Dairy Council spending a considerable sum researching the link between dairy consumption and weight loss and coining the '3–every–day™' slogan. The 2005 revised MyPyramid was criticised for being 'flawed' (Mitka 2005), despite a $2.4 million spend to create 12 individualised pyramids and daily calorie intake advice based on gender, age and activity levels. In addition and unlike its predecessors, the revised pyramid is also clear that physical activity and a healthy diet must be interlaced. The dietary guidelines, moreover, are limited in their applicability by the fact that people rarely compartmentalise their food intake and very rarely eat just one thing. The dietary guidelines thus act as a vehicle for communicating health and acceptable/optimal risk thresholds to a public deemed to be suffering a 'knowledge deficit' (Allum and Boyd 2002; Hansen et al 2003; Sturgis and Allum 2004).

In the UK, dietary guidelines are overseen by the FSA and coalesce around the Eatwell Plate (Figure 6). In theory, the advice in both MyPyramid and the Eatwell Plate should be broadly similar and this is mostly the case (see also Painter et al 2002). The Eatwell Plate does, however, differ from the food pyramid in the generality of its advice. For example, people are advised to eat 'plenty' of fruit

Figure 6: The FSA's Eatwell Plate

The eatwell plate

Use the eatwell plate to help you get the balance right. It shows how much of what you eat should come from each food group.

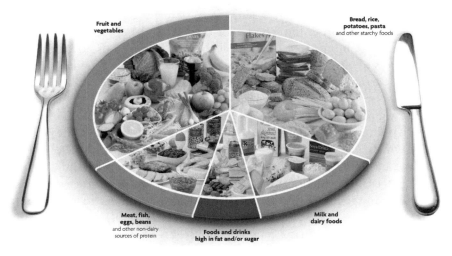

Source: Produced by Department of Health in association with the Welsh Assembly Government, the Scottish Government and the Food Standards Agency in Northern Ireland (www.food.gov.uk/images/pagefurniture/ewplatelargefeb10.jpg)

and vegetables and 'plenty' of starchy foods, 'some' dairy and non-dairy sources of protein and 'just a small amount' of fat and sugar. The US advice is far more prescriptive and, within a 'model' 2000 Kcal a day diet, suggests 6 oz of grains, 2½ cups of vegetables, 2 cups of fruit, 3 cups of milk/dairy (low fat or fat free) and 5½ oz meat and beans. It is notable that 'unhealthy' foods or 'discretionary calories' from fat and sugar appear on the Eatwell Plate as part of a suggested diet, whereas they form a tiny component of MyPyramid and are set apart from those foods that are recommended. A further difference is that the Eatwell Plate is conceived at a population scale and is highly generic in its recommendations, whereas MyPyramid has several versions (such as for children and pregnant women) that personalise its messaging, albeit to a limited extent. Such personalisation of risk has been demonstrated as essential for individuals to change their behaviour (see for example Edgar et al 1988 for a discussion of risk personalisation and HIV/AIDS).

The FSA's desire to communicate risk in a way that is universally accessible, regardless of brute luck, is evidenced by its drive to push through its mandatory traffic-light labelling scheme. The scheme intends to aid 'informed choice' by providing a neat visual cue as to the relative healthiness or unhealthiness of a product. Thus, fat, saturated fat, salt and sugar are labelled as 'low' (green), 'medium' (amber) or 'high' (red) according to integrated advice from the European Regulation (EC) No 1924/2006 on Nutrition and Health Claims, the Committee on Medical Aspects of Food and Nutrition Policy and the Scientific Advisory Committee on Nutrition. The labels are set out as per portion recommendations with any food providing over 30% of fat, saturated fat or sugar or 40% of the recommended maximum daily intake of salt labelled red. Unsurprisingly, the potential to vilify many packaged food products meant that the scheme was forcefully rejected at the EU level after intense lobbying by the food industry. However, in a move that mirrors the early years of the UK's fight against genetically modified organisms in the food chain, it was actually the supermarkets that independently signed up to the scheme for their white label products (Herrick 2005). While this demonstrates a great deal about the enormous power that the UK's 'Big Five' supermarkets hold over the political economy of food (Blythman 2004), it also exemplifies the growth in consumer demand for healthier food, as well as the importance of food labelling as a CSR strategy.

The dietary guidelines and advice serve principally as tools of behaviour change that exist within an educational paradigm of a preventative public health, the validity of which is deeply disputed in the case of both alcohol and obesity. The Pyramid and Eatwell Plate serve as models of sensible consumption, but lack the power (or paternalistic manipulation of choice) to ensure that these aspirations become reality. In the presence of persistent bad luck – as evidenced by widening health inequalities in both the US and the UK (Shaw et al 2005; Singh and Siahpush 2006) – diagrammatic representations of sensible behaviour do little to undo structural inequalities of the obesogenic environment and may instead reinforce the gulf between intention and action. This is made clear by the 2007 FSA Consumer Attitudes Survey. Between 2006 and 2007 there was a climb in the percentage of Britons aware of the 'at least five a day' (fruit and vegetable) message from 71% to 78%. However, the percentage of those actually consuming at least five a day was only 55% in 2006 and 58% in 2007. While any upward movement in this figure is positive, it sits uneasily with the fact that 87% of respondents said that healthy eating was 'important' to them, signalling that these efforts to encourage healthy eating are undermined by persistent inertia. However, there is some evidence that phrases such as 'five a day' have an influence on dietary choices. For example, among those who correctly identified the advice to eat five or more servings a day, 62% did so. Among those incorrectly identifying the advice, only 45% consumed an adequate quantity of fruit and vegetables. Despite the mismatch between knowledge and action, 63% of consumers still claimed that they had 'about the right' amount of information and 66% thought that what did exist was 'easy to understand'. Interestingly, only 50% said that labels influenced their buying decisions, a figure which deeply problematises foundational beliefs in informed choice.

These assertions of the ambiguous effects of information are further corroborated by Downs et al's (2009) study of strategies for promoting healthier food choices. In this they conclude that providing calorific values of foods has little impact on total calories consumed (and actually increased the number of calories consumed by dieters). By contrast, the 'asymmetrically paternalist manipulation of convenience' by putting high-calorie options at the back of the menu had a significant effect on total calories consumed. Not only does this show that city policies such as those in New York, where all prepared food retailers have to indicate the calorie content of their products on menu boards are unlikely to have a marked impact on total calorific intake, but that information saturation can often produce unintended consequences due to the innate irrationality of consumers. Thus, moulding sensible behaviour through guidelines and point of sale information such as labelling provides a tool, but stops short of provoking change when unhealthy choices remain so convenient. Dietary guidelines convey a lifestyle aspiration as much as they communicate risk. They also put responsibility firmly on the shoulders of the individual consumer and reduce the holism of a healthy lifestyle to a set of proxy indicators (such as portions of fruit and vegetables). Rather than being a general lifestyle choice, being sensible is thus segmented into quantifiable categories. Where does this leave luck? Healthy eating is cast as a sensible choice, but information alone does not create choice in situations where this has been undermined by persistent structural inequalities in, for example, food retailing quality and cost. Such advice is then merely a navigation tool that skirts over poor luck, assumes a willingness to change and elevates 'lifestyle' to a panacea for all ills.

Market growth and sensible behaviour

Sensible behaviour is an engine of market growth in that *appropriate* consumption mediates between discipline (self-denial) and pleasure (self-indulgence) (Smith Maguire 2008). Thus, in political economic terms, a healthy lifestyle is rarely about consuming *less*, but about consuming *better*. Government agencies such as the UK's Department of Health and the US Department of Agriculture may develop dietary guidelines, but because these are open to intense scrutiny by industry coalitions and consumers themselves, their advice is often subsumed under or entangled within commercial marketing messages. In the rush to comprehend the system of food provision and the social conditions under which people make dietary decisions, the role of food manufacturers in fostering demand for tasty but obesogenic products has been largely overlooked until recently. The focus on childhood obesity in both the UK and the US has brought the products and processes of the food industry into sharp focus, given the supposed and particular vulnerability of children to marketing messages (Linn 2000; Nestle 2000; Seiders and Petty 2004; Story and French 2004; Harris et al 2009). The result is a system which provides the choice so coveted in neoliberal discourse, while simultaneously creating desire for the 'wrong' choices. As the UK's 2007 Foresight Report notes, obesity might thus be understood as the 'perverse outcome of constantly expanding "choice"' (Government Office for Science 2007: 17). Offer expands on this irony when he writes, 'obesity shows how abundance, through cheapness, variety, novelty, and choice, could make a mockery of the rational consumer, how it enticed only in order to humiliate' (2007: 169). Furthermore, since marketers are happily aware of the malleability and fallibility of human consciousness (see Bernays 1947), the repeated apparent inability of consumers to choose healthily has paradoxically revealed a glaring gap in the market that has been filled by weight loss, 'healthier' and functional products. As the Foresight Report further notes: 'In modern societies, there is a psychological conflict between what people want (e.g. fatty, sweet foods) and their desire to be healthy and/ or slim. Mixed feelings and beliefs about healthy lifestyle choices complicate individual choices' (Government Office for Science 2007: 49).

This 'ambivalence' (Room 1976; Bell and Esses 2002) not only curtails efforts to be sensible, but also creates a void that can be filled by 'healthful' products promising a quick-fix route or bolt-on for better health. The proportion of household income spent on food has been in gradual decline for the past 40 years and currently stands at 10% in the UK. While there are marked differences between the proportion spent on food by low-income households (23%) and high-income households (15%), the story is of a steady fall in spending matched and facilitated by a general fall in the real cost of commodities such as fats, oils, sugars and starches, which comprise the core ingredients in processed food. At the same time, the cost of fruit and vegetables, the mainstays of sensible eating, have climbed in the US and the UK. Cost and availability are clear structural barriers (opportunity costs) to healthy diets and can preclude even the best of intentions. As a result, and as a mainstay of CSR, food manufacturers have started to expand and reformulate their product ranges to satisfy consumer demand for healthy diets (remember that 87% of those surveyed by the FSA's Consumer Attitudes Survey claimed that healthy eating was important to them). In this burgeoning political economy of food and drink, health has emerged as an 'aspirational commodity'

—

(Curtis 2004) that can easily be bought. As Harris et al note, it is important to question the 'extent to which the food industry shapes the definition of what is acceptable and desirable to eat and the role it plays in a rapidly evolving food environment' (2009: 212). Healthy living is thus not simply defined by the medical or public health community (Seiders and Petty 2004), but rather is a constellation of actors that, increasingly, are the same food and drink industries held up as culpable for the present 'crisis'.

We know very little about 'how consumers determine obesity risk and make trade-off decisions in various purchase contexts, specifically, the roles of cost and convenience in product decisions' (Seiders and Petty 2004: 164). It is clear, though, that cost and convenience act as major purchasing incentives and disincentives, depending on the perceived necessity and desirability of the product in question (Whelan et al 2002). This has given great scope for new product development that melds (low) cost and convenience (lower opportunity costs) with promises of health improvement and personal risk reduction. One clear example of this is the rise of 'functional foods' as the latest products of the burgeoning food technology industry (Heasman and Mellentin 2001). These merit brief scrutiny for they represent targeted efforts by the political economy of food to tap into and bring into being particular consumer 'health orientations' (Dutta-Bergman 2005a, 2005b). Thus, motivated (or health-orientated) consumers are more likely to seek and be armed with information and find products to satisfy their demands. By contrast, a consumer without this orientation is unlikely to take an *active* role in seeking information or health solutions. Both consumer types (and the manifold shades of grey in between them) have a place in the political economy of food and drink, but it is the enfolding of health orientation into commercial techniques of health communication that has become a powerful marketing and CSR tool. Not only do these products offer a way by which discipline and pleasure can coexist, but their reconciliation also aids in actively sustaining and promoting market growth.

The American Dietic Association defines functional foods as 'any modified food or food ingredient that may provide a health benefit beyond the traditional ingredients it contains' (Heasman and Mellentin 2001: 5). Functional foods are further distinguished from regular foodstuffs in legal terms by the fact that they make a 'claim to improve wellbeing or health' (Katan 2004). This is a rapidly growing segment of the otherwise stagnant grocery market, with projected global sales in 2010 estimated at $167 million (Lang 2007) – carving out desperately needed novel niches for food manufacturers suffering in a stagnant grocery market. Kelloggs Optivita™ cereal, for example, is branded on the principle that its consumption will have a positive health effect by reducing the risk of certain conditions; Optivita™ contains high levels of oat beta glucan (oat bran) and is sold on the basis of the 'soft claim' that it can *actively help* lower blood cholesterol and thus the risk of heart disease. Functional and fortified products are marketed on the back of 'implied health claims' that link ingredients and health outcomes or 'biomarkers' (Katan 2004). Examples of functional foods with health claims currently approved in the EU and the US include calcium-enriched juices (reduce the risk of osteoporosis), folic acid-enriched bread (reduce the risk of neural tube defects) and reduced-sodium products (reduce the risk of hypertension). Functional foods and the rise of the branded weight-loss food industry illustrate the business potential inherent in the delivery of a product that simultaneously identifies a problem and then offers a convenient solution. Indeed, in the case of Optivita™, its marketing discourse highlights that the decision to eat the cereal is, in effect, a positive choice for your health. The US advertising rhetoric acknowledges that there is a confusing surfeit of voices advising people what to eat, but armed with the knowledge that this product *could* help lower cholesterol, the decision making is left to the individual. At the root of functional foods is therefore the repositioning of choice as an individual responsibility and duty. In short, why pick regular yoghurt when faced with the one that might also help improve the vague domain of 'digestive health'? Making this choice is thus cast as a positive step for the self and for the family. In the process, no concessions are made in this win–win situation – the pleasure of consumption is thus magnified by the satisfaction of such an easy and delicious path to self-discipline.

As with almost all realms of health and consumption, underlying these products is the assumption that 'information is a precondition for real choice' (Gabriel and Lang 1995: 36). As Lang and Rayner (2005) have instructively noted, the pressing need to develop a coherent food and health policy in the UK, where four major companies control over 90% of food retailing, means that any study of obesity prevention must draw on political and economic aspects as well as sociological and psychological theories governing the interaction of the state, market and consumers; within this, choice is often an empty promise. Sociological and historical studies of changing social relations since the 1950s have highlighted the paradox of choice (Schwartz 2004; Salecl 2010) and now chart its recent rise as a rhetorical device legitimising neoliberal structural and policy reform (Jordan 2005, 2006; Clarke et al 2006; Price 2006; Clarke 2007; Harvey 2007; Greener 2009). Interestingly, the rise of obesity has coincided with a dramatic reconfiguration of the role of choice in both the political economy of food and political language itself. With the average supermarket having 25,000 different food products and a further 20,000 launched and/or failing annually (Lang and Heasman 2004), 'choice' assumes a new magnitude. Ehrenhalt (1995) argues convincingly that much of the current feeling of social malaise and loss of interpersonal connections can be traced to living in a society that presents us with not only a huge array of choices to make, but also a seemingly unending amount of information that we must process to optimise decision making. There is a perverse reverse logic in this system; a healthy diet rests on *resisting* the temptation of choice on which the political economy of food is built (Government Office for Science 2007). The job of food manufacturers is therefore to widen the range of foods within consumer repertoires by creating demand for new products through marketing, while the goal of public health is to encourage healthy lifestyles by enabling people to exercise informed choice and to demand the 'right' kinds of foods. For many

—

people, health thus becomes an outcome of the ability to withstand the very pull of media-generated desire, rather than a normative state.

Cultivating the self-control and willpower needed to ensure good health in such 'toxic food environments' (Brownall and Battel Horgen 2003) assumes the ubiquity of choice. The level of popular criticism directed at the political economy of food has reached unparalleled levels in the UK and US (see for example Blythman 2004; Lawrence 2004; Pollan 2006). Not only is the food retail market segmented along class and cost lines – the difference between economy retailer Wal-Mart and upscale organic Whole Foods in the US is clear evidence of the divide – but there is mounting feeling that better health through better food *should* cost more. This idea taps into the more holistic notion of health, where the integrity of the whole food chain is as important as the quality of the final product. Thus being sensible as an active lifestyle choice and strategy to manage the tension between discipline and pleasure becomes a much broader political project of ensuring distributive justice in the food system. Consequently, activists, academics, journalists and the public are now questioning the morality of the present political economy of food and asking if there is scope for viable, local alternatives to global systems of trade. The way in which the media have long equated obesity with global fast food, aided no end by a string of litigations against the corporate giants, has produced a vociferous counter-movement championing an alternative vision of sustainable food production and retailing. However, Tim Lang has long noted (1999, 2003) that the food industry's lobbying power with respect to the state makes the development of health-directed food policy a significant risk for governments courting fickle corporate affections. As Andrew Lansley's speech indicates, this aspiration of copartnership working is unlikely to change any time soon. Food is a deeply contested element of healthy lifestyles and rendered all the more so by the expectations and aspirations set by the market. Indeed, as Schwartz suggests:

> The 'success' of modernity turns out to be bittersweet, and everywhere we look it appears that a significant contributing factor is the overabundance of choice. Having too many choices produces psychological distress, especially when combined with regret, concern about status, adaptation, social comparison, and perhaps most important, the desire to have the best of everything – to maximise. (Schwartz 2004: 3)

Reconciling pleasure and discipline requires attention to choice, but often those choices cause distress and heighten ambivalence. This ambivalence is especially problematic when current trends in the political economy of food are set against efforts to curb obesity rates. Essentially, functional foods and their ilk 'allow people to eat and drink more healthily without radically changing their diet' (Lang 2007: 1016), but instead of 'technical fixes', 'big changes in diet are needed' (ibid). To make these changes would require the kind of structural intervention that goes against a neoliberal governmentality that foregrounds the *promise* of choice at the expense of actively *delivering* the means of having it. This disjuncture between

—

ideological aspiration and the structural conditions needed to realise these will be discussed in the next chapter.

Conclusion

This chapter has drawn on the example of obesity in order to explore the first and second contentions underpinning this book, namely that in order to be sensible, people need to be able to overcome the effects of their brute luck and that being sensible is an active tool of reconciliation between some of the core tensions besetting neoliberal economies and societies. It has first argued, drawing on the increasing number of studies in the critical obesity studies canon, that obesity is a particularly contentious epidemic in the biomedical sense. As a result of the aetiological uncertainties of obesity, many governance efforts rely on commonsense suggestions about healthy lifestyles that, instead of distilling the complex and contested scientific 'facts' about obesity, actually rehearse stereotypes and social fears about difference and abnormality. As Gard and Wright (2005) have suggested, the assertions that modernity and Western lifestyles are culpable for population-scale body weight rises, reveal as much about social and cultural unease as they do about the aetiology of obesity. It is also crucial to be mindful that 'obesity is an utterly plastic social issue and one's orientation to it is much more a matter of visceral belief than cerebral truth' (Bauman 2005: 98).

This chapter has explored how being sensible in the context of contemporary landscapes of obesity governance has invoked sensible behaviour in three key ways: First, as an active strategy of risk minimisation; second, as an active choice that might overcome the effects of unalterable bad luck; and third, as a tool of mediation between discipline and pleasure that points to new areas and opportunities for market growth. Being sensible in order to mitigate and manage the risk of obesity involves both a general adherence to the commonsense principles of a healthy lifestyle (eat better and move more), but it also involves assimilating conflicting renditions of the aetiology of obesity. However, this is inconclusive as a form of risk communication and leads to prevailing discourses of 'control' by knowing your risk through knowing your BMI, without ever changing the 'default option' as suggested by the kind of libertarian paternalist thinking so popular among both the US and UK administrations.

As an active strategy of overcoming luck, being sensible becomes a technique of self-empowerment or a route to the kind of self-efficacy highlighted as essential for widespread behaviour change (Central Office of Information 2009; Cabinet Office 2010). Yet, as studies in the UK have shown, awareness of sensible guidelines does not always translate into purchasing and consumption behaviours. The dietary guidelines and labelling may provide information, but they do not undo brute luck and only create the illusion of choice. The tools and techniques promoted as encouraging and facilitating sensible behaviour thus evade luck and serve as a yardstick against which to judge an individual's determination to overcome luck. Where sensible eating guidelines are adhered to, there is still a lingering tension

—

between the discipline needed to resist the temptations of the tastiest products in the supermarket aisles and the short-lived pleasure that these will bring. The ambivalence between a prevailing sentiment that it is good to be healthy and purchasing choices (and body weights) that suggest otherwise, creates new market opportunities. Thus, feeling the need to be sensible, but without the willpower to adhere to a complete lifestyle change is fuelling a market for functional foods and healthy options of existing brands. These products marry convenience and choice while, once again, leaving the political economy of food untouched.

It is therefore clear that being sensible as an *active* lifestyle choice sanctions the current status quo of voluntary codes of self-regulation of the food industry and minimal legislation. Yet, the 2007 Foresight Report and the most recent NICE advice on preventing cardiovascular disease both assert the need for fundamental legislative and structural changes. However, the UK's obesity policy now seems afloat on a sea of uncertainty, with Lansley stating that he 'freely admit[s] that none of us have all the answers. But, it's clear that we have to find a new approach – to think new thoughts. We need a paradigm shift' (Lansley 2010). By contrast, there is great forward momentum, leadership and financial investment coming from the US into community-scale obesity prevention programmes. This is where the domain of sensible behaviour buttresses luck in ways that go beyond the empty neoliberal rhetoric of choice and into the arena of sustained action. When considering the relationship between the prevailing social, cultural, consumption and built environments, it may be the case that being sensible will be far more likely if it is rendered *inevitable*. There is an increasingly vociferous school of thought that argues that choice is counter-productive, self-control is rarely possible and that ensuring the common good might necessitate more than just the provision of information. The wide constellation of stakeholders now governing obesity are becoming more mindful of the ways in which ecological thinking might produce policy solutions that not only render sensible behaviours *inevitable*, but also have a far more holistic effect on individual and population health. It is to this ecological frame of reference that the next chapter turns.

FIVE

The incidentally sensible city

> Health and wellness reflect the nature of the interface between ourselves and the environment . . . The illness we get may be seen as telling us what is wrong in that interaction. (Wilkinson 2005: 8)

> Preventative population-level interventions having to do with the built environment and the food environment may lead to health benefits for the entire population, not just the obese population; and some interventions may reduce body fat among the obese population even without large concomitant changes in weight. Enhanced efforts to provide environmental interventions may lead to improved health and future decreases in the prevalence of obesity. (Flegal et al 2010: 241)

Introduction

This chapter explores the nature of what has been termed the 'obesogenic' environment (Swinburn et al 1999). It does so in the context of the manifold and variegated efforts that try to address national and local rates of obesity in two cities in the US and UK: Austin, Texas and London. The comparison of these two national and urban settings is crucial, if only to dispel the assumption that America is distinctly and particularly obesogenic (Lang and Rayner 2007). In so doing, the chapter also aims to provide a counterpoint to related assertions that the UK 'looks like America in every way . . . The question we all need to ask ourselves is, do we really want the world to look, feel and taste just like America?' (Spurlock 2005b, n.p.). The assumption that America represents the UK's destiny may be common, but it is also highly improbable. However, and as Marvin and Medd have suggested, the turn to the exemplar of the US is useful in order to 'see where the rest of the world is going' (2006: 314) and, therefore, the kind of future health we might expect. However, this may be wishfully simplistic thinking; as geographic approaches to health remind us at the most fundamental level, the landscapes of risk that characterise the US health experience cannot and will not be a universal endgame.

The obesogenicity of an environment is defined by Swinburn et al as 'the sum of influences that the surroundings, opportunities, or conditions of life have on promoting obesity in individuals or populations' (1999: 564). In contrast to environments that pose barriers to the achievement of a healthy body weight, the authors suggest that there is a need for 'leptogenic' environments that 'promote healthy food choices and encourage physical activity' (ibid). However, defining the causal pathways through which obesogenic environments operate (and, therefore, the best ways to proceed in designing leptogenic environments) has been mired by conflicting evidence, scalar inconsistencies in research findings, institutional inertia and the politics of implementation. Population-scale shifts in average BMI point to the importance of environmental influences and to the necessity of bringing an 'ecological' perspective to bear on the question of preventing further rises in prevalence (Egger and Swinburn 1997; Reidpath et al 2002; Pepin et al 2004; Pickett et al 2005; Sallis et al 2006; Lang and Rayner 2007). This necessitates a shift in thinking away from the idea of individual risk towards the concept of living with a profusion of risks, often imperceptibly embedded in our everyday surroundings. The fact that these often may not even be perceived as risks means that policy makers have started to turn to environmental modifications in order to circumvent individual choice-making and instead encourage physical activity or adherence to dietary regulations by creating contexts that facilitate such lifestyle modifications (Townshend and Lake 2009). Aspiration and application often remain infuriatingly distinct in obesity interventions. This is despite the agreement that making healthy lifestyles an *incidental* outcome of certain environments – rather than the result of the uncontrollable, unpredictable and erratic decision making discussed in the previous chapter – may be the most productive and progressive way forward given the clear difficulties in persuading people to adopt healthier behaviours and the limited governmental appeal of health-focused legislation (such as so-called fat taxes).

This perpetual dilemma means that urban policy and public health demands are (by necessity and invention) now reconnecting in new ways and with mixed effects in order to work towards fashioning a more sensible city. Returning to the third contention set out in Chapter Two, addressing the obesogenic environment marks out a clear spatialisation of public health policy, that, in turn, can mark out those residents of 'fat places' as particularly culpable and irresponsible. While this might seem antithetical to the population-scale concern of the ecological paradigm undergirding environmental thinking in obesity prevention, there are clear social consequences to this way of thinking that will be further explored through the case studies in this chapter.

To this end, this chapter first offers a critical exploration of the concept of the obesogenic environment in order to background an empirical analysis of the efforts to create healthier places (and, by extension, people) in London and Austin, Texas. It will draw on situated case study examples and primary interview material to examine the endeavours to create better cities *in the name of* healthy lifestyle promotion and obesity prevention. In London, the promotion of 'active travel' (for example walking and cycling) has been one of the clearest ways in which obesity prevention and urban policy agendas have coalesced in trying to instigate a 'modal shift' among commuters. In Austin, attention has instead concentrated on the particularly risky nature of certain, racially segregated urban neighbourhoods and smaller-scale, incremental ways of addressing these in the context of the city's aspirations to become America's 'fittest'. While Austin reveals the difficulties inherent in getting beyond individual behavioural explanations of obesity risk, London demonstrates the will to skirt individual risk and concentrate on using health as a vehicle to push through urban improvement objectives. Interestingly, in neither case are the effects of such efforts being measured or evaluated, despite the international hunt for evidence-based obesity prevention policies (Macintyre 2003).

Obese city

While the existence of a 'dramatic increase in [obesity] prevalence over the past decades' (Feng et al 2010: 175) has been the subject of ardent debate (see the 'Point-Counterpoint' section of the *International Journal of Epidemiology* 35, 2006, for perhaps the best example of this), there is, nevertheless, evidence of a 'population-scale shift towards larger body mass indexes' (Feng et al 2010: 176). This shift in the normal distribution of body weight among both the adult and child population has been noted in a large number of countries, including the US (Ogden et al 2007), the UK (Rennie and Jebb 2005), Australia (Thorburn 2005), New Zealand, Canada, Mexico, and the Gulf States. In addition, rising obesity prevalence is now noted in a host of low-income countries (Prentice 2006), where issues include a concern with childhood obesity in China and evidence of strong correlations between obesity rates and rapid urbanisation in India (Yajnik 2004), where a 'nutrition transition' from low-fat, high-fibre to high-fat, low-fibre diets characterised by an increase in meat consumption (Popkin 1999, 2003) has taken place over the past two decades. While obesity was previously confined to the richest sections of society in low-income countries, it is increasingly the case that adiposity and malnutrition now coexist even among the poor (Webb and Prentice 2006) in urban areas.

The result of this generalised population-scale rise in obesity prevalence is a growing awareness that exploring the interrelationships between people and places, first, is crucial if public health policy rhetoric is to deliver on its promises and, second, represents a dialectic that is exceptionally difficult to disentangle. It also points to the fact that the traditional epidemiological and public health distinction between contextual (area) and compositional (people) explanations for health outcomes cannot meaningfully be considered in isolation (Macintyre 2007). Indeed, as Macintyre highlights, *who you are* is a more significant predictor of health and health-related behaviours than *where you live*. However, place of residence is correlated to diet, physical activity, smoking and alcohol consumption, ensuring that when it comes to fostering a healthy, sensible populace, individual behaviour is almost always entangled with the cultural and social norms of locale. This is even more the case in areas of deprivation and disadvantage where poor-quality environments, it has been argued, may 'amplify' – and thus compound – individual disadvantage (Macintyre et al 1993). The 'deprivation amplification' thesis has, since the early 1990s, served as an exceptionally important conceptual tool to analyse the effect of environmental 'bads' on individual deprivation (and thus health outcomes). However, its authors have more recently concluded that the picture is, predictably enough, far from simple (Macintyre 2007). While the thesis was based on the assumption that 'only the physically "local" matters in terms of the health-damaging and health-promoting features of the social and physical environment' (Cummins 2007: 1), urban studies theorists, geographers and sociologists have long argued that people are influenced by (and in turn influence) environments far beyond their own neighbourhoods (see for example Matthews 2008). As Cummins et al have suggested, 'place is relevant to health variation because it *constitutes* as well as *contains* relations and physical resources' (2007: 1825) and is thus fundamental to the formulation of causal pathways from environmental determinants to individual health. In this case, the authors argue for a 'relational' understanding of place, in which mobile individuals may take behavioural cues from far more distant locales, situations, people and norms, complicating causality in terms of the environmental determinants of health.

While very few countries now remain untouched by fears over obesity (World Health Organization 2004), research on the nature of the obesogenic environment is still overwhelmingly concentrated in the US (Feng et al 2010). In these studies, the environment (most frequently conceptualised at the scale of the neighbourhood) is either an 'effect modifier' or a 'direct mediator of individual behaviours' (Black and Macinko 2008: 13). As such, the environment either acts on preexisting behaviours to influence their effects (for example the desire to take a long walk in the park is curtailed by a forbidding and unsafe-feeling environment and a short-cut is instead chosen) or as a direct mediator (for example no park exists). Environmental determinants are most commonly differentiated as pertaining to either the built/physical environment or the sociopolitical environment. The physical environment is then further subdivided into those features that influence the propensity for healthy eating and those that influence the likelihood of physical activity uptake. The sociopolitical environment can be further broken down into a concern with social influences on obesity and the political/policy context that characterises the landscape of both risk and prevention. Table 2 summarises the main environmental determinants of obesity (after Booth et al 2005; Cummins and Macintyre 2006; Lake and Townshend 2006; Black and Macinko 2008; Smith and Cummins 2009). These synthesise and offer up crossnational comparisons of what has been rightly described as a 'highly complex scientific literature' from 'a large number of disciplines' (Feng et al 2010: 175) in a field that is 'still in its infancy' (Black and Macinko 2008: 14). This infancy, it has been suggested, might explain the 'many inconsistencies' in the literature and the persistent difficulty in establishing causal relationships between environmental risk factors and health outcomes (ibid) in any geographically or culturally generalisable way (Cummins and Macintyre 2006).

The research and review literature on the environmental determinants of obesity is surging. This is unsurprising given the current policy interest in the field, but still makes for complex reading. As Table 2 illustrates, many of these determinants have thus risen to the status of assumed predictors for high obesity rates, even as research findings can offer somewhat counter-intuitive narratives

—

Table 2: Environmental determinants of obesity

Physical environment		Sociopolitical environment	
Food	**Physical activity**	**Social**	**Political**
• Fast food outlet density/proximity • Distance to grocery store • Grocery provision and price (food deserts)	• Neighbourhood deprivation • Neighbourhood walkability/ connectivity • Access to amenities (leisure facilities or open space) • Urban sprawl (residential density and usage mix) • Transport provision • Perceptions and attitudes towards the use of urban space • Neighbourhood safety (actual and perceived)	• Cultures of consumption • Cultural value of physical activity • Socio-economic status • Social networks and external influences • Personal safety • Ethnic residential segregation	• Agricultural policy (e.g. subsidies) • Trade policy • Policies towards industry (e.g. regulation or laissez-faire) • Advertising policies • Fiscal policies • Competition laws • Transport policies and priorities

Source: Adapted from Smith and Cummins, 2009

of environmental bads. For example, despite evidence suggesting that access to health-promoting resources is actually better in more affluent neighbourhoods, a study by Pearce et al (2007) in New Zealand has countered this by showing that greater access is actually found in more deprived neighbourhoods, a situation that mirrors that found in Austin. The spate of studies on 'food deserts' in the wake of the 1995 report of the Low Income Project Team of the UK government's Nutrition Task Force (Cummins and Macintyre 2002a; Whelan et al 2002; Wrigley et al 2003; White et al 2004), have also called into question the idea that better availability and access to healthy foods (e.g. fresh fruit and vegetables) in deprived neighbourhoods will necessarily have a marked impact on dietary health and, therefore, the risk of obesity. Instead, as Cummins and Macintyre (2002a) have argued, food deserts have risen to the status of 'factoid' – where highly conflicting and contested evidence has been repeated to the extent that it has risen to the status of incontrovertible fact. Furthermore, as a recent study in Glasgow found, large supermarkets were more likely to be located in deprived areas, and yet there was no difference in the price of food in affluent and deprived areas (Cummins and Macintyre 1999, 2002a).

While the existence of 'food deserts' is deeply contested in the UK, inadequate access to healthy food remains a significant problem in the US, where residentially segregated African American and Hispanic inner city neighbourhoods frequently suffer from a complete lack of adequate grocery retailing (Morland et al 2002). As a result, transport-poor residents in those areas are reliant on higher-priced convenience stores that rarely stock foodstuffs that even come close to satisfying the dietary guidelines. Detroit is a prime example of this 'grocery void' as the city's last chain supermarket fled the city in 2007 (Hargreaves 2009), leaving only those in the overwhelmingly white suburbs. The recession has hit Detroit harder than anywhere else in the US and rapid rises in food insecurity rates, combined with acres of empty and vacant lots left by residents abandoning or destroying now-worthless homes, has transformed the landscape of food provision in the city. Yet, Detroit is now courting a new kind of attention, for its urban gardening projects (Harris 2010), which are increasingly addressing gaps in welfare provision for acute food insecurity as unemployment rates climb even among the white middle classes. Such entrepreneurial fervour has been cast as a model for cities and the rise of urban gardening does demonstrate that people can provide solutions to food insecurity even in the absence of realising the 'panacea by large supermarket' suggested by the food deserts literature. Interestingly, urban gardening would also be the kind of activity that public health practitioners would support in efforts to prevent obesity, given the inclusion of 'yard work' and gardening in the US and UK's physical activity guidelines respectively (Department of Health 2004c; United States Department of Health and Human Services 2008).

If the food environment brings geographical and cultural discrepancies to the fore, research examining the physical activity environment also suffers from a similar degree of discord. As Sallis and Glanz contend, there are currently 'more questions than answers about the role of physical activity environments in explaining racial, ethnic and socioeconomic disparities in physical activity and obesity' (2009: 131). Table 2 sets out some of the major areas of 'active living' (Sallis et al 2006) research, namely neighbourhood walkability/connectivity, access to amenities for physical activity (for example sports facilities or open, green space), urban sprawl (for example car usage, neighbourhood density and land use mix) and public transport provision. Aside from these structural factors, studies have also investigated (to a far lesser extent given the methodological difficulties), the influence of perceptions and attitudes towards urban space on physical activity uptake as well as the impact of personal safety (both real and perceived) on the propensity to exercise and feelings of wellbeing (see Airey 2003). However, just as with the food environment, recent research has demonstrated very few areas of concordance in the relationship between the built environment and physical activity uptake.

Black and Macinko's (2008) review highlights how, regardless of environment, those of a lower socioeconomic status and/or lower educational attainments are more likely to be sedentary. They add, somewhat doubtfully, that 'decreased neighbourhood opportunities *could* contribute to these trends' (ibid, emphasis added). One of the more compelling findings is that of the effects of neighbourhood 'walkability' – a composite measure of density, street connectivity, land use, aesthetic measures, crime, traffic, retail and provision for walking and

—

cycling. A study undertaken across two neighbourhoods in San Diego, California showed that those living in neighbourhoods characterised by a high degree of walkability took, on average, an extra 52 minutes of exercise a week and also had lower BMIs (Saelens et al 2003). Similarly, a study in Perth, Australia showed that those neighbourhoods with greater access to *attractive* open space had higher rates of activity than those with poor access (Giles-Corti and Donovan 2002, 2003). However, the same study showed no association between access to formal sports facilities and activity rates.

A more recent study in Chapel-Hill, North Carolina investigated the difference in BMI and activity rates among household heads in a new urbanist community (a dense, modified grid, mixed-use and mixed tenure community) and a traditional suburban community (low density, cul-de-sacs, curvilinear streets, residential, single-family homes) (Brown et al 2008). The study found that while residents of the new urban community had slightly lower BMIs on average than their suburban counterparts, this was explained by more 'utilitarian walking' rather than any greater level of planned physical activity. The far higher degree of walkability of the new urbanist community thus had an indirect effect on BMI through enabling more trips to be made on foot rather than by car. Significantly for the argument put forward here, the authors conclude that 'utilitarian trip-making may have an impact on social cohesion and community support which, in themselves, could lead to improved mental and physical health outcomes' (Brown et al 2008: 982). The broader, holistic value of addressing the environmental determinants of health, even in the absence of any definitive evidence as to their effects, will be revisited later with respect to the case studies.

Studies of the environmental determinants of health may be increasing in number, but:

> The body of research thus far is somewhat inconclusive. There certainly seems to be a relationship between physical activity and the built environment, though what factors within this relationship are paramount and which are peripheral is not agreed on. The relationship between diet and physical environment seems even more elusive and by the same token, the relationship between all three remains unexplained. (Townshend and Lake 2009: 913)

The difficulties in establishing causal relationships are further compounded by methodological limitations, which, in turn, destabilise the evidence base for obesity prevention policies. First, most studies are cross-sectional rather than longitudinal and are thus unable to divine changes over time and to establish clear causal relationships between risk factors and outcomes (for example walkability and BMI) (Cummins and Macintyre 2006). Thus, and as Moon (2009) has further argued, establishing causality within this field is fraught with problems. This is further compounded by the issue of residential self-selection (Frank et al 2007; Brown et al 2008; Townshend and Lake 2009). Given that some (but far from all) residents can exercise housing preferences, it is possible that environmental attributes are as much a reflection of the needs, wants and desires of those residents as they are responsible for shaping their behaviours. Thus, several authors have pointed to evidence that people with high BMIs self-select into car-dependent neighbourhoods and people with lower BMIs choose more walkable neighbourhoods (Lee et al 2009). This problematises the assertion that urban sprawl has a *causal* effect on obesity (see also Sui 2003 for a more sociotheoretical perspective on this debate). As Black and Macinko write:

> These inconsistencies have led some to posit that the observed associations between the health of neighbourhoods and the health of people living in them are artefactual. That is, neighbourhoods do not determine the health of residents; instead, individuals, based on their own preferences for physical activity or access to healthy food, sort themselves into neighbourhoods that provide desired services. (Black and Macinko 2008: 14)

While self-selection is an almost impossible confounding factor to control for, studies are also limited by their ability to derive consistent (through both time and space) measurements for these environmental determinants and often rely heavily on proxies (such as sedentarism measured through the proxy of TV viewing). There are also problems in defining 'neighbourhood', which has been of particular concern to both geographers and sociologists (Cummins 2007; Cummins et al 2007; Matthews 2008). While studies often rely on administrative (and survey data) borders such as ward or census tract, individuals rarely conduct their everyday lives within such neat parameters and their environmental cues can come from geographically disparate sources. Yet, inculcating this complexity and fluidity within epidemiological study design has proven to be both methodologically and conceptually problematic. Furthermore, studies are also limited by understandings of individual environmental interactions and, therefore, why some people are more vulnerable and others more resilient to 'obesogenic' environmental features. For example, is socioeconomic status the most important protective trait, or might certain cultural habits and values have a greater effect? As Macintyre et al highlight, 'one of the [problems for this type of research] is the difficulty of capturing in words, let alone in figures, a sense of what these places look like and feel like' (1993: 231). Given the methodological design of these studies, it is unsurprising that very few pause to consider what their places of study are actually *like* – an undertaking that might, in some cases, facilitate explanation more thoroughly than establishing correlations. The question of how to understand and represent 'place' in research has recently received some welcome attention (Cummins et al 2007), reinforcing the importance and value of the kind of qualitative approaches that form the empirical bulk of this book. Most important, the authors argue, such qualitative approaches are essential if policy interventions are to be effective and meaningful.

It thus seems counterintuitive that, given the predilection for evidence-based policy, the significant contradictions within the existing evidence base discussed earlier and the outspoken criticism of a situation where policymakers 'have been slow to recognise the seriousness of [obesity]' (Lang and Rayner 2007: 167); it is still the case that 'policy and practice are moving rapidly . . . to address aspects of the obesogenic environment' (Townshend and Lake 2009: 909). That such policies are being pushed forward *in spite* of the contradictions between epidemiological study results demonstrates the broad allure of the environment as a target of intervention. Of particular concern has been addressing those aspects of urban form and design that *might* enhance the adoption of healthy lifestyles and, in the words of one interviewee in London, provide a "value-added bolt-on to existing policy" (local government, interview, 2005). This has proved politically popular because improving the food and physical activity landscapes represent a win-win situation for urban regeneration and redevelopment strategies. Conversely, by working environmental features such as the provision of cycle parking and pedestrian access into planning conditions for urban regeneration plans, much of this work has actually been led by fields outside public health. The research on which this book is based found that the urban governance of obesity expands far beyond public health. Instead, the 'cacophonous' nature of obesity cuts across almost all urban policy agendas (Lang and Rayner 2007) and, as a representative from the Texas Department of Health and Human Services (TDHHS) in Austin suggested: "The issues about obesity are staggering as it crosses every possible area. The things that are forcing, that encourage people, to keep them from having a healthier lifestyle are so pervasive" (interview, 2006).

These policy crossovers are evident when approaching obesity from both a behavioural and environmental standpoint. Yet, these domains, as Sallis and Glanz remind us, should not be dissociated:

> Diet and physical activity interventions that build knowledge, motivation and behaviour change skills in individuals without changing the environments in which they live are unlikely to be effective. Similarly, merely changing the physical activity or the food environment may not be sufficient for a substantial change in behaviour. (Sallis and Glanz 2009: 126)

A sensible city is, consequently, ineffectual without sensible citizens and vice versa, despite the manifold difficulties in conceptualising, delineating, measuring and bringing forth either. Yet, due to governmental delineations of policy responsibility (which coincidentally are not the same between countries), the tendency is to focus interventions on one sphere of activity or the other. Even when policy addresses the environmental determinants of obesity to make sensible behaviour incidental (and thus factor out the inconvenient and unpredictable individual choices discussed in the previous chapter), the realms of behaviour and environment remain inseparable. This produces a new urban politics of health where certain people can 'make a place appear unhealthy' (Black and Macinko 2008: 14). However, certain places (within the episteme of ecological approaches to obesity) can also make people *appear* unhealthy, regardless of their actual health status. Disentangling these strands is a complex, but important, undertaking. Thus, in order to think through this complex interaction empirically, this chapter now turns to the case of Austin to explore the ways in which obesity governance interlaces individual and environmental explanations of health outcomes, revealing, in the process, some of the pragmatic and conceptual tensions at the heart of contemporary health interventions.

Austin and the fit city

> 'It's one of those things you can't really legislate, you can't tell people to be more active . . . It's still a question of personal responsibility. I guess there's nothing at the state level we could have done to change that person's mind about his lifestyle . . . People view any intervention by government, at any level, as infringing on their personal rights.'
> (adviser to the Governor's Council on Physical Fitness, interview, 2006)

Austin lends itself to further empirical exploration in the context of ecological readings of obesity risk and prevention for three reasons. First, Texas may not have the highest prevalence of obesity of any state in the US, but at 28.7% in 2009 it is firmly in the second tier of obesity prevalence severity, behind the nine states which have prevalence rates greater than 30% (see Map 2). In addition, Texas exhibits marked variations in obesity rates between racial groups, with recent data from 2006–8 highlighting a division between prevalence rates for non-Hispanic whites (23.5%), non-Hispanic black (37.8%) and Hispanic (32.3%) (Pan et al

Map 2: Obesity prevalence by state in 2009

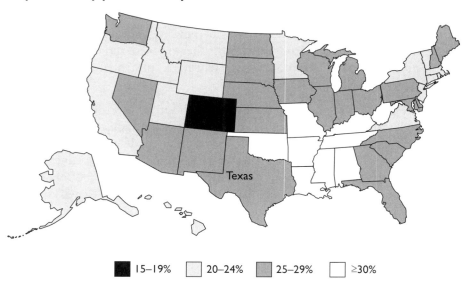

15–19%   20–24%   25–29%   ≥30%

Source: CDC and BRFSS data at www.cdc.gov/obesity/data/trends.html

2009). The obesity rate among Hispanic Texans is the second highest of any state in the US (behind Tennessee) and of particular note given that almost 37% of the state's population is Hispanic. With a population of 24 million in Texas, this equates to over 9.14 million obese Hispanic Texans. By contrast, while over 36% of Tennessee's Hispanic residents are classified as obese, this only equates to 244,443 people. Texas is demographically particular and the public health challenges facing the state may well presage others at a time when 'Latinisation' (Davis 2000) is broadening beyond the US border states and major cities (Murdock et al 2002). Second, Texas is one of 25 states in the US that currently receives federal funding for obesity-prevention programmes, demonstrating not just that a problem exists, but also that there is a state-level will to address this. Thus, from 2005 to 2010, Texas was able to use its Nutrition, Physical Activity and Obesity Prevention Program (NPAOP) funding to implement a range of local-scale interventions across the state. This Texan dedication to the cause was further reiterated by Governor Rick Perry in his assertion that:

> Building a healthier Texas is one of the top goals of [this] administration. A healthier Texas is about much more than putting money into public assistance programs. It starts with the personal responsibility each Texan must assume for their own health. (Office of the Governor: Texas 2004)

Third, Texas is obese in the popular imagination. The state's unofficial slogan – 'everything's bigger in Texas' – is underpinned by a vast, hot, humid landscape grown on oil money and a certain pride that whatever any other state might achieve, Texans will better it and then supersize it. Austin, the state capital, is the counterpoint to this stereotype, where fit and fat coexist in tense and fascinating ways and a host of entrepreneurial go-getters in this economically successful city try to do their bit to address obesity, often with mixed results.

In 2006, Austin had a population of 709, 893 (US Census Bureau 2010, www. census.gov). Between 2000 and 2009, the population of Travis County grew by 26% and, from 2000 to 2006 the city of Austin by 7% (US Census Bureau 2010). The population now stands at 760,000. Travis County is one of the most economically prosperous and fastest growing urban centres in the US with IBM, Motorola, Dell and a host of other high-tech companies lured there by a strong graduate pool from the University of Texas, Concordia University and Austin Community College. With over 40% of Travis County residents holding at least a bachelor's degree (the Texas average is 23%); it is clear why the area is a magnet for firms seeking skilled labour. Austin is also staunchly Democrat and socially progressive in a state with a Republican governor and famously conservative politics. The liberal politics also seem to translate into a high-earning city with average per capita income of $25,883 in 2000 (over $6,000 more than the Texas average). In 2009, 51% of the city's residents self-classified as non-Hispanic white and a further 33% as Hispanic, slightly below the Texas average of 37%. The city is thus demographically and socioeconomically distinctive and has long lured its relatively young population on the basis of quality of life and job opportunities.

Austin is anchored and built around Town Lake to the south of downtown – a stretch of the Colorado River with parkland covering 509 acres. The city also has three other major parks: Zilker Park (351 acres); Barton Creek Park (1,022 acres); and Walter E. Long Metropolitan Park (3,802 acres). In all, the city's Parks and Rec Department (PRD) oversees 16,682 acres of land, comprising 206 parks and 26 greenbelts and 43 public pools. It therefore comes as little surprise that the residents of Lance Armstrong's hometown take great pride in the quality of the city's open space and the opportunities for recreation that this affords. It is worth noting that Austin is not without its environmental problems and, while green spaces may characterise the city in one sense, it is also (in)famous for its traffic. The two-tiered Interstate-35 bisects Austin, shaping the city as it skirts just to the east of downtown and plays a key role in the geographical imaginaries and everyday life of Austinites.

The I-35 also serves as a real and imagined boundary between Austin and East Austin beyond. Officially, East Austin is the neighbourhood delineated by Town Lake to the south, Airport Boulevard to the east, and the I-35 to the west (Map 3). However, residents frequently refer to any area east of the I-35 as East Austin, a sweeping term delineating difference and usually expressed through phrases such as 'over there' or 'the other side of the tracks'. The Austin/East Austin division serves, at a basic level, to mark the poor from the rich side of the city. However, this imaginary is increasingly being challenged by gentrification associated with the East 11th and 12th Streets Urban Renewal Plan and neighbourhood conservation plans. While East Austin may now be a 'hipster haven' (Smithson 2009), there remain marked socioeconomic and demographic disparities between the two parts of the city. Furthermore, in public health terms, East Austin has become something of a philanthropic Mecca in ways that fuse environmental and behavioural readings of obesity risk in noteworthy ways. In short, if Austin is the sensible side of the city, where health outcomes are assumed to be generally good, East Austin is repeatedly cast as the badly behaved neighbour (Herrick 2008) with obesity interventions that both reflect and actively recreate this characterisation.

Austin is an excellent illustration of how 'obesity has to be seen not just as a technical, food, physical activity or healthcare problem, but a challenge for what sort of society is being built' (Lang and Rayner 2007: 167). This is especially the case in a city where a highway forms a boundary between an average income of over $34,500 to the west and $17,400 and a poverty rate of 14% to the east (US Census 2010). It also marks the start of a zone where gentrification is increasingly displacing residents from central East Side neighbourhoods into cheaper, more distant ones, with a clear impact on lifestyle. Austin is also an exception in Texas for making it into the coveted *Men's Fitness* (*MF*) fittest city list. This is all the more impressive given the propensity for Texan cities (such as Houston, Dallas, Fort Worth, El Paso, San Antonio) to dominate the fattest city league. The city's exceptional status also explains one interviewee's assertion that "what works in Austin will not work in El Paso" (TDHHS, interview, 2006) and the related belief that "Austin is in a better place as we have a lot of green space where people

Map 3: Map of Austin with East Austin indicated by the shaded triangle and downtown by the shaded rectangle

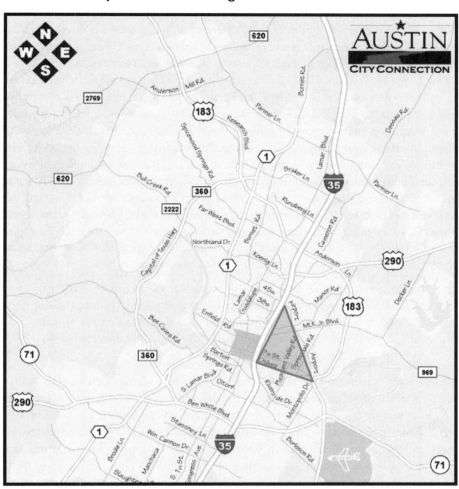

Source: www.ci.austin.tx.us/help/austinmap.htm

can be active and we have a culture, in terms of running activities" (Governor's Council on Physical Fitness, interview, 2006). However, when the research began in 2006, the new 'motivation' category in the fit city rankings had pushed Austin down into 25th place. When Mayor Will Wynn was reelected in 2006, he promised Austinites that he would make the city the nation's fittest by 2010 and gathered together a specially selected 'Mayor's Fitness Council' to push through the necessary changes, thus ensuring the city would at least rise in the 'mayoral and city initiatives' category. However, moving beyond initiatives in name only, this section explores the rationale and practices of one such constellation of initiatives, gathered under the umbrella provided by the HealthierUS initiative.

Taking Steps to a Healthier Austin

The recognition that there is a correlation between deprivation and obesity (Booth et al 2005) and the visual cues that link deprivation to particular environmental traits means that, as one interviewee on the Mayor's Fitness Council pointed out, improving the city's 'fitness' means "hitting a certain part of the city" (interview, 2006). Indeed, when the CDC granted the Steps to a Healthier Austin programme $2 million over five years in 2005, it set its intervention area as 20 contiguous zip codes east of the I–35 (see Map 4). In basic terms, Steps delivered funding for community interventions to address the risk factors for obesity, diabetes and asthma with the overriding aim of reducing health disparities more generally. The Steps funding provided for several full-time staff and facilitates coalition building among a broad range of 'community consortium' members, including the Parks and Recreation Department (PRD), Austin Independent School District, the American Heart, Lung and Cancer Associations, TDHHS, Capital Metro, sports store RunTex, the YMCA, the Sustainable Food Center and several churches, including the huge El Buen Samaritano complex. The discussion here will focus on just one of Steps' seven community-based objectives:

> To work with Austin's Parks and Recreation Department (PRD) to facilitate the planning and construction of walking and hiking trails in the intervention area and promote the use of existing city resources, such as recreational centers and parks, to increase physical activity (Steps to a Healthier US 2005)

BRFSS data commissioned by the Steps programme shows that in East Austin in 2005, 55% of white people were moderately physically active, while only 43% of Hispanic people met this target. Similarly, 18% of white people and 48% of Hispanic people were inactive. However, while the Texas state average for overweight and obesity was 64% in 2005, rates in East Austin were a less concerning 57% among white people, 62% among Hispanic people and 68% among black residents. However, while the disparity between white and Hispanic overweight and obesity rates may only be 5% and both fall below the state average, these figures mask a significant difference in rates of physical activity uptake (Austin/Travis County Health and Human Services Department 2005). In 2005, 55% of white Austinites were 'moderately physically active', compared to only 43% of Hispanic citizens meeting this target. And, while 18% of white residents reported engaging in no leisure-time physical activity in the past 30 days, almost 48% of Hispanic people fell into this category. The conclusion often drawn from this disparity is that, given that lifestyle is a matter of culture as much as education, it must be some facet of Hispanic culture (and lack of education) that leads to relatively high rates of sedentarism. Interviewees in Austin thus repeatedly conceptualised the aetiology of obesity through a conflation of culture, lifestyle and behaviour filtered through the lens of racial difference.

Map 4: City zip codes with Steps intervention zip codes shown below

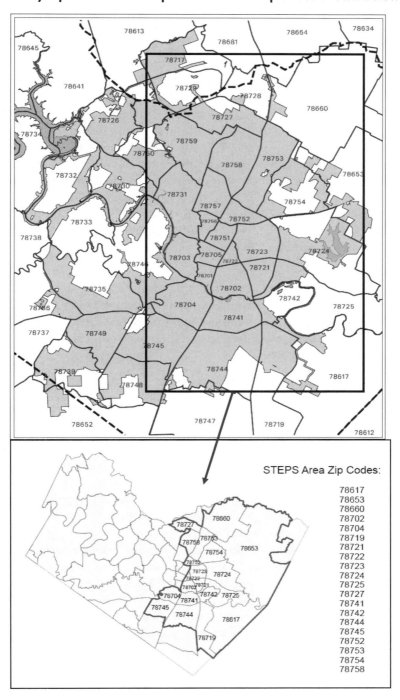

STEPS Area Zip Codes:

78617
78653
78660
78702
78704
78719
78721
78722
78723
78724
78725
78727
78741
78742
78744
78745
78752
78753
78754
78758

Source: Map, personal correspondence, 2006

Such assertions of difference were partly legitimised through the effects of racialised residential segregation that renders such disparities and deprivation legible in the built form of the city. This divide then sanctions the opinion that: "We certainly have a large Hispanic population, you know Hispanic populations have been more prone to high levels of obesity and that's related to diet and other cultural things . . . you know, they don't exercise" (state government, interview, 2006). This idea was further reinforced by a TDHHS obesity prevention strategy leader's opinion that Texas's unique challenge is "ethnic diversity" as "they [minorities] share more of the burden of obesity' and, therefore, 'a lot of our problems have to do with the [minority] culture" (interview, 2005). Environmental thinking in obesity prevention offers up the potential to make better cities (as Flegal et al's 2010 quotation at the start of this chapter highlights), but in order to do so, practitioners have to get beyond the idea that culture alone explains both health disparities and visible differences in the city's fabric. Given that Austin, like most US cities, has high levels of residential segregation, culture is racially, socially and spatially patterned. This means that interviewees repeatedly conflated cultural stereotyping with place of residence:

> 'Austin is always touted as the fittest city but I know that isn't true about those who live east of I-35. I know it's a lot harder for them to take advantage of some of those opportunities when they are just worried about living from day to day.' (Governor's Council on Physical Fitness, interview, 2006)

Such preconceptions about life in Austin's 'other side' often get elided to form a picture of Hispanic risk factors for obesity that guide targeted interventions, even in the absence of the full cultural comprehension or empathy of those charged with improving health outcomes: "There are many more life challenges over here [the East Side] . . . it's just not easy, you know? And again, I don't really know why that is . . . it might be some cultural things I don't understand" (Austin PRD, interview, 2006). For example, interviews with those focusing on getting residents of the Steps intervention area to increase their physical activity participation rates were of the (reasonably patronising) opinion that, "these people [in the intervention area] are the beginners' and 'we just want to get them moving and to stop their kids from playing videogames" (interview public health promotion, Austin, 2006). Thus, it is clear that 'in the matter of health, culture matters' (Hayes-Batista, cited in Suarez-Orozco and Paez 2002: 234). More than this, though, the discursive construction of obesity as problematic in Austin and the concomitant pragmatic attempts to address behavioural risk factors show the degree to which culture is both an explanatory narrative (cause) and cultural modification used as a vehicle to improved health (solution), even as those in the Steps coalition extolled the virtue of environmental thinking. This is especially true in Austin where Hispanic culture, frequently and simplistically reduced to Mexican cuisine and the assumption that "the interest [in fresh fruit and vegetables and exercise] just isn't there" (community intervention programme, interview, 2006), is afforded

—

causal significance. This belief in the explanatory power of the knowledge deficit model is in stark opposition to claims that Steps' overriding goal was to think about health in environmental terms and to get those in public health to change the way they think. As the director of Steps noted: "A lot of people in public health . . . who've gone through different training, different social work backgrounds, have a hard time making that leap from, you know, giving people information to actually making environmental changes" (interview, 2005).

However, money was not spent on 'actually making environmental changes' or asking, "what are the structural, organisational, community and policy decisions that are influencing people to get more or less obese?" (TDHHS, interview, 2006). Instead, the Steps coalition fell into the trap suggested by the TDHHS director:

> 'We underestimate the influence of environment on behaviour. We place a lot of focus on the individual and we put a lot of weight there and a lot of weight therefore on interventions that focus on the individual. That might be 5 or 10% of it and the other 90% might be out there . . .' (TDHHS, interview, 2006)

As such, $210,000 of the Steps budget was spent jumping onto the social marketing bandwagon by employing a local marketing firm to design a wellbeing umbrella brand. The result, 'I thrive' aimed to motivate people on the East Side to, in the words of their commercial, 'Love what you do. Live all you can. Thrive'. While great faith is placed in social marketing to deliver the kind of cultural shift needed to normalise healthy lifestyles (Lefebvre 1992; Hastings 2002; Maibach 2002; Williams and Kumanyika 2002; Centers for Disease Control 2005; National Consumer Council 2005; Jebb et al 2008), the approach is not without its critics (Herrick 2007; Robinson and Robertson 2010). In Austin, interviews conducted when the campaign was just being rolled out in 2005 were characterised by unbridled enthusiasm for the project (it is worth noting that such enthusiasm around social marketing to address obesity was also high in the UK at that time as the National Social Marketing Centre was inaugurated in 2006). However, by 2006, there was palpable tension between those at the TDHHS steering the NPAOP and Steps, with the former wishing that Steps would just "know that we are here" and "keep us up to date with what's going on" (TDHHS interview, 2006). Steps' own marketing manager was more stinging in his criticism, branding the campaign "a waste of $210,000" and, although the website was "very nice looking", there "should be more going on" (interview, 2006). The general inefficiency of the marketing message was clear as other interviewees were unaware of the campaign, despite all working in the field of obesity prevention in Austin.

Steps claim its devotion to the socioecological framework when designing interventions to encourage healthier behaviours, yet the I Thrive brand did nothing to reduce the structural barriers to being healthy. The choice of the verb 'thrive' therefore seems misplaced given that the income and health gap between East Austin and the rest of the city may make thriving a superfluous goal. The belief that "people are not empowered by their environment over [in

East Austin]" (public health advertising agency, interview, 2006) marks another socio–spatial assumption – that East Austin, by virtue of the fact it is the poorer, Hispanic side of the city must therefore lack recreational facilities. While there is a clear disparity in the number of supermarkets in Austin and East Austin (see Map 5), the same cannot be said of the provision of opportunities for physical activity. As the maps from Austin's PRD clearly show, the provision of pools (Map 7) and playgrounds (Map 8) (as *MF* indicators of city fitness) are as prolific

Map 5: Major food retailing in Austin

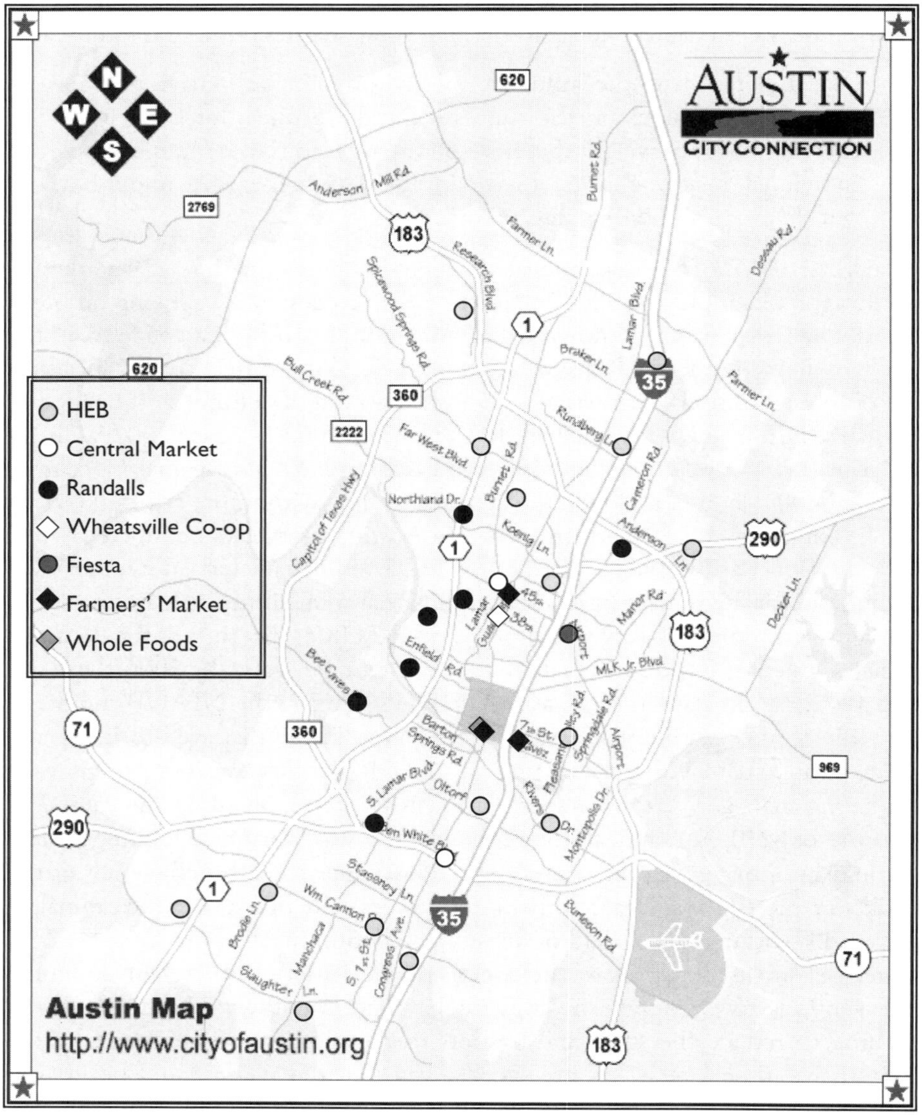

Source: Mapped from retailer online store locator tools, 2006

in East Austin as in the west of the city. There is, however, a paucity of recreation centres on the East Side (Map 6), perhaps reflecting the area's rapidly changing demographic as gentrification tightens its grip. Yet, with little data on usage rates or the demographic profile of consumers, underuse is often assumed rather than known, with the PRD itself asking, "why aren't these people coming? Is it education? Is it the hours? I don't know yet" (interview, 2006).

The example of Austin demonstrates how, despite huge enthusiasm and a city full of go-getters (and philanthropists such as Susan Dell), public health interventions to address obesity still rely overwhelmingly on a series of 'technical fixes' overlaid with individually held cultural stereotypes, norms and preconceptions. In effect then, "fitness is chosen because it's easy . . . it's easier to say than we're going to make the nation the healthiest by eradicating poverty and racial injustice" (interview, TDHHS, 2006). Yet, encouraging fitness does little to alter long-term health outcomes as the host of partners that form the Steps consortium "have

Map 6: Location of recreation centres in Austin

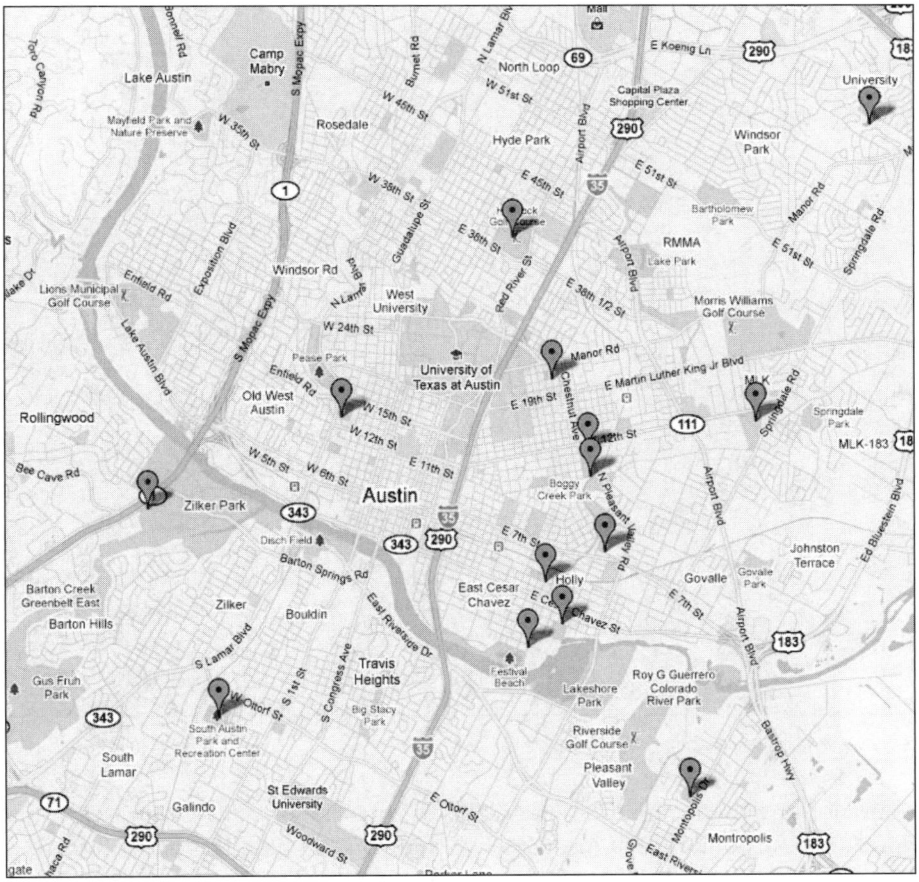

Source: www.ci.austin.tx.us/parks/rec_centers.htm

Map 7: Location of pools in Austin

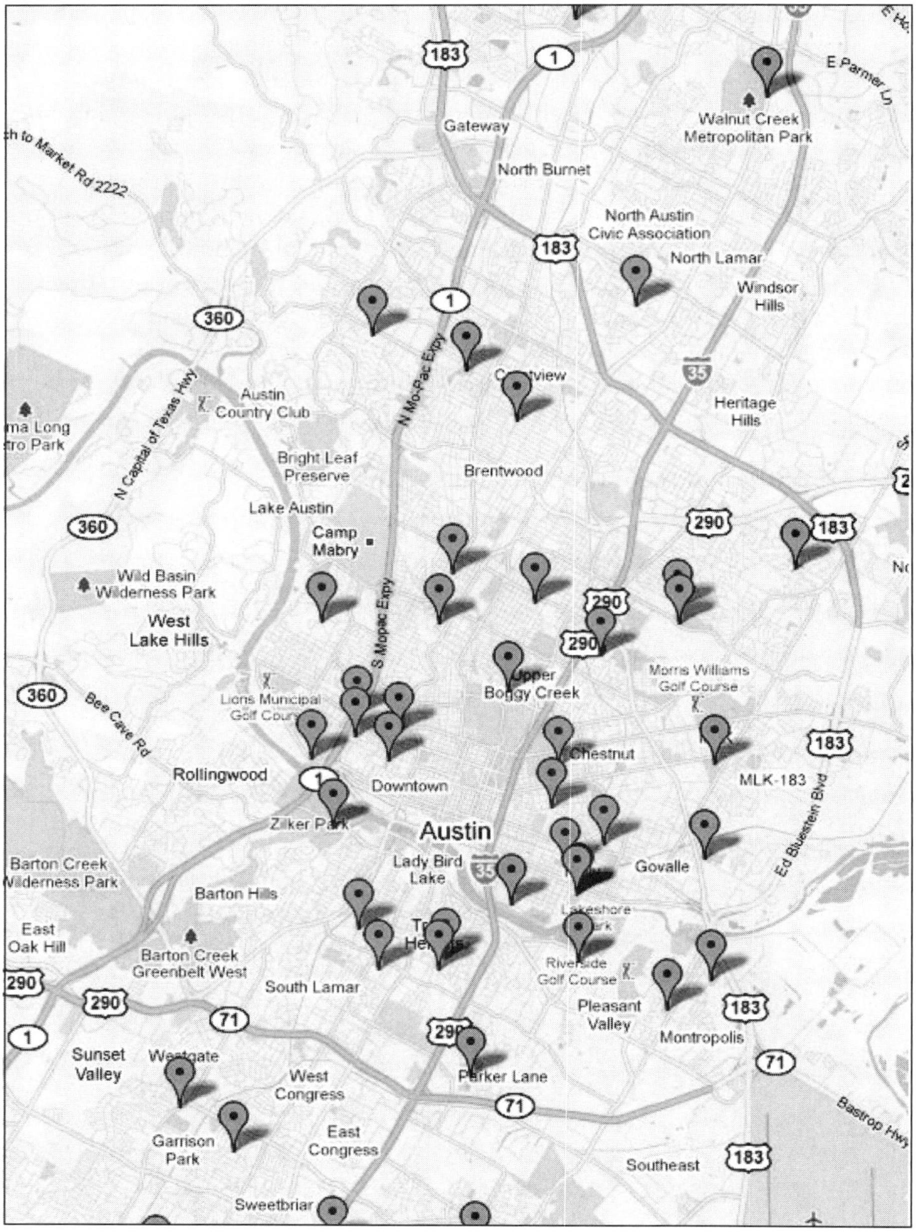

Source: www.ci.austin.tx.us/parks/poolmap.htm

done nothing to change the system" (ibid). Furthermore, "when on top of that you lay obesity and lack of insurance . . . and you just have this perfect storm of bad demographics and bad policy resulting in a really unhealthy society" (TDHHS, interview, 2005). Austin may occupy a coveted place on the fit city list, but it

Map 8: Location of playgrounds in Austin

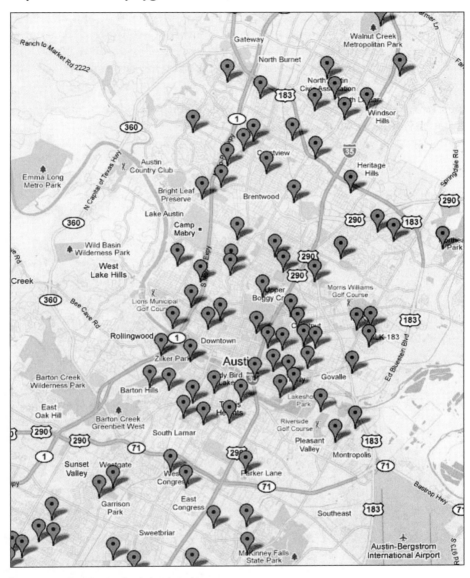

Source: www.ci.austin.tx.us/parks/poolmap.htm

still suffers health disparities, high rates of sedentarism, low rates of fruit and vegetable intake and high rates of obesity and overweight among all racial groups. The residents of East Austin may be more deprived than those on the other side of the I-35, but the reasons why they suffer poor health outcomes are spatially and structurally complex and extend far beyond their local neighbourhood. The perception of East Austin as a deprived 'space of difference' among those charged with improving health outcomes has little to do with baseline data, but rather with visceral reactions to a neighbourhood that is evidentially poorer (see Figure 7) and has higher crime rates than the city average (66% of total indexed and non-indexed crimes in Austin in 2009 occurred in the Steps intervention area (City of Austin Police Department 2009)). Thus, for those that may only venture to East Austin on occasions, it might take just one car break-in to taint the

Figure 7: East 6th Street looking towards downtown – dive bars and a paucity of pedestrians

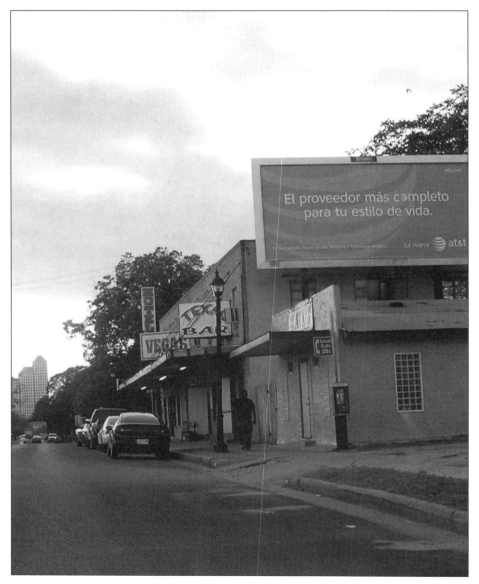

Photo, author's own

neighbourhood's existing image and cement stereotypes of place, deprivation and safety. Indeed, as Macintyre et al suggest, health promotion policies are based on:

> [the] principle that if working class *people* could become like middle class *people*, then their rates illness and premature death would become more like those of middle class people. An alternative approach would be to try to make working class *areas* more like middle class *areas* by improving the social and physical environment. (Macintyre et al 1993: 229)

Austin demonstrates that, within the limitations of funding and the residual conservatism of many in public health, thinking often remains at the level of trying to explain why at-risk individuals do not act in more middle-class ways, without asking which facets of middle-class life could be of benefit to their health. London offers up a different perspective on obesity prevention, skirting the issues of cultural difference and the spatially but actually socially targeted interventions seen in Austin, asking instead how environmental upgrading might offer up incidental health improvements.

London and active travel

Austin's Steps programme reveals the unwillingness and inability of those in public health to effect real environmental changes and the tendency to recourse instead to racial, cultural and environmental stereotypes in their discursive rationalisations of obesity prevention. This section offers up a contrasting example, drawing on the case of London to consider environmental modifications to address obesity. This section will thus examine the example of 'active travel' or 'non-motorised transport' (walking, cycling and running for instrumental purposes and the activity associated with public transport use) promotion in London. In particular, it will explore implementation efforts in the inner London boroughs of Camden and Islington, in order to provide a geographically comparative case study area to Austin. Active travel promotion is not a new phenomenon, but its popularity has grown in policy circles in recognition of the manifold benefits it promises (for example addressing climate change, congestion and individual health). However, in recent years, the rhetoric of health has become a de facto discourse in active travel promotion even as its undertaking has remained firmly within the remit of borough councils' environmental, transport and planning teams (Ogilvie et al 2004). As a result, active travel promotion in London exemplifies the third contention of this book – that the melding of transport, public health and environmental agendas has recast obesity risk in overtly spatialised terms. In so doing, it also presents a particular reading and vision of both the incidentally sensible city and the hope for equally sensible citizens.

London, with the UK's most comprehensive public transport system, two successive mayors dedicated to the cause of active travel and low levels of individual car ownership (UK Census 2001, www.census.gov.uk) is a particularly good site for exploring the operationalisation of environmental interventions to improve health. Furthermore, the recent call for health strategies to take London to the 2012 Olympics (NHS London 2009) and the Mayor's 2010 Health Inequalities Strategy's (Mayor of London 2010) focus on 'healthy places' make tackling obesity in the city even more pressing. This is further reinforced through the elision of health strategies with other objectives such as economic vitality, social cohesion and the vibrancy of public space. Consequently, measures to address obesity in London are inextricable from broader mayoral policies to invest in urban regeneration and infrastructural improvement, promote civic pride and create a 'global city' with a high quality of life. London clearly demonstrates that health is no longer compartmentalised at a policy level, but is rather edging into almost every domain of governmental rhetoric and practice and is a requirement of most grant applications. Health is also transforming a growing host of non-governmental organisations who are drawing on this powerful discursive currency to update and promote their own agendas and attract funding:

> 'Well, I think that health has become higher level in transport over the years. It's either second or third in our priorities in our bids. That wasn't something that was in any TfL [Transport for London] criteria. It's gradually worked its way in there as people have realised that's a good way to market trying to change travel behaviour, trying to market personal benefit. Health is something that improves their business case.' (Camden sustainable transport planner, interview, 2010)

Unlike many European cities where cycling is the norm, London has a long way to go. In Copenhagen, for example, rates of cycling exceed 34% of all commuting journeys (City of Copenhagen 2002). By contrast, the modal share of commuting journeys undertaken by bike in London is less than 3% (Transport for London 2010). The UK has seen a fall in the distance cycled per year for travel purposes (see Figure 8) and in 2007 the average person spent less than one minute per day cycling for travel purposes, while the time spent walking fell to 10 minutes (Figure 9). However, even as participation rates have fallen, over 40% of people polled still thought they could have made a journey of less than two miles just as easily on foot or bike as by car (Figure 10). More optimistically for the future of active travel promotion, over 75% of respondents in 2005 agreed that walking was 'a good way to stay healthy', over 70% 'felt safe' walking in local streets, and over 75% agreed that their local area was 'pleasant to walk in' (Figure 11). The basic preconditions for walking thus seem to be in place and, indeed in 2009, 76% of people stated that they walk for at least 20 minutes more than three times a week (Figure 12). While there is cause for quiet optimism about walking rates, cycling remains exceptionally low, with the frequency of trips tailing off as people get older, and remaining stubbornly low among women (Figure 13). Despite this and the limitations of the national-scale data, London seems to be bucking the national trend with the events of the 7/7 bombings, the increasing cost of public transport and the rising visibility (and vocality) of cyclists pushing

Figure 8: Changing distances walked and cycled relative to 1996 levels

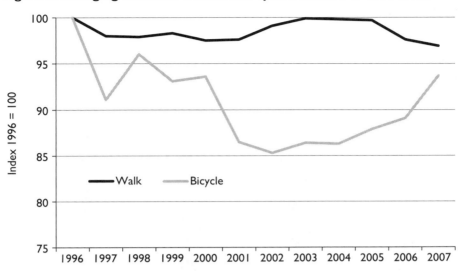

Source: Department for Transport (2009)

Figure 9: Average minutes per day per person spent cycling or walking for travel purposes 1995/97–2007

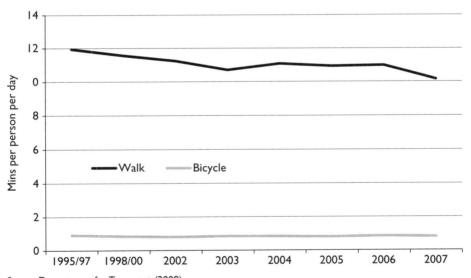

Source: Department for Transport (2009)

forward a 114% increase in cycling rates from 2000–9. Camden has emerged as a shining light in the hope for a cycle-friendly London as 10% of all journeys in the borough are now by bike (Travel Survey 2009, personal communication). The momentum behind active travel is growing and 25% of Londoners recently proclaimed that they were actively considering taking up cycling in the next

Figure 10: Those agreeing that walking and cycling possible over short distances 2006–09

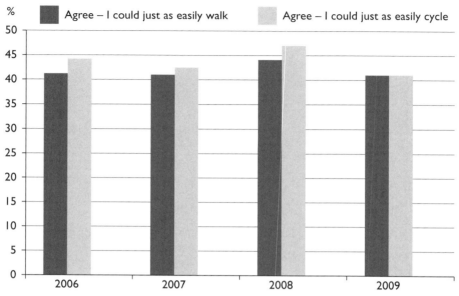

Source: Department for Transport (2009)

Figure 11: Opinions on walking, 2005

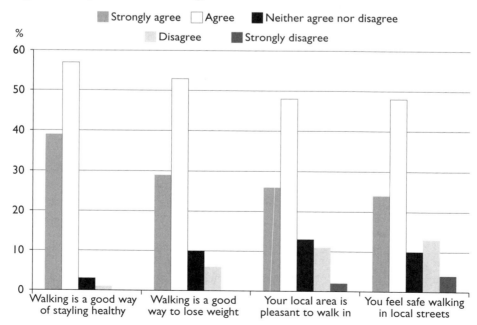

Source: Department for Transport (2009)

Figure 12: Variations in bicycle use by age and gender 2007–09

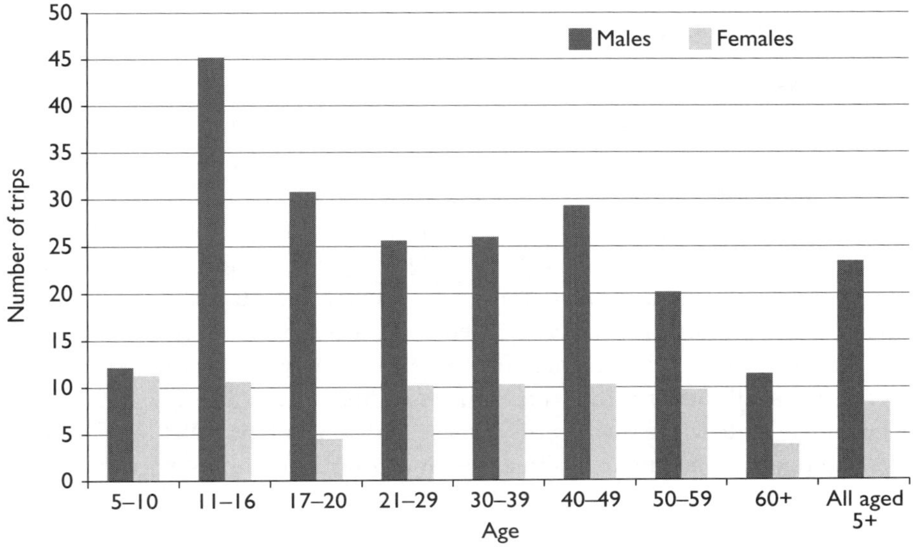

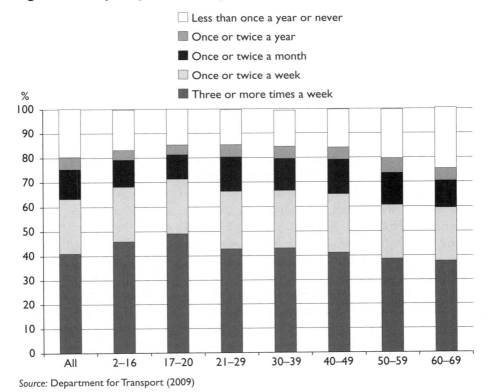

Source: Department for Transport (2009)

Figure 13: Frequency of walks of greater than 20 minutes by age, 2009

Source: Department for Transport (2009)

12 months (Transport for London 2010). A series of repeat interviews in 2010 suggests that the groundwork being laid when fieldwork was conducted in 2006 is now coming to fruition.

The potential significance of a low uptake of active travel for obesity rates is made clear by Bassett et al (2008) in their comparison of cycling rates in the US and Europe. In 2000, Europeans cycled an average of 187 km per year, while Americans managed only 40 km a year. This activity equates to 43–80 Kcal per day for Europeans (or 5–9 lbs of fat per year) and only 20 Kcal per day (2 lbs per year) for Americans. In policy terms, physical activity promotion has been repeatedly cast as a 'best buy' (Morris 1994) for public health. With walking and cycling counting as moderate physical activity and current UK guidelines advocating 30 minutes on five days a week (Department of Health 2004a), active travel offers up an accessible, equitable route to, in the words of one interviewee, "getting a health benefit from something you might be doing anyway" (central government, interview, 2006). It is thus a win–win situation that goes beyond meeting the national public health target of getting 2 million more people active by 2012 (Department of Health 2009) as well as London's target of lifting 150,000 people out of inactivity and getting 300,000 people more active. It also spills over into aspirations for the kind of cultural and environmental change set out in the 2005 Choosing Activity White Paper:

> We need a culture shift if we are to increase physical activity levels in England. This will only be achieved if people are aware of, understand and want the benefits of being active. Opportunities will be created by changing the physical and cultural landscape – and building an environment that supports people in more active lifestyles. (Department of Health 2005b: 6)

London Mayor Boris Johnson has a very visible penchant for cycling and a level of enthusiasm that would most likely ensure that London would score highly in the *MF* 'mayoral and city initiatives' category. In 2010, Transport for London launched its Cycling Revolution London document to coincide with the city's new £23 million cycle super highways and its Barclays cycle hire scheme. In the report, Johnson declared his desire to see London become a 'cyclised city – a civilised city where people can ride their bikes safely and in a pleasant environment' (Transport for London 2010: 3). More than this, the mayor further proclaimed a belief that cycling is 'the best way to get around our city, and arguably the single most important tool for making London the best big city in the world' (ibid). These opening statements are compelling for several reasons. First, the notion that the cyclable city represents the epitome of civilised living – a discourse that has much in common with the fascination with European civilised drinking that will be discussed in Chapters Seven and Eight. Second, that cycling should necessarily be associated with and facilitated by a 'pleasant' environment (Sport England 2008c; National Institute for Health and Clinical Excellence 2009) and that, therefore, increasing rates of active travel will necessarily mean infrastructural as well as aesthetic upgrading. Third, that cycling infrastructure and the culture surrounding cycle use are now essential vehicles for realising broader urban improvement objectives. There is now a feeling that big cities *need* to enable a better quality of life and that cycling might be one politically painless route towards this. Indeed, with other cities following Paris's Vel'lib scheme (Copenhagen, Barcelona, Lyon, Vienna, Oslo, Brussels to name a few), cycling is increasingly becoming a *de rigeur* element of the 'good city'.

Cycling fetishism aside, the social and spatial delineation of obesity risk in London is far more complex than in Austin due to the city's characteristically tight, street-scale interlacing of socioeconomic and demographic characteristics. With policy documents such as the Cycling Revolution strategy differentiating explicitly between the needs of inner and outer London residents, it is unsurprising that the most recent HSE London boost data (2006) also uses this geographic scale of analysis. It also differentiates between the health status of the residents of spearhead and non-spearhead primary care trusts (PCTs) (those in the bottom deprivation quintile) as a measure of deprivation. The recent publication of the data boost results (Coyle and Fitzpatrick 2009; Coyle et al 2009) shows that 16.5% of Londoners were obese and 34.2% overweight. Given that the average for overweight in England was 22.7% for men and 32.2% for women in 2004, it would be fair to ask whether lower rates of obesity are a facet of London's environment (context) or its residents (composition). It is therefore notable that there was no statistically significant difference between rates in spearhead and non-spearhead PCTs, nor in rates by socioeconomic status or deprivation quintile. It is worth highlighting that rates of obesity in London were significantly lower in inner London (13.5%) than in more suburban outer London (18%), suggesting that easy access to public transport networks may play some role in reducing obesity risk.

The same data boost results also demonstrate a gradient in obesity rates by age, with 16- to 34-year-olds having the lowest rates (8.7%), climbing among 34- to 55-year-olds (17.9%) and again among those aged over 55 (25.8%). There are also marked differences between prevalence by race, with 22.4% of black and 16.7% of white Londoners obese. Rates of overweight are highest among British Asian Londoners at 37.3% and it is also worth noting that obesity rates among Asian people are higher in spearhead (17.2%) than in non-spearhead PCTs (13.8%). The fact that differences between obesity rates in inner and outer London are more significant that variations between socioeconomic groups and spearhead/non-spearhead areas does not, however, help establish causality. In turn, this does little to clarify which environmental modifications might induce sensible behaviour. It thus remains unclear whether the forces of self-selection are at work, or if there are some specific features of the inner London environment that reduce the risk of obesity. The inherent difficulties in establishing causality also plague obesity prevention policy development and deployment and are just as marked when physical activity and fruit and vegetable consumption data are considered.

The pattern of physical activity uptake in London also shows a similar social and spatial patterning. 58.4% of Londoners were inactive in 2006, while 26.7%

exercised for less than three hours a week and only 5% for one hour a day. Rates of inactivity also demonstrate statistically significant correlation with socioeconomic status, with 49.9% of professional and managerial workers inactive, 60% of intermediate groups and 70.8% of routine and manual workers. Importantly for the implementation of active travel policies, physical *inactivity* is significantly lower among those living in the least deprived quintile (50.8%) than in the most deprived (66%). Furthermore, 20.1% of those living in the most deprived quintile exercised up to three hours a week, while among those living in the least deprived quintile the figure climbed to 33.7%. When fruit and vegetable consumption (as a proxy for dietary health) is considered, there are no statistically significant differences between inner and outer London and spearhead/non-spearhead PCTs, but marked variations by individual PCTs are evident. For example, 60.9% of Camden residents consume five or more servings a day, compared to only 37.9% in Bexley. There are also significant differences by racial group, with 62.8% of Asian, 62% of Chinese, 49% of black and 48% of white residents meeting the five a day target, deeply problematising notions of risk based on ethnicity. Among those living in the most deprived quintile, 7.9% consume less than one serving a day, while only 1.9% of those in the least deprived wards did so, suggesting that socioeconomic factors might play a far more significant role.

With such complex and inconsistent patterns of health behaviours and obesity prevalence, it is unsurprising that active travel has emerged as a catch-all solution to improving health, without the need to establish causal relationships between risk groups, high-risk environments, health behaviours and outcomes. The discursive shift from 'green' to 'active' travel also reflects a changing vision and construction of the citizen-consumer. 'Active', according to Camden's transport planner suggests individual benefits and agency rather than the self-sacrifice associated with green living (interview, 2005). It also recognises that encouraging people to adopt healthier lifestyles in a consumer society involves communicating personal benefits in a language that alludes to improved control, ownership and short-term gain. More than this, health is also rhetorically and pragmatically powerful, as demonstrated in the quote from the transport planner quoted earlier. However and more than this, encouraging people to take to their bikes or feet to achieve the mayor's latest target of increasing trips made by active travel by 400% (on 2001 figures) by 2026 also means matching these rhetorical promises with the kind of environmental changes –those that improve the perception of the safety of cycling and also reduce bike crime (see Figure 14) – that render such rhetoric a possibility rather than a promise.

Unlike many other cities in the UK and the US, London does not lend itself to anti-car messaging. Indeed, with over half of Camden and Islington households without a car (UK Census 2001), messages centred on car use will clearly have little effect on activity rates in central London, especially given that the congestion charge already provides adequate financial disincentive to driving, and that parking is virtually impossible in daylight hours. TfL's support for active travel stems from the need to ease congestion on the tube and buses in central London (Transport for

Figure 14: London cycle thefts per year 2000–08

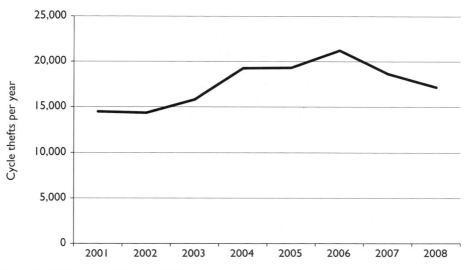

Source: British Transport Police data 2009

London 2005: 6). It therefore provides limited funding for small-scale, commuter and workplace-targeted borough initiatives to promote walking and cycling and reinforces this through practical tools such as TfL's online travel planner, allowing commuters to choose cycling and walking as travel options. As Camden's transport planner points out, this mapping technology is crucial to the success of active travel as "understanding distances is key to a modal shift" (interview, 2006). Indeed, he goes on to state, "London is the victim of the tube", suggesting that the way in which the tube map obscures geographical reality, confusing any conception of the relative location of places and the distances in between – and how commuters feel compelled to get value from their weekly travelcards – is one of the most fundamental barriers to walking and cycling in the city. Thus, much of the activity in active travel is actually around designing workplace and school 'travel plans' and developing maps that enable commuters to make an informed choice as to the relative time efficiency of either walking or cycling.

In line with the mayor's revised role in meeting the PSA physical activity targets, TfL have also produced a series of high-profile cycling promotion campaigns. Its 2006 cycling promotion posters proclaimed (Figure 15) 'Extend your life. Cycle' with the ambiguous strapline 'You're better off by bike', hinting that 'better' might not just be limited to health. Its 'London: Made for Cycling' poster (Figure 16) recreates the city's skyline with cycling accoutrements and makes the reader rethink the cityscape in a new language. However, it does not expressly cast cycling in the language of better health, but rather recasts London in the language of better cycling. It is notable that research conducted for TfL showed a marked change in the public perception of its marketing materials in 2006. The proportion of those associating the adverts with health and fitness climbed from 22% in September

Figure 15: Transport for London cycling promotion campaign poster, summer 2006

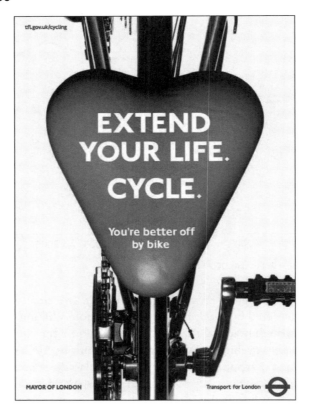

Source: TfL 2006

Figure 16: Transport for London cycling promotion campaign poster

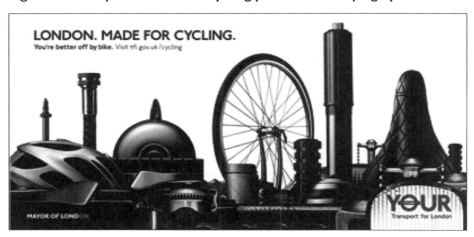

Source: TfL 2010

2005 to 41% by April 2006 after a change in rhetoric (TfL, private communication, 2006). Acting alongside TfL's pan-London promotional strategy, Camden and Islington put lifestyle messaging to work, designing concrete local infrastructural improvements enabling people to walk and cycle easily and safely and then using the rhetoric of health benefits both to justify the expenditure and to raise public awareness. By 2012, London aims to have 66,000 extra cycle parking spaces and Section 106 agreements (that allow local authorities to enter into a planning obligation with a landowner or developer when planning permission is granted) and community infrastructure levies also help fund extra parking provision around key transport nodes such as bus and tube stations by holding private developers responsible for their provision. Furthermore, schemes such as Cycle to Work allow employees get tax relief on a new bike and, combined with workplace travel plans and new planning guidance that asks workplaces to provide shower facilities ensures that cycling is increasingly viable.

Local provision of cycling routes, wider pavements, signage indicating walking times, Clearzones (urban redesign to address air quality and congestion), healthy travel initiatives (partnerships with local business to ensure the provision of, for example, cycle parking and showers) and school schemes such as 'Walk on Wednesdays' are now being combined with work undertaken by PCT's Active Health teams. This coworking is now a needs–must issue at a time of rapidly shrinking funding. Yet, despite the rhetoric on joined-up thinking, transport planners and the PCT still work in different ways and have different aims:

> 'I mean, that's the difference between what the PCT do and what we do, because we are targeting commuters and the PCT have got target areas in the boroughs and their residents. Obviously the people that we talk to and the businesses we talk to, they could be coming in from all over, from Kingston . . . but we do do community events as well. But most of our stuff is about the commute. What we have had is health advisers come to our walking and cycling events and do BMI testing. I think its works fairly well and it adds value to what we do as an event, particularly from the walking which is more accessible particularly for safety and the need to own a bike. They also get advice about healthy eating. It gives more of a lateral value to things that we might not cover.' (interview, Active Travel Planner, 2010)

The idea is that getting people to walk and cycle as part of their daily commute fits the assertion that 'thirty minutes of moderate walking a day will only be achieved by helping people build activity into their daily lives' (Department of Health 2003: 43). Despite these concerted efforts at modifying the environment and raising people's awareness of the significance and possible benefits of these modifications, there is still a notable lack of any work to measure or gauge behaviour change apart from that measured through transport surveys and informal feedback from promotional events. As one transport planner explained:

A: 'We did 20 events last year, which was the biggest ever.'

Q: 'With success?'

A: 'Well, it's hard to know how you measure … attendance on average was about 300, which is good. It's difficult because you can have a busy event and then you have less quality contact with people there.'

Q: 'What about measuring behaviour change?'

A: ' That's a difficult one …'

Q: 'Is it a question of money? Time?'

A: 'Well, we've been doing it more, we've been doing surveys this year at our events to find out what people draw from the event, how did they travel initially and how are they likely to travel in the future. So it helps us understand how potentially they might change. Obviously we don't know if they do change as we never see them again. The way that we measure it really at a borough-wide level is traffic surveys. We also do travel plans with businesses so we can monitor those and see what effect they are having. Again that's the disparity between us and the PCT as they are looking at personal health in the borough … we're looking at setting up some more community initiatives, I think it would be good to tackle some of those issues as well. But the PCT are already working on active health, so they can benefit from some of our initiatives. It's also about being cost effective.' (transport planner, interview, 2010)

In contrast to Austin, the idea of risk groups within active travel rhetoric and implementation is underdeveloped, with promotion activity to induce behaviour change targeting general commuters, rather than specific at-risk 'communities'. When asked whether such measures might ameliorate health and social inequalities in Islington, the sustainable transport planner dismissed the relevance of the issue by replying that 'hard to reach' groups were not their domain as, "we've got a cultural team for that kind of thing" (interview, 2006). Indeed, in a more recent interview, it was felt that such targeted interventions were the PCT's domain. Such general application is in stark contrast to the work being undertaken in Austin and, in many respects, is refreshing in its inclusivity even if it means that active travel promotion results in existing cyclists cycling more rather than converting new recruits. This is turn begs the question asked by an interviewee at the Ramblers' Association – "is health really a motivating factor? Maybe enjoyment is the bigger draw" (interview, 2006). Despite the paucity of data on individual motivations for cycling uptake, promoting active travel still makes sense given that walking and cycling are good for health, the environment and also good for London. Active travel is thus an attractive policy option largely as it tries to argue why walking and cycling are *better* and *easier* choices, while providing the infrastructure (bike lanes and improved pedestrian crossings) that offer a visual enticement for greater use. As one interviewee argues, "the health thing is a good way to get those dubious people involved" (interview with active transport planner, Camden, 2010). In health terms, active travel is powerful as the health benefits can be incidental to the financial, time or stress savings of not taking public transport, but remain regardless of the motivation for undertaking a modal shift. Thus active travel is amenable to promotion across a broad range of registers dependent on the prevailing social and cultural concerns of the day. Yet, the specificities of language aside, the health benefits will always remain incidental, thus avoiding the particularly British aversion to more prescriptive, nanny statist health promotion exercises.

Conclusion

This chapter has explored, in conceptual and empirical terms, the limitations to the aspiration of rendering sensible behaviour incidental to certain environments. The considerable research now being undertaken on obesogenicity and the selective fervour with which ideas about 'healthy places' are infusing a plethora of public policy realms are indicative of the manifold attractions of thinking environmentally rather than behaviourally in efforts to reduce obesity. However, while this area of research is expanding, the highly conflicting evidence base concerning the correlations and causal relationships between environmental determinants, physical activity, nutrition and BMI between different countries, cities and neighbourhoods demonstrates the limits to the kind of tick-box, tool-kit thinking so often seen in urban policy. The search for causality is also in stark contrast to sociological, anthropological and geographical theorisations of the city and the urban condition, in which it is understood that people and places interact in multiple, complex and dynamic ways. This is no less the case when it comes to health behaviours. Theories of health must therefore be inculcated within urban theory if policies are to be better (and more equitably) deployed. As Sui suggests, 'If the fat body becomes an obsession for health reasons and narcissism alike, it cannot be returned to a more sustainable size and shape as long as the city remains outside of theories of health' (2003: 82). Moreover, the healthy city is increasingly being recognised as a place where being active is good not just because it might reduce BMI, cholesterol and the risk of heart disease, but also because there is a hope that it may build social capital, trust and cohesion and, therefore, make better places. Thus, as Sui further suggests, 'a healthy city is not just a city where people are healthy, but rather a city where the impulse to escape has been counter-balanced by social cohesion' (ibid).

Public fears over the rise and rise of obesity are intertwined with a persistent concern over the type and quality of places in which we live. They are also therefore inescapably bound into discourses of the people who live in those places with 'risky' environmental traits, as the example of Austin clearly shows. As this chapter has discussed and demonstrated, ecological frameworks offer an attractive alternative to behavioural explanations of obesity, not least because they hold the promise of policies that offer up benefits that extend far beyond public health. In reality, and as the cases of both London and Austin demonstrate, there are practical and financial limits to the kind of environmental modifications that those seeking to address obesity can and will undertake. Moreover, there also seem to be limits to the ability of those implementing policy to think beyond eliding behavioural, cultural and environmental explanations for unhealthy lifestyle behaviours to thinking in more active ways about the creation of new and better places. In London, strategies to increase 'incidental exercise' by supporting, developing and promoting active travel have deliberately avoided targeting specific risk groups and have instead focused on commuters. By contrast, the array of programmes falling under the Steps to a Healthier Austin coalition's remit have done nothing to alter East Austin's environment even while singling it out as both disempowering and pathogenic. There can be little doubt that environmental readings of obesity risk hold the potential to reframe how we think about personal responsibility and individual choice with regards to health – as considerations of luck egalitarianism in the previous chapter explored. However, in reality they rarely seem to achieve this and instead fall back on behavioural explanations of low activity levels and poor food choices.

In the case of obesity, the environmental determinants of the health paradigm clearly represent a missed opportunity. It seems that, unless there are other reasons for implementing environmental changes (for example climate change, safety, city prestige), public health improvements remain little more than an attractive bolt-on or a rhetorical necessity for funding. This situation is further reinforced by the paucity of an evidence base on which to legitimise structural investment at a time of scarce state resources. Cycling and walking data in the UK are collected at a national level and, apart from showing very general trends, offer little of any relevance to London. Furthermore, even where data are collected at a borough scale, they just show cycling traffic *through* the borough and do not demonstrate modal shifts among borough residents. There is also a paucity of evidence as to whether investment in cycling and pedestrian infrastructure actually results in higher physical activity rates. Such selective use of data was also characteristic of practitioners in Austin, who instead relied on cultural assumptions to back up their readings of environmental risk. Yet, without a two-way process of listening to and understanding a community's environmental determinants of health, there is little reason to believe that interventions will achieve an impact. As Ogilvie et al suggest, 'Interventions that engage people in a participative process and address factors of personal relevance may be more effective than those that simply aim to raise awareness or impose changes in the physical and economic environments' (2004: 767). In neither Austin nor London were obesity prevention efforts the outcome of an engaged participative process, but rather a general consensus of actions that would be in the public's best interests. Better places cannot be imposed from above, but must instead emerge from dialogue and consensus if they are to have equitable and just outcomes, especially when they are read through the lens of public health aspirations.

SIX

Events and the lucratively sensible city

The evidence of the potential health gains from active lifestyles is clear. We now need a culture shift to achieve these goals. Changing inactive lifestyles and levels of inactivity presents a tremendous public health challenge – a challenge we must rise to if we are to improve health. The solution does not lie in any single innovation. Nor does it lie in advances in medical science. Current levels of physical activity are a reflection of personal attitudes about time use and of cultural and societal values. (Chief Medical Officer 2004: iii)

Introduction

This chapter changes tack slightly to consider a particular point of intersection between physical activity, the built environment and behavioural readings of health: the event. More specifically, it draws on the phenomenon of mass participation running events (MPREs) to explore how 'event thinking' has permeated the governmental and non-governmental aspiration of creating a more active populace. In contrast to the previous chapter's focus on *incidental* physical activity such as walking and cycling, this considers efforts to promote and encourage the uptake of sport as leisure. Defined by the Council of Europe's *European Sport Charter* as, 'all forms of physical activity which, through casual participation, aim at expressing or improving physical fitness and mental well-being, forming social relationships or obtaining results in competition at all levels'(1992: 15), sport is increasingly being cast as a solution for an array of social, cultural, economic and developmental ills. At the same time, urban events are also being seen as a 'panacea for the contemporary social and economic ills of cities' (Waitt 2008: 513). As such, sporting events are far from politically innocuous. Yet, one has only to look at the interplay of sport and British imperial ambition (Stoddart 1988; Majumdar 2006), apartheid (for its justification, eventual unravelling and more recent efforts to eradicate its legacy) (Booth 2003) and communist ideologies (Riordan 1999, 2001) to see that it has long been used to realise political ambition. This chapter thus dwells on the salience of sport in relation to the governmental aspiration of increasing participation.

Sport England's 'value of sport monitor' lists seven domains where sport is thought to 'deliver benefits across a wide range of public policy agendas' (Sport England 2010a). These include crime reduction and community safety, economic impact and regeneration of local communities, education and lifelong learning, participation, physical fitness and health, psychological health and wellbeing, and social capacity and cohesion. The depth and breadth of this list make clear the great hope being placed on the ability of sport to deliver where other instruments have failed. Furthermore, it also demonstrates that the sporting agenda now goes further and deeper than obesity prevention alone, even though controlling obesity has clearly imbued sport with renewed significance. The value of sport has not been lost on the United Nations, whose Sport for Development and Peace initiative recognises the role that the 'intentional use of sport' might play in realising the Millennium Development Goals (Kidd 2008). This idea is perhaps even better reflected in the French translation of the concept – *le sport au service du développement et de la paix* – where the notion that it might be put 'to the service' of a series of disparate ends succinctly sums up the level of expectation currently being placed on sport across a broad register of governmental domains.

Events are significant to this exploration of efforts to create sensible people and places, primarily as they provide a platform from which to examine the politics of participation – how it is defined, measured, the strategies used to encourage it and the legitimisation of its importance – and its intersections with the broader domains of responsibility, choice and behaviour change considered throughout this book. This chapter asks how the relationship between urban space and individual and group behaviour is both mediated and shaped by events. It therefore not only adds to our understanding of the significance of the emergent phenomenon of MPREs, but does so in the explicit recognition that they have been subsumed beneath analyses of sporting mega-events (see for example Roche 1992, 1994; Hall and Hodges 1996; Hiller 2000; Andranovich et al 2001; Burbank et al 2002; Cornelissen 2004a, 2004b; Matheson and Baade 2004; Nauright 2004; Hall 2006; Horne and Manzenreiter 2006a, 2006b; Cornelissen 2008; Pillay and Bass 2008). Such 'hallmark events' include the Olympics (Newman 2007; Gold and Gold 2008; Walton et al 2008), the Football World Cup (Cornelissen and Swart 2006; Pillay and Bass 2008; Cornelissen 2010), the Rugby World Cup (Jones 2001; Van Der Merwe 2007) and the Commonwealth Games (Carlsen and Taylor 2003; Smith and Fox 2007). Yet, while mega-events may dominate the corpus of work on sporting events, they nevertheless form a fascinating body of literature that critically approaches the multitudinous ways in which events crosscut themes such as urban development and regeneration (Gratton and Henry 2001; Smith and Fox 2007), the construction and creation of 'legacy' (Dyreson 2008; Girginov and Hills 2008; Gold and Gold 2008), their economic contribution (Atkinson et al 2008; Walton et al 2008), civic boosterism (Cornelissen 2004b; Cornelissen and Swart 2006; Waitt 2008), the sport–media–tourism complex (Nauright 2004) and their use in and by public policy (Burbank et al 2002; Pillay and Bass 2008). As such, while empirical analyses of mass participation events are a relative rarity (Nettleton and Hardey 2006), they are nonetheless conceptually significant for what they reveal about contemporary urban politics, governance and their growing role in realising political ambitions. Moreover, they also speak to the second contention of this book: that events materialise sensible behaviour in reconciling the tensions internal to neoliberal economies discussed in Chapter Two.

———

Thus, to explore the strategic role now played by sport and the event, this chapter will first examine how and why the instrumental and intrinsic value of sport has been operationalised in policy discourses and strategies in both the US and UK. It will then turn to the MPRE and explore the genesis of this event format and, therefore, some of the reasons for its current ubiquity. MPREs represent distinct political economic formations that inculcate public sector *goals*, private sector *means* (such as marketing, publicity, global reach) and voluntary sector *needs* (such as charity fundraising). In this way they have particular aspirations, means and ends that are as much about 'taking part' as raising money and catalysing the adoption of healthier lifestyles to prevent morbidity. However, despite the purported synergies between these goals, tensions remain even where events are historically deeply embedded in particular communities. As such and in order to explore the tensions between these political economies and the sporting aspirations of politicians, the chapter will turn to two empirical examples: the ways in which multiple, smaller-scale MPREs in Austin are being woven into the narratives and enterprise of health promotion; and the role played by large-scale events such as the Great North Run (GNR, held annually in Newcastle-Gateshead) in promoting and achieving participation. Both cities are known for their MPREs and they therefore offer a clear insight into the politics of hope that views sport as a route to inculcating an ethic of responsibility, motivation, participation and, therefore, the self-efficacy that can facilitate the adoption of healthy behaviours. In other words, successful MPREs are helping to fashion a lucratively sensible city in many ways, but, as ever, the question remains of who benefits and how.

Participating in the mass sporting society

In their critique of the cacophony of current obesity policies 'fissured by significant ideological distinctions', Lang and Rayner suggest that scenario planning may help 'galvanise the necessary inter-sectoral work' that they view as currently lacking (2007: 173). MPREs are strategically located at the intersection of two such scenarios: 'policy as usual' and 'business (almost) as usual'. In the first, initiatives are encouraged in the absence of full-scale legislative change that would address, for example, food advertising. Within this scenario, sporadic events such as fun runs are given priority over 'policy delivering daily physical activity' and 'vast attention is given to prime sporting events, like the Olympics, where elite athletes compete and others watch' (Lang and Rayner 2007: 174). This paradigm, they suggest, exemplifies an ideology of 'individualised, personalised health' (ibid). In the second scenario, in a language mirroring the words of Andrew Lansley discussed in Chapter Four, 'governments abandon state responsibility to shape responses to obesity' where the focus is on 'individual solutions serviced by the food and sports industries' (ibid). Here also, 'Corporate Social Responsibility is the core policy ethos' and a 'substitute for government leadership' (ibid).

In this reading, choice becomes a commercial offering and industry is welcomed as a partner in fulfilling public health ambitions. MPREs are squarely positioned in the space left by government retrenchment from 'sport as welfare' (Gratton and Henry 2001), instead promising a highly commercialised route to the realisation of policy goals. Yet, the commercialisation of MPREs allow race organisers to parody the language of governmental objectives as marketing strategy, while coating their delivery in a attractive and lucrative veneer of performance, drama and spectacle and personal achievement. These events are somewhat unique in relation to the governance of health and lifestyles in that they also quite literally and figuratively exemplify what Rose and Miller have famously called 'governing at a distance' (1992: 173). In this case, such events may have a role to play in realising government sports participation targets and policies, but often they only loosely and quietly involve state actors. On the other hand, the familiar, government-led behaviour-change language of motivation, self-efficacy and (both instrumentalised and intrinsic) participation have also become marketing techniques used by MPREs to ensure growing consumer participation.

However, while participation is a central defining feature of the MPRE, participation as a governmental objective is not consistently defined in relation to physical activity and sport. It is worth noting, therefore, that the most recent *Sport England Strategy 2008–2011* sets out plans to 'create a world-leading community sports system' (Sport England 2008c: 8) in order to realise the target of 45% sports participation by 2020. This is measured through national indicator (NI) 8, or the percentage of people in any one area participating in sport at moderate intensity for at least 30 minutes on at least three days a week, and recorded through Sport England's Active People Survey (APS). This indicator excludes walking and cycling undertaken as active travel and only includes recreational walking and cycling. There is a curious mismatch between NI8 and the CMO's advice to engage in physical activity 'at least five times a week'. The APS consequently paints a more optimistic picture of participation than might be the case had the CMO's prescriptions formed the basis of NI8. In the US, the President's Council on Fitness, Sports and Nutrition has set the slightly tougher 'challenge' to adults to engage in moderate physical activity for 30 minutes a day on five days a week. The US national guidelines on physical activity recommend that for 'substantial health benefits', Americans should engage in 75 minutes of vigorous intensity aerobic activity and for 'additional and more extensive health benefits' this should be increased to 150 minutes a week. The addition of an explicit recommendation for vigorous activity represents an update on the previous 1995 Recommendation for Adults on Physical Activity and Public Health. This explicit distinction between vigorous and moderate activity thus marks out a specific strategic role for sport in meeting the US's ambitious targets. However, it also reveals disparities in the level of expectation that are being placed on individuals in these differing notions of responsible and sensible lifestyle choices.

The US guidelines are thus in sharp contrast to those of the UK, where the CMO is at pains to suggest that 'physical activity does not need to be vigorous to confer protection from cardiovascular disease' and that moderate intensity activity 'is sufficient to achieve benefit' (Department of Health 2004c: 4). Instead of physiological benefit, vigorous activity is linked to 'psychological well-being' where the participant is 'already accustomed to this type of activity' (ibid: 6). Moreover and again in contrast to the US stance, vigorous activity is cast as a source of potential and unexpected personal risk for the uninitiated. This disjuncture mirrors the inconsistencies and discrepancies in epidemiological studies of the relationship between activity intensity, type and amount and cardiovascular disease risk, with medical (and thus national policy) divided on whether vigorous activity is needed to confer additional health benefits (Morris et al 1990; Tanasescu et al 2002; Yu et al 2003; Swain and Franklin 2006) or whether moderate level activity suffices (Shaper et al 1991; Wannamethee and Shaper 1992; Wannamethee et al 2000). While biomedical research may be replete with internal contradictions, there still remains a tacit international consensus that physically active lifestyles are associated with reductions in the risk of CVD, stroke, hypertension, type 2 diabetes, osteoporosis, obesity, colon and breast cancer, anxiety and depression (Haskell et al 2007: 1082). National guidelines may differ, but it is interesting to note that the WHO's guidelines for adults matches those of the US. Furthermore and of note for this chapter is Haskell et al's (2007) suggestion that jogging is an example of vigorous activity. In the UK, jogging is the country's fifth most popular sport with 6.6% of people taking part at least four times a month (Table 3). While these numbers may seem relatively small, MPREs also seek to convert those 15.1% of people who 'regularly' undertake health fitness activities. Thus, in its popularity and significance for health, running and jogging (understood here as recreational and used interchangeably) is automatically conferred a particular role in public health policy, to which this chapter now turns.

Table 3: Top 10 sports activities (undertaken at least four times in the past month)

Activity	2009/10 (%)
Health, fitness, gym or conditioning activities	15.1
Swimming or diving (indoors)	14.7
Cycling (health, recreation, training, competition)	10.5
Football (include 5-a-side and 6-a-side) (outdoors)	6.7
Jogging, cross-country, road running	6.6
Snooker, pool, billiards (exclude bar billiards)	5.8
Keep fit, aerobics, dance exercise (include exercise bike)	5.7
Cycling (to get to places, i.e. work, shops)	4.4
Golf, pitch and putt, putting	4.1
Swimming or diving (outdoors)	3.6

Source: Taking Part Survey 2009/10

Note: Recreational walking is excluded from this data set. Had it been included, it would have been the most popular activity.

Physical activity, events and mass participation

In many respects, MPREs represent the latest incantation of the 'physical hygienist' movement (Gillick 1984), in which the art of wellbeing was promoted as a palliative for all manner of modern ills. While the tone might have changed since a 1975 letter to the editors of the *New England Journal of Medicine* in which the authors 'advocate the hobby of marathon running for everyone [suffering from heart disease]' (Bassler and Scaff 1975), jogging has evolved from being a concern of the eccentric few to become a mass pastime (Gillick 1984: 383). Popular running for fitness emerged in the late 1960s and early 1970s as a middle-class, educated, male pursuit to reduce the risk of heart attacks. However, it should be noted that 'the inspiration for jogging was primarily popular rather than medical' (ibid: 376) and by the 1970s the 'flagellantist delusion' of the 'jogging craze that was beginning to grip the country' (Berking and Neckel 1993: 68) had been cemented by legendary figures such as Jim Fixx (author of the 1977 bestseller *The Complete Book of Running*). As the 1970s wore on, jogging became not only more popular in the US and elsewhere, but also broadened its appeal to women as the tone of the language describing its benefits shifted from cardiovascular health, to psychological wellbeing. It is thus no coincidence that the 1970s gave birth not just to handbooks on running, but also to the running shoe, running clubs and the road race. Running is the quintessentially sensible pastime – in terms of those who are statistically most likely to partake (white, professional, highly educated) and the reasons for which they do so (a continuum from preventative strategy to palliative care to aesthetic concern). Running indeed makes a virtue out of sensibleness.

The rise and rise of running as a popular pastime is inextricable from the expansion in the frequency, geographical range and the marketing inventiveness of MPREs. Such events represent, on the one hand, a clear instance of what Conrad has called 'wellness as virtue' in which the 'pursuit of health and fitness becomes a "good" end in itself. Independent of the results, merely engaging in wellness activities is a virtuous activity' (1994: 397). On the other hand, they represent the epitome of an instrumentalist vision in which 'merely engaging' is insufficient and instead, health, fitness and participation become a means to an end. Such 'achievement running' or 'a world of numbers, ranks, hierarchy, records and a sense of certainty' (Bale 2004: 25) thus drives participation. However, in more recent years, the running boom has undergone a demographic shift away from middle-aged men fighting off the excesses of the boardroom to include more women and older amateurs. These newer runners are looking for an 'accessible ultimate challenge' (Olberding and Jisha 2005: 193) and are drawn to MPREs for a particular set of reasons. These include the race destination, the ancillary attractions, entertainment along the route, the contents of the race registration 'goodie bag' and first aid support (ibid). Such consumers have high demands which may put them at odds with those more attuned to their inner 'achiever' and concerned with bettering their personal best. Thus, in a rhetorical sense, the appeal to participate is driven by the twin desire for the qualitative thrill of the experience and quantifiable evidence of self-improvement. As a consequence, these events have genuine mass appeal. They therefore hold the potential to be valuable tools for individual behavioural change at a time when government spending and welfare cuts have created a provision vacuum ripe for commercial endeavours.

The emergence of the MPRE has been shaped by the modernisation of marathons and, in particular, the evolution of the New York Marathon under the guidance of its founder Fred Lebow. From a race with 100 competitors lapping Central Park in 1970, the New York Marathon has metamorphosed through the fame bestowed on it by Frank Shorter's 1972 Olympic marathon victory and by the inclusion of women, attracting the sponsorship of Olympic Airlines and the reworking of the route to take in the landscapes of all five boroughs and, with it, TV coverage, prestige and greater prize money. The conjunction of elite runners, sponsorship, appearance fees, large winnings and media coverage with a scenic backdrop, an ethic of inclusivity and personal narratives of motivation, perseverance and triumph among the 'masses' therefore characterise the contemporary MPRE. The numbers of participants in these events far exceed those of marathons alone for, as Tables 4 and 5 show, New York Marathon's 38,096 finishers in 2009 pale into insignificance compared to Sydney's 'City to Surf' race at 76,254. It is perhaps obvious that the shorter the race, the greater its mass appeal and mass accessibility. It is also clear that the more scenic the race's backdrop or the more compelling the race cause, the greater the event's appeal for the growing band of 'running tourists' who scour cities for the most alluring races. In 1982, the Association of International Marathons and Distance Races (AIMS), which certifies race lengths and also provides a promotional platform through its widely distributed magazine, had just 28 members. By contrast, in 2009 it certified over 270 road races of varying lengths in destinations ranging from Antarctica to Kigali (Rwanda) and San Francisco. While MPREs remain predominantly a phenomenon of the Global North, an increasing number in the Global South are making it into the

Runners' World '20 international races to do before you die' list, including the Great Ethiopian Run, the Comrades (ultra) Marathon in South Africa and the Inca Trail Marathon. While two of these may be far from 'fun runs' in terms of length, it is worth noting the global diffusion and profusion of these race formats.

With the exception of the JP Morgan Chase Challenge, which is a corporate event and thus has a unique and exclusive set of participants, the most popular races are over 10 km in length. To run or jog such a distance requires

Table 4: Number of finishers in the world's top 10 marathons in 2009

City	Total finishers 2009
New York	38,096
Berlin	35,786
London	34,417
Chicago	31,343
Paris	28,846
Tokyo	27,386
Boston	21,963
Honolulu	20,058
Washington DC	18,219
LA	17,311

Source: individual marathon websites

Table 5: Number of finishers in the world's top 10 MPREs (including marathons) in 2009

Race	City	Distance (km)	Total finishers
City to Surf	Sydney	14	76,254
JP Morgan Chase Corporate Challenge	Frankfurt	6	73,719
Lilac Bloomsday Run	Spokane, WA	12	61,298
Cursa El Corte Ingles	Barcelona	12	60,088
Vancouver Sun Run	Vancouver, BC	10	59,179
Peachtree Road Race	Atlanta	10	55,000
Great North Run	Newcastle	13	54,100
Bolder Boulder	Boulder	10	54,040
Goteborgsvaret	Gothenburg	13	53,700
Bridge to Brisbane	Brisbane	10	45,265
NY Marathon	New York	42	38,096

Source: Individual event websites

some training for the moderately fit, but for the nominally fit, it necessitates a fitness regime or what the Great North Run's organisers recognise as a 'twelve week communication plan' (Nova International 2010). Therein lies the discursive hook and appeal of the MPRE, that, unlike the 'cultural symbol of almost superhuman endurance' that is the marathon (Reischer 2001: 25), completion of a shorter MPREs is achievable. However, fatigue-free completion (a novel sensation for many) is not necessarily to be taken for granted. The act of participation thus poses an array of emotions: uncertainty and excitement, motivation and conviction, pride and shame, pleasure and pain. It is the fact that such races 'belong in the city . . . the measure against which the strength of will, endurance, speed and determination of the runner had to prove themselves' (Berking and Neckel 1993: 68) that ensures their wider import and commercial success. Put simply, MPREs are often only as popular as their geographical backdrops, with particular attention paid to the visual choreography of the race route. This materiality also has pragmatic consequences and these often mark the domains where the private interests of race organisers butt up against the public concerns of the state agencies that are obliged to close roads, divert public transport, offer medical services, street cleaning and an appropriate police presence.

The limited literature on MPREs and urban marathons focuses almost exclusively on the dialectic between the event and the self. However, while the 'self-transformative' (Reischer 2001) appeal of these races is a clear element of their enduring popularity, rarely are these events analysed from the perspective of their organisers and those state agencies who are called on to support the race in infrastructural terms (for example traffic management, litter collection, first aid). In addition, only very rarely is it asked whether these races actually deliver the broad benefits of sport and the behavioural transformations that they promise. The research on which this chapter is based explores those charged with materialising and operationalising the complex dialectic of private and public goals that mark out sport understood in instrumental terms. In so doing, it approaches MPREs as particular political economic and experiential formations that have definitive spatial and temporal dimensions. Given the specificity of events – even as they tend to share certain common characteristics – MPREs in Austin and Newcastle are explored in the context of the urban politics of mass sporting participation that they reveal. In this the two examples will be used to explore critically the nature and internal contradictions of participation itself – who takes part, how and why? And, perhaps most crucially, can event participation ever have demonstrable health effects?

Fun-running city: Austin, Texas

As the previous chapter explored, Austin is a city that takes great pride in its culture of physical fitness. Indeed, with two of the city's residents – Paul Carrozza (founder of RunTex, Texas's largest chain of running shoe stores) and Susan Dell (wife of Michael Dell) – sitting on the President's Fitness Council, it should be expected that the city is wholeheartedly committed to fitness. So it comes as little surprise that not only is Austin home to a host of mass participation sporting events, but that these have also actively been taken up as catch-all health improvement tools. As one interviewee from the food retailing sector suggested "Austin is a unique town . . . the mayor, Kay [founder of the Marathon Kids programme], they're all very interested in this obesity issue" (interview, 2006). As in Newcastle, the story of fitness promotion through MPREs in Austin is one that would not exist without a cast of inspirational and visionary individuals that have brought them to fruition and, moreover, continue to ensure that they consistently evolve to meet participants' changing demands and expectations. Every year there are over 130 MPREs in and around the city, and the number increases year on year as an ever more diverse range of events are inaugurated. At present, runners of all abilities can choose from Austin's annual marathon or Statesman Capitol 10k to less gruelling events such as the annual 'Pet Fest 5k and Dog Jog'. Fun runs are nothing new to Austin – the Capitol 10k is in its 33rd year – however, as the 'war on obesity' has raged, these events have assumed a new significance and role. In spite of the fact that they are undeniably popular among Austin's significant running community, opinion as to the instrumental worth of such events remained deeply divided among interview respondents in Austin. This section will therefore seek to draw out the tensions between the public health and social policy expectations placed on these events and their use as part of a wider place branding and promotion strategy. The key question that remains to be resolved is whether MPREs, however popular they may be, do anything to make city residents fitter in any sustained and sustainable way.

South of downtown, the Colorado River bisects the city, creating a huge lake ideal for recreation. A 'hike and bike' trail circles the perimeter of Town Lake for 10 miles, through Zilker Park to the West and into East Austin. Despite a torrid summer climate in which temperatures rarely dip below 100° F, running and cycling are big business for the city. This culture is particularly notable as it is in stark contrast to other Texan cities where, a representative from the TDHHS suggested, even walking "is just something that's not done" as "if you were walking down the street someone would probably stop and ask you if you wanted a ride" (interview, 2005). Austin is also home to the nation's largest privately owned running shoe store chain, RunTex; its owner, Paul Carrozza, holds coveted places on the President's, Governor's and Mayor's Councils on Physical Fitness. He is also a personal friend of the former president, a fact that is obvious on entering his office and seeing the walls emblazoned with letters from George Bush and a framed pair of the ex-president's old trainers complete with a personal note thanking Paul for his advice, friendship and shoes. Austin thus has an enviable pedigree in wanting to be crowned the nation's fittest city and also actively capitalises on its built and natural environment in designing, marketing and hosting its suite of MPREs.

The centrality of Carrozza to Austin's plethora of obesity prevention efforts also clearly demonstrates how, in the words of one interviewee, "a lot of people are now in the game of obesity in this state" (TDHHS, interview, 2006). While the use of the adjective 'game' to describe obesity hints at the strategic clashes over limited obesity prevention funding that occur in Austin, it also demonstrates the breadth and creativity of health promotion efforts in their transposition from the public to the private domain. Moreover, both hope and scepticism are now being placed on the private domain of obesity prevention, with some interviewees suggesting that any real change will not necessarily be public sector driven. Indeed, "the people that can carry the message are not government types . . . things move quickly when they happen" (TDHHS, interview, 2006). More than this, though, Carrozza's presence also represents the interweaving of the cults of personality and celebrity with more sober public health goals. This is especially true as commercialised events, rather than individual or community interventions, increasingly start to shape our repertoire of solutions to public health challenges such as obesity and its co-morbidities.

RunTex sponsors and advertises almost all the charity runs taking place in the city and its environs, the aim being, in Carrozza's words, "to get the haves to raise money for the have-nots" (interview, 2006). For him, MPREs serve a public health function in a number of ways. First, they act as a means of raising funds for health-centred charities and programmes through participant sponsorship. Thus, the idea is to get the white, middle-class, active residents west of the I-35 to raise money for East Austin-based non-profits such as Marathon Kids, which provide services and work with schools to help overcome some of the barriers to participation. Second, Carrozza believes that "getting ready for the event is part of the solution for the have-nots". Thus, participating in training programmes in preparations for a MPRE – where they are undertaken by participants from disadvantaged backgrounds – provides the necessity and motivation to be physically active. Third, the act of taking part in the event helps "bring those

East Side kids into the mainstream" as "exposure is what public education is all about" (Paul Carrozza, interview, 2006). Thus, MPREs are characterised by a series of stages that trace the decision to take part, the preparation for the event, the event itself and its legacy in terms of any longer-term changes in lifestyle. Interestingly, the synergies between the multistage value of MPREs and the 'Stages of Change' model (Prochaska and DiClemente 1986; Prochaska et al 1993) so popular in health promotion thinking are clear. The tales of personal triumph that characterise MPREs tap into individual consciousness at the pre-contemplation and contemplation stages (when individuals start to recognise a problem and a need to change), but come into their own in the complex processes that characterise the gap between contemplation and maintenance. Essentially, MPREs facilitate behaviour change by using the spectacle of the 'masses' as a vehicle for enhanced self-efficacy through messages that are personal and resonant. In other words, they can create an ethic of 'if they can, I can'. This source of motivation is also the case in Newcastle and will be further discussed in the next section.

Carrozza's assertions demonstrate the niche that events have come to fill in the public health domain; something that is actually far more evident in Austin than in Newcastle where, as this chapter will later explore, events such as the GNR are often relatively agnostic towards the specificities of local public health needs, despite placing great rhetorical store on the importance of healthy lifestyles. Instead, in Austin, there is an assumption that solutions might come from a variety of sources and that governmental channels often lack the same mechanisms. They also demonstrate the effective limits to government intervention in obesity; as one interviewee asserted, "I guess there's nothing at the state level we could have done to change that person's mind about his lifestyle . . . that's the dilemma" (Governor's Council on Physical Fitness, interview, 2006). Indeed, as another interviewee further corroborated, "[health and fitness] is one of those things you can't really legislate, you can't tell people to be more active" (Governor's Council on Physical Fitness, interview, 2006). This is key to the popularity of MPREs: they are not prescriptive, but rather their explicit encoding of narratives of individual choice, motivation and self-betterment resonate well with a general aversion to nanny statist interventions. As "people view any intervention by government, at any level, as infringing on their personal rights" (Governor's Council on Physical Fitness, interview, 2006), MPREs are successful as they empower through offering specific support and training structures for the event. Austin is not alone in trying to overcome the unwillingness of people to change their behaviour and in recognising that:

> 'People don't want to be told what they can eat. People don't want to be told that they have to exercise. People want to take a pill and so it's going to take a long time I think to really get people to change. I mean the norms have to change.' (TDHHS, interview, 2005)

MPREs thus hold strategic value in a situation where people are increasingly demanding quick fixes such as bariatric (weight loss) surgery and are unwilling to comprehend that lifestyle changes represent a long-term shift in thinking, rather than a quick fix. In behavioural economic terms, the event provides a ready-made 'choice architecture' (Thaler and Sunstein 2008) in that it offers incentives (early enrolment discounts, lower race fees for returning competitors) to lure competitors and seek to break down the gap between the short-term costs of 'investment goods' such as exercise and the tendency to discount delayed benefits such as improved fitness. In this case, gratification through the event itself exists in a clearly delineated time period known as 'race preparation and training'. Further, MPREs ensure participant buy-in through emotive rhetorical tools such as pledges. While the pledge has long been a feature of political rhetoric (the Pledge of Allegiance or Martin Luther King's 'I have a dream' speech are cases in point), it is increasingly being used to signify solidarity and compliance with a host of social causes, the most notable of which in recent years has been abstinence among young people in the US (for example True Love Waits). The pledge has also become a feature of one of Texas's largest races, where participants are asked to sign up to the promise that:

> I pledge to myself and my loved ones to increase my daily activity level, and to make healthier choices each and every day. I want to lead a long and active life, free from preventable disease, so that I can enjoy my family, friends and community. Incorporating more physical activity into my routine is my first step. I aspire to have true Texas willpower, and I will ask my family and friends to support me – and to join me – In my pursuit of a healthier life. Let it be known that I accept the Governor's Challenge to spend at least 150 minutes a week engaged in physical activity. I have joined Texas' movement for a healthier tomorrow (The Texas Round-Up Pledge, 2006, www. getfittexas.org/GetFitTexas/Governors-Challenge.aspx)

The Texas Round-Up (TRU) is worth dwelling on in order to explore some of these assertions in more detail. The TRU was founded in 2002 by Paul Carrozza, former Mayor Will Wynn and Governor Rick Perry with two central aims: to address obesity and to become the biggest 10 km race in the state. In 2006, the race had 6,000 participants, of which the majority were government employees incentivised by a rare four hours of leave and a free health check. Participants are also encouraged to join in a six-week training programme to prepare them for the challenge ahead. The training programme was still under development at the time of interview and, as an organiser asserted, was "based on what we think sounds good . . . not science" (interview, 2006). While they had plans to 'acquire' science through partnering with the Texas on the Move coalition and the Cooper Institute, at that time the training programme was more a generic commitment to healthy lifestyles. Moreover, reflecting the inherent time weaknesses of MPREs, "it should ideally be a year-long commitment, but six weeks is more plausible in practice" (TRU organiser, interview, 2006). Further, with the event sponsored by Pilgrim's Pride chicken – which the race organiser dutifully described as "not the best, but at least it's healthy" – as well as fast-food chain Wendy's, Wal-Mart and Michelob Ultra, the event's healthy credentials remain slightly problematic.

Even as the TRU offers some real benefits to city and state employees, interviewees remained sceptical about the reach of MPREs in terms of behaviour change. It was repeatedly said that MPREs were not a catch-all solution and that they did not encourage participation among the most vulnerable or inactive groups. Specifically, the races were seen as particularly excluding African Americans. As one interviewee categorically stated, "black people don't run 5ks" (Steps to a Healthier Austin, interview, 2006). She went on to say that Austin's black residents would be far more likely to throw a block party and have an exercise class there. More than this, though, she suggested that the simple reason of intricate and expensive hairdressing among black women meant that exercise and sweat were often avoided for fear of wasting money and spoiling the hairdresser's good work. While such insights may just be anecdotal, it is nevertheless clear that the excitement and spectacle of talking part in MPREs may provide the impetus to participation, but that this remains partial and far from the degree of inclusivity really needed to effect widespread behaviour change.

The disparaging attitude towards MPREs often found among those working in public health is exemplified by the withering comment, "we're trying to get kids to walk . . . not to do fun runs" (public health marketing company, interview, 2006). It was often suggested that that MPREs were superfluous to the real concerns of promoting sport and fitness at a far more basic level. Yet, the success of school-based programmes such as Marathon Kids, which, after 15 years and the support of the Dell Foundation and Whole Foods, has now expanded beyond Austin into eight other metro areas, demonstrates that mass participation formats can have success. The programme sets children the goal of running or walking 26.2 miles, starting with a 'Kick-Off Celebration' event and culminating in a 'Final Mile' celebration. The programme's success comes from the excitement of inclusion, of being part of an event and of working towards a challenging and meaningful goal (the value of completing the marathon distance). The enduring popularity of Marathon Kids demonstrates the allure of the MPRE format and, even though the programme's organisers never carry out official evaluations – preferring instead a more ad hoc approach where "we pretty much know how many kids start the programme and how many finish, but we just have anecdotes" (interview, 2006) – the annual increases in the number of kids enrolled shows that even anecdotal information has its place in Austin's cacophony of obesity prevention and sports promotion efforts. It also demonstrates the emphasis placed on enrolment and finisher numbers, with less importance being put on the demonstration of any sustained impact on behaviour or lifestyle change. Thus, as the discussion of Newcastle shall explore, because events are time limited, their horizons are also conceptually limited. It is here that the tensions between commercial need and public health demands cause friction.

Great running in Newcastle-Gateshead

Austin and Newcastle share a passion for MPREs. However, while Austin combines a plethora of small events with a few larger-scale prestigious races, Newcastle's race diary is subsumed by the world's largest half-marathon – the Great North Run, which had 54,000 entrants in 2010. The GNR is instructive not just for its sheer scale and fascinating pedigree, but also for the ways in which the event blends both sports and cultural promotion. More than this, the GNR is of exceptional importance to the regional economy of the North-East, with the race weekend packing out hotel rooms for miles around.

The GNR also exemplifies the ways in MPREs are increasingly seeking to enhance their brand value and event reach by surrounding the race in a comprehensive programme of associated sporting and cultural events. In the case of the GNR, this now extends to the showcase Great North Games, which take place on an exhibition track situated along the Quayside between the Baltic and Sage Gateshead, and the GNR Cultural Programme, which has been running since 2005. As a result, the GNR is now as much the kind of large-scale urban festival discussed by Waitt (2008) as it is an elite and mass running race. Newcastle and its sister city, Gateshead, have long made an impression on the athletics scene. The Gateshead Harriers Athletics Club has produced some of the UK's finest athletes, including Mike McLeod and Steve Cram, who both won silver in the 1984 Olympics in the 10,000 m and 1,500 m respectively. The Gateshead stadium has also played host to international athletic meetings, and the Great North Way – a 1-mile route along the Quayside – has become the UK's first permanent interactive timing system, allowing any jogger with a chip and the appropriate download to monitor their training. Moreover, as the home of former Olympic athlete and world record holder, Brendan Foster, Newcastle has also inadvertently given the world the commodified mass participation running event. From humble beginnings in 1980, Foster's sports marketing company, *Nova International*, now boasts a portfolio of 18 branded adult and junior Great Run events across the UK, Ireland, Ethiopia and Australia. In the UK, Great Run events have over 150,000 entrants annually and the Great Ethiopian Run claims to be Africa's largest road race, with 35,000 (official) entrants.

From 12,000 participants in 1981, the GNR's 54,000 entrants now follow the very same half-marathon course from its famous start on the A167 Central Motorway, crossing the Tyne Bridge before making the long journey out to the finish on the coast at South Shields. Through Nova, the events are also a platform for showcasing new and existing athletic talent and ensure that the elite, club and celebrity runners garner sufficient TV coverage to attract sponsors and thus return a profit. The BBC, Sky Sports and Channel Five cover the event and, as Nettleton and Hardey (2006) contend, this ensures the spectacle of the *mass* participation. As such, the GNR is a clear instance of 'the collective event of those individual strivings that require the city as a social space' (Berking and Neckel 1993: 71). This notion of individual strivings marks a key characteristic of MPREs – the explicit tension between the 'lonely battle with oneself' (ibid: 73) and the collectivity of mass participation. MPREs as experiential and visceral happenings are greater than the sum of their parts, but are also given meaning by the stories, motivations and narratives of those individuals as well as the complete synonymity of the event with the North-East region. Yet, the question of whether Nova's flagship event aids or abets the uptake of sport in its home city is one that warrants further discussion because of two issues. The first issue is Nova's statement that 'we want people to be active, so we are asking people to take to the streets' (Take to the Streets 2010). The second is Nova's colonisation of smaller mass participation events as they develop their Great Swim, Dance, Walk and Cycle portfolios.

In 2008, 59% of the GNR's participants were men, whose modal age group was 30–39 and 41% women, with a modal age range of 20–29 (Figure 17). This gender split resonates with national picture for sports participation (Figure 18), in which women's uptake is consistently lower than that of men. However, it demonstrates a slightly different age profile in that, on average, participation decreases with age (Figure 19), while MPREs seem to hold particular appeal to men in their 30s, a time when sports involvement might ordinarily tail off. Of the race competitors 27% came from less than 50 miles away and 30% from less than 100 miles (Figure 20). However, 21% travelled from the South-East (251–301 miles away), suggesting that while the race remains a relatively local event, its reach and popularity extend far further. The North-East still remains a central factor of the GNR and consistently features local celebrities to start the race, with musician Sting and TV presenters Ant and Dec appearing in recent years.

Figure 17: GNR participant age by gender

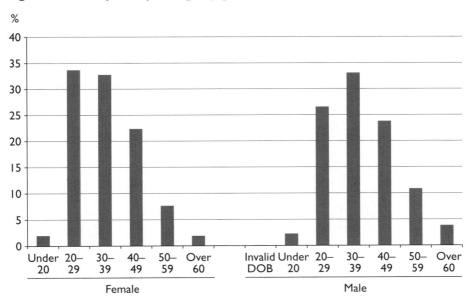

Source: Nova International, personal communication (2008)

Figure 18: Average adult participation in sport by gender in England defined by NI18 – 30 minutes of moderate activity on at least three days a week

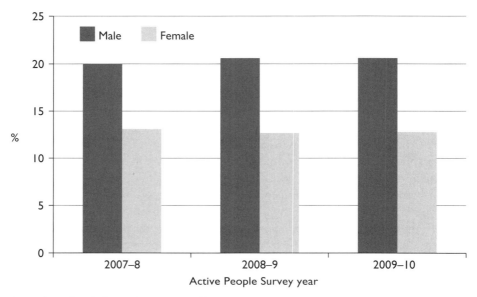

Source: Active People Survey, Sport England, 2007–10

Figure 19: Average adult participation in sport in England by age, defined by NI18 – 30 minutes of moderate activity on at least three days a week

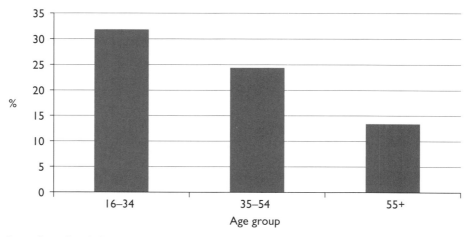

Source: Active People Survey, Sport England, 2007–10

Figure 20: Distance of participants' home postcodes from Newcastle–Gateshead in 2008

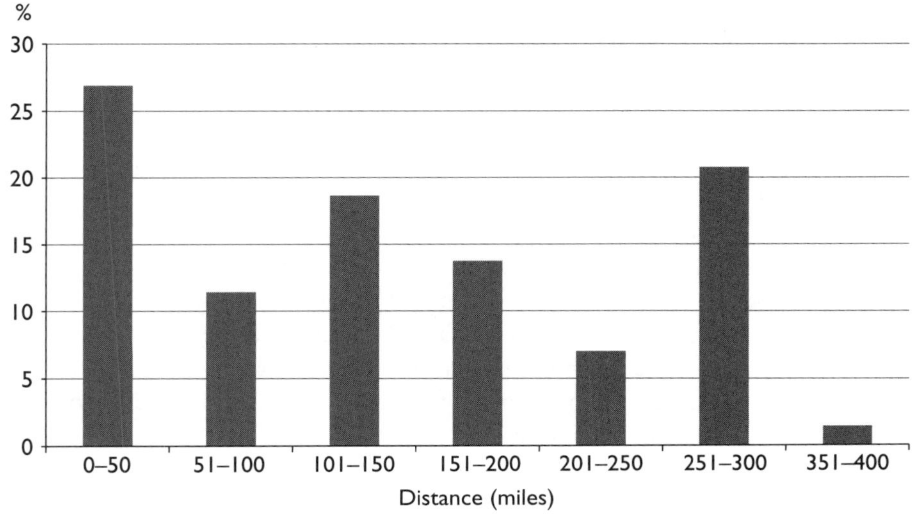

Source: Nova International 2008

Great Run events are associated with over 400 charities and raised over £28 million for a huge array of causes in 2009. Charities and MPREs are inextricable (Nettleton and Hardey 2006), and it is increasingly the case that the only way to ensure a place in the GNR is through taking up a charity place. Charities pay a significant fee to Nova (depending on whether they choose a bronze, silver, gold or platinum marketing and hospitality package), plus an additional fee per place. In return, runners have to guarantee that they will raise a certain amount through fundraising – usually in excess of £1,000 – with the individual bearing the responsibility for making up any shortfall. Even where tickets have been procured through the hugely oversubscribed ballot, they are £46 a head. Given that 61% of participants have travelled more than 100 miles to the event, this means a significant outlay for accommodation, transport and an array of associated costs. It also means that being more active comes at a significant financial cost; an irony, given that running is ostensibly free.

The 'fit' of the GNR with the city's aspirations for a more active populace is emblematic of a wider antagonism between the potential reach and capacity of such a large-scale event and the limited financial means of local authorities. Interviews among race stakeholders in Newcastle revealed that the GNR suffers a surprisingly uneasy relationship with the city's health and physical activity promotion agenda. Briefly to place this in context, physical activity uptake (30 minutes on five days a week) among men in the North-East is slightly higher at 24.6% than the national average (23.8%) and, at 20.8% slightly lower among women than the national average (19%). However, at a city level, while uptake among Newcastle's men is higher than the regional average (26.7%), the rate among women (15.7%) is significantly lower than both the regional and national average (Sport England 2010b). Consequently, while the North-East does not, in general, have significantly lower physical activity participation levels than other regions, there still remain large pockets of social deprivation that demand dedicated promotion work and investment.

To this end, there has been impressive forward thinking in the city, with the country's first gym for children and young adults at the Lightfoot Centre, a new pool completed in 2000 in the East End, hugely popular walking groups and a host of free or reduced-price leisure activities targeted at residents in the most deprived areas. At the same time, Nova has been championing its Take to the Streets website, which aims to increase physical activity participation through a range of online tools: activity search engines, training plans, blogs, forums, activity logs and a downloadable mobile phone application that logs your training. The disjuncture between the community-centred health promotion undertaken by the city council and the technologically integrated marketing and promotion undertaken by Nova is notable and marks an arena of particular uncertainty about the ability of the GNR to inspire participation among those deemed most vulnerable. One interviewee from a local authority summed up this unease over the race cost:

> '£42 [the fee in 2009] is a lot of money when you get a T-shirt which has been produced for a couple of quid maximum . . . Yes, a lot of people have been priced out, definitely they have. I mean people, when we stupidly signed up four weeks ago, they said they wouldn't have done it as there's cheaper runs, but people who are actually runners have said to me I can go and do an alternative run, you know what I mean. So I think there's a bit of that because it's a lot of money isn't it?' (interview, 2009)

The high entry fee also meant that interviewees saw the event as doing little to address the significant health inequalities in the city and North-East.

> 'I've mainly worked in areas of social deprivation in my career in sports development, there's not many of the families will be paying 40 quid or 80 quid or 120 quid if there's three of them, to do the Great North Run, 'cos they can't afford it. I find it's more of a middle-classy and upwards event, 'cos it costs.' (Sports Development Newcastle, interview, 2008)

This problem was compounded by the fact that "a lot of the people who do it come from areas where people know about health and about what they should be doing in terms of their lifestyles to improve their health" (ibid). While there is no specific research on the socioeconomic background of race participants, there was the general perception among those interviewees involved in sports development that the race fees were a significant barrier to participation and, therefore, the event *must* be not only middle class, but a haven for the already sensible. While clearly an unsubstantiated assumption (and indeed one interviewee was quick to assert that his was "just a gut feeling"), such an assertion of MPREs' innate middle-classness does correspond to writings exploring running as a form of class embodiment (Abbas 2004). A recent thesis shows that 43% of runners in the 2009 New York Marathon were first-timers (Loughren 2009), suggesting that either runners are increasingly shopping around for new and exciting events or that such events are viewed as a one-off experience before moving onto cheaper and less prestigious events. However, Nova's continual search for opportunities to strengthen its brand equity suggests that participants are demanding more and more in an increasingly competitive MPRE field (Olberding and Jisha 2005). In the case of the GNR, this now includes pre- and post-race hospitality, onsite massage, high-quality food and drink, promotions and a rigorously efficient transport system. The run may have reached capacity, but Nova's aspirations are great and the diversification of the race weekend into high-profile cultural events (such as specially commissioned plays, installations and exhibitions in local venues) clearly demonstrates the need to add value to MPREs continually as,

> 'It's very hard for the run itself to grow any more as an event and weekend. It's really packed. There's a lot going on and they can't get any more entries into the run – it's colossal. So, I think there was an interest in broadening their reach, they wanted to be the immediate brand that everybody thinks of. So people say big sporting event, Great Run.' (GNR Cultural Programme, interview, 2009)

As a result of this aspiration, "the cultural programme is about finding another way to reach into other peoples' consciousness" (ibid) in a way that ensures the popularity of the race weekend, but does not necessarily encourage further sports uptake. While the GNR has most likely reached its ceiling on race entrants, opinion remains divided as to whether the event draws people into sport, or whether it conflicts with local-scale efforts already being undertaken.

When respondents at the local authority level were asked whether the GNR had helped increase sporting uptake or catalysed any of the wider social, cultural or economic goals of participation, the response was mixed. Respondents felt that, "it puts lots of money into the local economy . . . and it gives a sense of community and a sense of pride and probably to the region" (Newcastle Leisure Services, interview, 2008), but remain less convinced of the event's sustained impact. Some interviewees expressed disbelief that a single event could motivate sustained physical activity participation:

> 'I think for most people it's something that just happens once a year . . . I think it is useful, but I can't honestly say that it has a huge impact on anything we do for the rest of the year really.' (Newcastle Leisure Services, interview, 2008)

Ultimately, interviewees concurred that the activities of the city and those of the GNR serve very different markets, but that this should not preclude them working together in the shared goal of increasing activity. Yet, some stakeholders expressed anger that they had never been able to use the GNR to promote their efforts, something that would be powerful given that "we do actually work with people who have a real need to be pointed in the right direction to do things that they can afford in terms of physical activity" (Newcastle Leisure Services, interview, 2008). Despite repeated assurances of efforts to work with the GNR, there was still a feeling that "[we] have underutilised the public health potential of the GNR . . . it hasn't featured very prominently in any of our plans and increasing participation locally", especially given that "as a PR exercise in physical activity, it's so powerful . . . we should exploit it more and tie in some of our local interventions more" (Newcastle PCT, interview, 2008). Yet, ironically one of the reasons why the local authority were "not milking it enough" (ibid) was the very temporality that makes MPREs meaningful. As was explained, "everyone's too busy . . . there are too many other pressing priorities. Something that comes around once a year and is not part of mainstream work tends to get shoved to the bottom of the pile" (ibid).

Despite the acknowledgment of the GNR as a valuable and underutilised resource, there was still concern that the GNR's scale and marketing capacity threatened to eclipse far smaller events such as a significant number of local fun runs organised by the local authority sports development team:

> 'But again, being local authority we maybe don't always have the capacity and the budget for that sort of marketing thing, whereas Brendan's company or private sector would probably go, "That's what we're gonna do . . . and we can do it 'cos we've got the cash and we don't have anybody to answer to." Whereas I come back to, you know, the website thing, if I say, "You can find our community fun run on Newcastle City Council website," they go on the home page and go, "Oh no." Whereas if you go to a Nova one or Newcastle United one, whatever, it's all completely different.' (interview, physical activity promotion, Newcastle, 2008)

This marked divide in the ability to create an exciting, professional and branded 'commodity' has often left smaller events flailing. The GNR is not the only fun run in town and the sports development team have invested significant time and effort in a series of 3 km and 4 km fun runs through different neighbourhoods. These were seen as offering a much better return on the council's investment in terms of sporting uptake as:

> '3 km or 4 km ones tend to be the more popular. So I mean whether, if you could have, I suppose the question again, in terms of value for money, the money I've put into the Great North Run, in terms of participation, if I did fifty 3 k runs I bet I'd get more people running than the Great North Run, from Newcastle.' (sports development, interview, 2008)

Such assertions also raise valid questions concerning the most appropriate means of achieving the ends of greater sports participation with all its related positive externalities. The value of smaller neighbourhood fun runs may, in actual fact be more holistic due to the way that they engineer feelings of pride, inclusion and acceptance among local residents:

> 'Every year you see a lot of, "Oh, I was here last year." And the good thing is you get your mams, your dads, kids, and then babies in pushchairs, people, and a lot of them don't run, they'll just walk it, and they're all two-mile courses, 'cos we don't want to kill anybody. And we just say, "You can toddle, you can run, you can walk, you can jog." All get a T-shirt at the end of it, they get a healthy meal, and there's always like a little community festival at the end of each one. And they're always well received and well attended . . . Well, that's what gives people a bit of pride, going, "Oh, we're having one here in Walker." It's, "We actually can have one." But it used to be people standing at their garden gate, clapping people through and all that, engendering a bit more community spirit, if you like, but that doesn't happen now because we cannot afford to run on the roads because they have to close them.' (Newcastle Leisure Services, interview, 2008)

As the interviewee above suggests, such fun runs have also faced structural barriers in the shape of the police cost of closing roads. The proposed solution has to be to transfer these small events to the Quayside, but this negates the community building and pride that comes from hosting even small-scale annual events.

It is thus perhaps the case that, as one interviewee asserted, "[the GNR] doesn't benefit the city as much as it should do. And when I'm talking about the city, I'm talking about the residents of the city, the people who actually pay their council tax to pay Nova" (Newcastle Leisure Services, interview, 2008). With the local authority paying a large annual sum to Nova in return for promotional banners along the course, there is a need to get a good return on this investment. Yet, it was felt that "simply getting a load of ads on the route doesn't do anything. It actually doesn't benefit the city as at all . . . as, guess what, everybody knows it starts in Newcastle" (Newcastle Sports Development, interview, 2008). Instead, a more joined-up promotional effort was thought to be needed in order to inspire people to take up sport. For example, this might be achieved through "the use of their elite athletes and trying to get them to inspire people, because that's what we find is that . . . you've got to inspire people and you've got to reinforce that with the right messages" (Newcastle Sports Development, interview, 2008). The inspirational potential of the GNR itself was hotly contested. On the one hand, one interviewee stated, "I don't think, I've never had anybody who's ever come to us who's said 'I watched the Great North Run' or whatever, 'and now I want to become physically active'" (Newcastle Leisure Services, interview, 2008). On the other hand, another disagreed saying, "it must do . . . it really is such an emotional event for the people taking part and the vast number of public that turn out . . .

It can only add value . . . and it could add a great deal more value" (Newcastle PCT, interview, 2008). Inspiration is one thing, but without the transformation of intention into action it was felt that "it really isn't a vehicle for helping us to deliver our targets [of increased participation]" as "it's the same people all the time doing it" (Newcastle Leisure Services, interview, 2008). Instead, it was felt that people needed structured, sustained and intensive ways in which to become more physically active and that these should be underpinned by manageable and realistic goals. To do this, you need

> 'A continually evolving series of initiatives, because if you just have one initiative it loses its allure. It's basically marketing, isn't it, you've just got to have something else happening to try and catch the people you haven't caught with whatever you did beforehand.' (Newcastle Sports Development, interview, 2008)

While interviewees concurred that the most effective route to sustained physical activity uptake among the most vulnerable was through community work, dedicated local staff (the majority of whom were volunteers, as highlighted by a local MP) and accessible facilities underpinned by clear incentives for participation. In the case of the local fun runs, these incentives were fairly low key and actually quite removed from sports promotion. As the interviewee explained, "I think the majority of the people kind of go because they always get a T-shirt and they always get like healthy food goodie bags, not brilliant, but they get it for nowt" (Newcastle Sports Development, interview, 2008).

   Nova might have the superior marketing, but those working for local authority and third-sector organisations involved in sports promotion bring a "kind of connections at a personal level with people and schools, community organisations" (Newcastle Leisure Services, Interview, 2008). However, despite their reservations as to the longer-term effects of the GNR, interviewees remained convinced that the event had an innately inspirational power:

> 'I mean, I think the Great North Run's great for raising the profile of physical activity and the area in particular, and I think I'm sure there's a spin-off when you hear the stories on the television; I mean, I was watching it yesterday and I was lying in tears when you hear of this young woman who had cystic fibrosis and who did the swim at Windermere and was doing the run and all these things, and you just think, my goodness. So I'm sure that must have an effect on people, even the people in the disadvantaged communities that we work with must say, "Well, God, they can do it, why can't I?"' (Newcastle Leisure Services, interview, 2008)

This assertion perhaps best sums up the appeal of MPREs: seeing and hearing stories of human endeavour by 'people like us' racing for themselves or a charitable cause that has personal resonance no doubt strengthens and increases self-efficacy. The effect on the masses, then, counteracts the often negative perceptions of sport as "an elite thing", which is then used "as an excuse to say, 'No, I don't want to get involved in that'" (Newcastle Leisure Services, interview, 2008). This is even as elite athletes are seen as being of central importance as inspirational figures and certainly feature prominently in tactics to ensure the sporting legacy – particularly among children and young people – of the 2012 Olympics. The contradictions in opinion even with those charged with achieving a common end of increasing sports participation is far from unusual and may be further reinforced by trying to get sport to *do* too much.

Conclusion

This chapter has critically examined the emergence, nature and significance of MPREs with regard to increasing sports participation and inducing the uptake of healthy lifestyles in both Austin and Newcastle. While both cities display unique experiences of MPREs and their public health role, they also demonstrate some clear commonalities. In essence, opinion in both cities remains divided as to the wider value of MPREs. In Austin and Newcastle, interviewees were quick to highlight that the events were good for the city's image, but remained unconvinced as to their ability to encourage sustained and sustainable lifestyle changes. These internal and transnational differences in opinion also clearly highlight areas of research weakness. In essence, as has been recently suggested:

> we lack precise understanding of the role of sport *in lifestyles*, the nature of the efforts/benefits ratio that underpins decisions to continue/discontinue sports participation and the extent to which participants view participation in terms of a social consumption or health investment good. (Sport England 2004: 79, emphasis added)

This gap in knowledge was evident in both case study cities; neither had conducted research into the reasons for the continuation or cessation of sports participation, especially after taking part in MPREs. Research has shown that very few marathon runners cease participating after their first event due to the considerable 'sunk capital' or time and effort invested in even completing the event. However, there may be reasons to hypothesise that those taking part in shorter races may be more likely to drop out because they have smaller amounts of sunk capital thanks to the significantly lower initial time and effort investment made in preparing for the event compared to a marathon (Clough et al 1989). In the same study, one of the reasons for dropping out was a lack of training and preparation as well as a relatively low degree of commitment to running. This would also lend support to the idea put forward by interviewees in both Austin and Newcastle that participation in MPREs for those new to sport usually followed a 'life event' (such as a death in the family or major health scare) that required a newly active lifestyle or had catalysed a drive to raise money for a charity associated with the event. As with other public health crises such as smoking or drinking, adherence to sports participation requires individual buy-in, which in turn depends on understanding of the value of a lifestyle change.

Sports promotion is essential to sports uptake, and the marketing prowess of events such as the GNR or TRU fundamentally eclipses far smaller, community-scale events. While state agencies and local authorities lack the money to engage in technological investments such as the kind of online training tools offered by Nova, they recognise that crossworking and data sharing may be the most productive way to increase sports participation. The suggestion that Nova's elite runners might want to come to local schools to meet students has clear merit and illustrates the potential that exists. In both case studies, however, there still remained the idea that MPREs were outside the sphere of possibility for the most deprived in the city, both financially and conceptually. While this may be true in part, I remain unconvinced as to the utility of assuming that participation is necessarily a middle-class preserve and therefore inaccessible to those on low incomes. This assumption runs counter to existing data on sporting participation, which show that even though rates are highest among those in managerial socioeconomic groupings (Figure 21), when split by ethnicity, rates are higher among non-white people than among white people in the UK (Figure 22). This problematises some of the assumptions around deprivation, ethnicity, class and risk that often tend to characterise more paternalistic readings of sports development work. As a consequence, it is clear that 'sports mega-events are a significant part of the

Figure 21: Sports participation by socioeconomic status 2007–10, defined as at least three sessions of moderate intensity activity three times a week

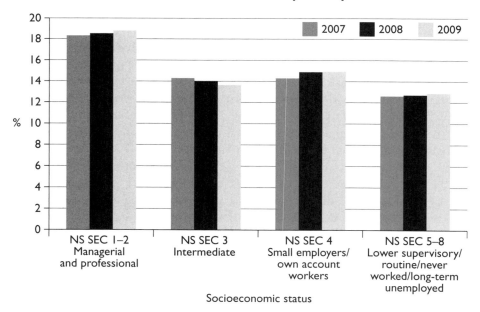

Source: Active People Survey, Sport England 2007–10

Figure 22: Average adult participation in sport in England by ethnicity, defined by NI18 – 30 minutes of moderate activity on at least three days a week

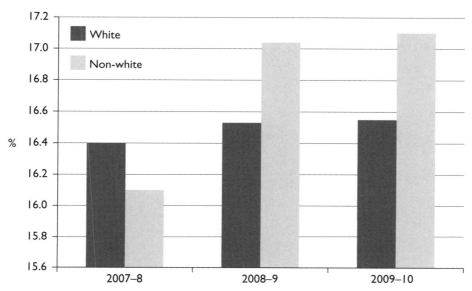

Source: Active People Survey, Sport England, 2007–9

experience of modernity, but they cannot be seen as a panacea for its social and economic problems' (Horne and Manzenreiter 2006a: 15). As spectacles with mass appeal that catalyse a training regime of sorts, MPREs do certainly have a clear role to play and will no doubt continue to grow in importance as the 'sportisation of society' (Abbas 2004: 172) continues apace.

SEVEN

The sensible drinker and the persistence of pleasure

We believe that England has a drink problem . . . it is not just a problem for a small minority, but a much larger section of the population (Health Select Committee 2010: 267)

Britain: the café society. What an agreeable idea it seemed at the time. Back in the days where the nation was still intoxicated by New Labour, our political leaders promised that they would transform not only our public services but our drinking culture . . . Britain is to café society what Iceland is to financial stability (Whitworth 2010)

Introduction

This chapter explores the ways in which drinking and drink epitomise the deep paradoxes inherent in efforts to govern consumption, especially in the UK, where alcohol has risen inexorably up government agendas since 1997. New Labour's efforts to both tackle alcohol-related harm and, at the same time, to reinvigorate city and town centres was underpinned by a drive to create and promote a 'new sensible drinking culture' (Department of Health 2007: 5) as part of the strong faith the government placed in the paradigm of both cultural and behaviour change (Cabinet Office 2004, 2008) discussed in Chapter Three. Historians of intoxication have clearly shown that the nation's drinking habits have long been of episodic concern to the British government (Kneale 1999; Berridge 2006; Plant and Plant 2006; Kneale and French 2008); however, the hysteria (that remains even after the departure of Labour from office) over the pervasive role of alcohol in British society appears to be qualitatively different from earlier incarnations. At root, the question of how and why alcohol has emerged as a significant contemporary 'problem' in the UK is inextricable from the manner in which quantitative shifts in consumption have occurred alongside qualitative upheavals in the social mores that serve to normalise drinking practices. Moreover, they reflect a growing appreciation that – just as with obesity – 'the issue comes down to the balance that a society chooses between a free market in alcohol products and regulation to limit the harm they cause' (*The Guardian* 2010).

Policy, media and academic studies of drink and drinking tend to focus on either the political economy of alcohol or its harms and costs. Only rarely do they pause to interrogate the points of intersection between these: the locations – both physical and psychological – where rights, responsibilities and freedoms meet in the creation of the sensible drinker. In order to think past this conceptual and empirical impasse, this chapter will explore how the manner in which drinking is framed by society at particular points in time and space is reflective not merely of presiding biomedical or public health knowledge of alcohol's health risks and/or benefits, but a far more normative sociopolitical vision of the role that alcohol *should* play in society in its very widest sense. The question of how alcohol is managed and regulated is therefore also a question of the kind of society and places that the management and regulatory process and rationale could and should induce. The alcohol debate is thus underpinned by and, in turn, produces a particular set of geographical imaginations, which will be further explored in the next chapter.

While the past century has been marked by periodic upheavals in normative judgements of alcohol's societal role (Valverde 1998), the past two decades are striking for the sheer magnitude and tumultuousness that the alcohol control debate has attained (Room 1984; Plant and Plant 2006). For this reason, this chapter will very briefly consider the role that alcohol has played in society over the past century, before developing what we might call, in Foucauldian terms, 'a historical awareness of our present circumstance' (Foucault 1982: 778). This is especially pertinent given that drinking so aptly typifies the extreme tensions between freedom and coercion that not only characterise the constant problematic of neoliberal governance discussed in Chapter Two, but also mark out the domains of self-governance where healthy, productive and engaged citizens might be created. Yet, because drinking skirts an exceptionally porous line between pleasure and danger and between the figures of citizen and consumer, the goal to inculcate an ethic of 'sensibleness' is fraught with conceptual and pragmatic difficulties (Measham and Brain 2005; Norris and Williams 2008). In order to explore how these hurdles play out in empirical terms, it is first necessary to explicate the techniques, mechanisms and tools through which sensible practices are delineated and crafted. Thus, the first step in developing the 'awareness' that Foucault highlights must be through a sustained and critical reflection on the codifications of sensible behaviour itself.

The sensible drinking debate

The drive to create the sensible citizen, capable of self-modified responsible drinking habits modelled on the fetishised and somewhat nostalgic vision of civilised (Southern) European café culture favoured by the Department of Culture, Media and Sport (DCMS) (Montgomery 1997; Roberts et al 2006; Tierney 2006), operates across two interacting domains of governance. The first concerns the realm of personal behaviour and the second, which will be considered in the next chapter, concerns the spatial as a tool of government. Drinking is a personal enterprise, but just as recent studies argue that obesity is a direct result of certain physical and psycho–social traits of 'obesogenic environments' (Smith and Cummins 2009), there is an emergent field of study arguing for the importance of drinking places and spaces in determining habits (Jayne et al 2006, 2008b, 2008c; Valentine et al 2007). As a result, the drive to inculcate sensible drinking habits to mitigate alcohol's notable health, economic, social and criminal costs has found two clear expressions and domains of action: the self and the spatial. This chapter will focus on the first of these in order to explicate the governance tensions inherent in trying to normalise sensible drinking, before in the next chapter expanding the focus to questions of how the spatial has emerged as a key governance tool.

In examining the question of personal behaviour, this chapter therefore takes on the challenge proffered by Nicholls, who asks, 'in our society of "binge drinking" . . . both liberals and critics of liberalism need to revisit these debates and learn from them in order not allow this critical social and political problem to fall into dangerous stagnation' (2006: 147). While there would seem to be little immediate danger of 'stagnation' in studies of alcohol, there is a concern that the debate over how best to disentangle the 'paradox of drinking responsibly' (ibid: 146) is becoming impossibly bifurcated, a situation that has direct repercussions for the political theatre's capacity to acknowledge the multiple arenas of overlap in the alcohol debate. On the one hand, a 'neo-temperance alliance' (Berridge 2006: 106), composed of those from addiction studies, public health, biomedicine and alcohol studies and highly influential at the WHO, calls for the reining-in of liberal approaches to alcohol regulation through supply-side strategies limiting availability and increasing price (Room et al 2005). On the other side sits a loose constellation of industry actors and cautious government officials calling for the coexistence of responsible drinking practices alongside a vibrant night-time economy through a laissez-faire ethic of copartnership and voluntary codes of industry (self-)regulation (Hadfield 2007). Thus, following from this and in order to map out the dynamics of this divided debate, this chapter asks *why* and *how* alcohol has now attained the dubious accolade of being a 'UK epidemic' (British Medical Association 2008). In so doing, it also hopes to counter the Health Select Committee's (2010) assertion that 'a much larger section of the [English] population' has a 'drink problem', by critically exploring the very construction and delineation of this categorisation.

As a consequence, this chapter also questions the conceptual utility of defining individuals as risky drinkers given the persistent myopia of the public's self-definition as such (Moss et al 2009). This disjuncture between perception and action is important to consider, given that, even while the public seems determined to pursue the 'freedom of intoxication' (Nicholls 2006: 146), the possibility of the concomitant 'freedom from regulation, discipline and order' (ibid) that this might have once meant has now been lost behind a slew of recent legislative changes under the rubric of tackling 'anti-social behaviour' (Norris and Williams 2008: 258; Rodger 2008) that have led to the increasing criminalisation of drunkenness in its many expressions. It is this disconnection between media reports of reckless abandon associated with the turn to 'binge drinking' facilitated by government liberalisation of licensing laws and the growing number and range of alcohol-related offences that this 'liberalisation' has both facilitated and necessitated. Thus, the arguments presented in the following two chapters are set in sharp contrast to the current regulationist tone of the UK's public health-driven alcohol control debate.

The chapter will start by asking where we have come from, before turning to where we are now. This will be done by taking up and exploring three contentions that have been guiding the alcohol control debate: that there is a difference between Southern and Northern European drinking habits; that binge drinking is an innately British trait, and that such behaviours are fundamentally new and, therefore, of legitimate public concern. These discussions draw on detailed health and behavioural survey data from the UK and Europe. In so doing, they highlight the limitations of our knowledge about drinking behaviours and, as a consequence, our ability to draw consistent conclusions about how best to manage drinking understood as a 'problem'. In the light of these explorations, the chapter then turns to a detailed critique of the construction and deployment of the tools and techniques of 'sensible drinking', before examining the ongoing disjuncture between public awareness and actions. As the most basic of public health mysteries, the persistent mismatch between awareness (in this case of sensible drinking messaging), understanding (of risks of drinking) and action (by moderating drinking), is one that often defies explanation. The chapter will therefore pause to consider why, despite evidence of high awareness of units by the British public, self-reflexive monitoring of drinking habits remains exceptionally low. This may well reveal the very limited allure of sensible behaviour and what has been termed the 'persistence of pleasure' (Measham 2004). The chapter concludes with a discussion of why pleasure is inextricable from the alcohol control debate, despite the complexity and inconvenience it clearly presents in public health calls for the tighter supply-side regulation of alcohol.

Our past drinking habits in context

The British have long enjoyed a drink. As Barr asserts, 'heavy drinking has always been part of the British character – one that has differentiated the inhabitants of these islands from their neighbours on the Continent of Europe' (1995: 25). This assertion is further reinforced by Norris and Williams who stress that 'as a Northern European country, heavy sessional drinking and drinking to get drunk have been an integral part of Britain's culture for generations' (2008: 259). Moving beyond the question of generalisation and stereotyping that these assertions encapsulate, they are an exceptionally prescient starting point for more detailed exploration of the well-rehearsed rhetorical battlefield that characterises the alcohol control debate. Such contestations over drinking are underpinned by a number of fiercely debated contentions, of which three stand out as being of particular salience and explanatory potential. First, is there a fundamental, demonstrable and continuing bifurcation in tastes and practices between Northern and Southern Europe? Second, to what extent are 'heavy sessional drinking' or 'binge drinking' – defined as such by the quantity of alcohol consumed within one 'drinking session'

(Measham 1996; Plant and Plant 2006; Herring et al 2008a, 2008b) – with the motivation of inebriation is an innately British trait? And, third, how far are such behaviours an established or a fundamentally novel phenomenon? Each of these questions, by itself, represents a complex set of interlocked debates that surround and characterise the wider alcohol control debate. A critical interrogation of these contentions should help explicate how and why codes of 'sensibleness' have become enshrined as a panacea for managing lifestyle-related harms to both the self and society.

North versus South

The notion that there is some fundamental and distinguishable difference between Northern and Southern European drinking habits has now risen to the status of received wisdom in discourses on alcohol. This wisdom was gradually solidified through the DCMS's aspiration of using licensing reform to bring forth Southern European drinking cultures and spaces from the ashes of British debauchery (Department for Culture Media and Sport 2005). In brief, the distinction between Northern (the UK, Ireland, Germany, Denmark and Scandinavia, the Netherlands) and Southern European (France, Greece, Italy, Portugal and Spain) drinking habits and traditions has frequently been explained in environmental terms, with the climate of the north far more suited to grain production systems, and therefore beer and spirit consumption and the vine-friendly climatic conditions of the south (Holt 2006) far more conductive to wine drinking. While this north/south, beer/wine distinction might once have been clear, the divide has gradually become more blurred as total alcohol consumption has seen a significant decline across Southern Europe since 1970, as shown clearly in Figure 23 and in marked contrast to the more mixed set of climbs and falls among Northern European countries shown in Figure 24. However, when Southern European drinking trends are broken down by drink type, it shows that between 1974 and 1992, beer consumption rose by 32% across the region, while per capita wine consumption fell by 42% (Gual and Colom 1997). This economic and cultural shift shows little sign of abating and confirms, when a marked rise in wine consumption across Northern Europe is brought into the equation, what might be called 'a homogenisation of European drinking trends' (ibid: S21).

This assertion of homogenisation is further backed up by Grigg (1998: 15), who writes of a 'tendency to convergence' in alcoholic beverage consumption trends across Europe. These shifts have been provoked by several factors: changes in the political economic structure of alcohol production and retailing across Europe that have tended to promote beer consumption over wine (due to its greater corporatisation) and lowered the relative cost of both; wider societal shifts that have increased the popularity of beer among the young; a fall in the occasions to drink wine as meal patterns change; greater health awareness and government legislation. In tandem, these have reduced the popularity of alcohol, deeply problematising reductionist assertions of a marked disparity between Northern and Southern

Figure 23: Southern European alcohol consumption 1970–2003

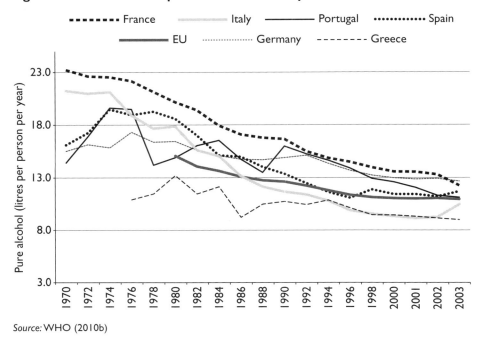

Source: WHO (2010b)

Figure 24: Alcohol consumption changes in Northern Europe 1970–2003

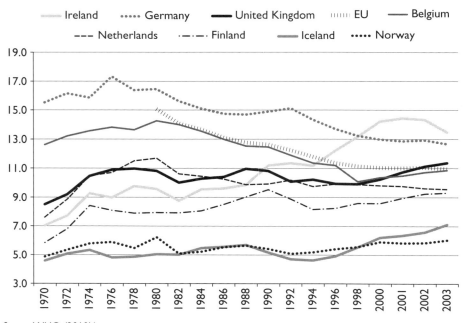

Source: WHO (2010b)

Europe. This also places at least one of the central assertions of the alcohol control debate on particularly shaky ground. If the gap between Southern and Northern European drinking habits are closing as beer becomes increasingly a drink of the south and wine a drink of the north, then the aspiration to adopt a Southern European café culture in the UK seems out of touch with contemporary cultural shifts at best, and seems to be a middle-class nostalgia for Tuscan wine-drenched holidays at worst. An interviewee from the nightclub trade sceptically alluded to this narrow and partial vision:

> 'People go to, it's very middle class but the people who run all the councils are very like that, all . . . you know, they're all very [puts on posh voice], "Hello!" If you go over to, I mean you'd have to imagine that none of them have ever been to Barcelona and seen what goes on there. I mean they have a vision of Europe which is a small province town or sort of a little bit of Tuscany, but have they gone out in Rome and seen it all kicking off?' (nightclub and bar company, interview, 2008)

This disjuncture between the partiality of the received wisdom discussed here and the unpalatable reality of an increasing convergence in European drinking trends thus warrants further discussion, in particular for what it adds to perceptions of 'sensible' drinking.

The British binge

> 'They decided to publish the alcohol harm reduction report in about 2001, that introduced this concept of binge-drinking, not in the *Oxford English Dictionary* sense of basically going out on a mission to get pissed, but overconsumption, which has muddied the waters horrifically. And it then managed to coincide with *The Daily Mail* and the others who got on a mission that we were all going to hell in a hand-cart and that Hogarth was alive and well, thank you, but living on every high street. The BBC sort of managed to get in on it with the *Panorama* programmes and if they could possibly take a shot of some girl mooning on the high street then they would, and then keep repeating it.' (alcohol industry trade association, interview, 2009)

The second assertion underpinning the alcohol control debate – that 'heavy sessional drinking' to get drunk is a thoroughly British trait – overlaps the first in its assumption that such behaviours are presumed absent elsewhere in (Southern) Europe. However, the 'pathological pattern of alcohol misuse' that Thomas Babor (2008: 455) suggests characterises British drinkers' propensity to binge and that forms the persistent stereotype described by the interviewee above is far from an agreed truth. In this vein, a recent Parliamentary Office of Science and Technology (POST) report claims that:

> Binge drinking [BD] is a common behaviour among young people in many Northern European countries. BD in the UK has gradually increased over the last decade and has typically been viewed as socially acceptable and a 'normal' youth behaviour: reversing this trend will require fundamental changes in the UK drinking culture. By contrast, BD is far less common in Mediterranean countries, some of which have an overall *per capita* alcohol consumption higher than that in the UK. Research suggests that drunkenness is seen as socially unacceptable in Southern Europe, particularly among women; family structure and dynamics, and historical factors may account for this difference in drinking cultures. (Parliamentary Office of Science and Technology 2005: 2)

In addition to distinguishing the British from their European counterparts, heavy sessional drinking is cast almost exclusively as a trait of those whom Measham and Moore suggest are routinely characterised as 'a small minority of "rough" youth and young adults' (2008: 284). This assumed synonymity between youth and binge drinking stems, in large part, from the problematisation by the UK government of such behaviours as an issue of public order rather than of public health. This perspective is further legitimised by the Alcohol Harm Reduction Strategy for England's overriding focus on the delivery of crime and disorder objectives, and the shunting of public health objectives onto *Choosing Health* (Department of Health 2004a). Moreover, the rise and rise of what Bell (2008) terms 'alco-tourism' has married public disorder and heavy drinking in a European setting, leading many to accuse the British of exporting their drinking habits across the Channel. Thus, while there can be little doubt that being British and binge drinking go hand in hand in the popular imagination, there is some evidence to suggest that the 'cultural homogenisation' in drinking habits discussed earlier now extends beyond just the total quantity consumed by other Europeans, to the *acts* and *nature* of consumption itself.

The faith in a tangible, fungible and visceral disparity between Southern and Northern European drinking habits is exceptionally persistent. Indeed, even a recent 'rapid response' in the *British Medical Journal* rehearses this common cultural stereotype in the alcohol control debate, despite its trenchant critique elsewhere (see for example Tierney 2006; Jayne et al 2008a) :'In Spain for example alcohol use has a different place within traditional culture than it does in the UK. For example it is much more associated with consumption of food rather than binge drinking for recreation' (Isaac and Domok 2010).

In marked contrast to this nostalgic, romanticised and thoroughly middle–class vision of Southern European responsible 'civility', the past decade has witnessed a surge in 'apéros géants' in France (Rosenberg 2010) and 'el botellón' (literally 'big bottle') in Spain, leading many commentators to bemoan the cultural pollution caused by the export (and thus undeniably clear attractions) of British drinking habits. There have also been rapid changes in youth drinking in Italy and Portugal; where once it might have been shameful to be drunk in public, attitudes among the young are changing (Beccaria and Prina 2009; Keeley and Bagenal 2010). The shifts in Europe have been tangible and not just for the crowds of thousands that 'el botellón' gatherings often marketed through Facebook regularly attract in Spanish cities in springtime. Indeed, the number of 15- to 24-year-olds hospitalised in France for alcohol-related conditions rose 50% between 2004 and 2007 (Crumley 2008) and the percentage of Spanish 15- to 19-year-olds reporting regularly getting drunk doubled from 22% to 44% between 2002 and 2004, with girls seeing the biggest shift in habits (Keeley and Bagenal 2010). The notion that heavy sessional drinking to get drunk is something innately and distinctly British is therefore becoming increasingly difficult to justify, especially among young drinkers. Yet, the pervasive tendency to pin the alcohol control debate on the assertion of definable and discernable national drinking habits among particularly culpable groups is surprisingly rare, despite the predilection for quantifying complex behaviours among those in alcohol studies.

A 'new' drinking problem?

The third assertion asks to what extent these 'exceptional' drinking traits are established and long standing or something novel that mark a clear (and thus justifiably worrying) shift in drinking cultures. Related to this, therefore, is the question of whether drinking patterns have changed over time in the UK and, if so, whether this shift should be cause for concern. It thus seems curious that historical data sources suggest that *consistently* heavy drinking has not been a British trait. The early 20th century, for example, was marked by exceptionally high annual consumption rates of almost 11 litres of pure alcohol a head, of which 70% was composed of beer (British Beer and Pub Association 2007; Health Select Committee 2010). The First World War and the establishment of the Liquor Control Board in 1915 brought a spectacular fall in the nation's alcohol consumption to roughly 3.5 litres per year as pubs reduced their opening hours and imposed strict pricing controls as prohibitionist campaigning gradually crept across the Atlantic from the US (Barr 1995; Berridge 2005; Nicholls 2010). While prohibitionist thinking never attained the same degree of popularity in the UK as it did in North America, the influence of broader temperance thinking and a slow post-war economic recovery meant that the nation's alcohol consumption did not really start to climb again until the early 1920s, when it gradually inched beyond 6 litres a head as a dramatic, nationwide pub improvement movement sought to capture the attention and wages of the middle classes. The increased appetite for drink was, however, relatively short lived as consumption fell back again to an all-time low in the early 1930s as the Great Depression led to dramatic falls in disposable income (Plant and Plant 2006) and brewers were forced to start advertising beer drinking to try and claw back some custom (Nicholls 2010).

The Second World War brought a far more permissive stance towards drinking than had its predecessor, with pubs seen as playing a positive and active role in the war effort through providing focal points for the community and, as Plant and Plant (2006: 21) suggest, providing a show of national unity against the invading Germans. However, despite the centrality of the pub and alcohol more broadly to the war effort, consumption remained at consistently low levels for two more decades as public drunkenness fell out of fashion with the working classes and alternative distractions in the newly built suburbs vied for public attention. The major generalised, upward trend in alcohol consumption started in the mid-1960s as real wages rose and the range and availability of alcoholic drinks started to expand, with new products such as Archer's Peach Schnapps and Bailey's tempting the middle classes, younger drinkers and growing numbers of female drinkers. The introduction of a plethora of alternatives to beer and their easy availability in supermarkets also coincided with a newly inclusive ethic in pubs. This upward trend in overall drinking since the mid-1960s has, however, been far from the general downward spiral into excess that many accounts have suggested (Room et al 2005; Babor 2008). Moreover, the misguided and somewhat patronising suggestion that the UK could and should 'return to its former status as a temperate nation' (Babor 2008: 455) is rendered both factually inaccurate and deeply problematic by the country's past history of inconsistent and fleeting trends with regards to its drinking habits.

Figures collated by the British Beer and Pub Association (BBPA), drawing on HM Customs and Excise data suggest that, contrary to screaming newspaper headlines suggesting our rapid descent into an alcohol-fuelled Hades, British alcohol consumption has remained reasonably steady over the past 20 years, and in the past five years has actually started to fall. As Figure 25 shows, per capita consumption stood at 7.9 litres per head in 1990, and rose steadily throughout the 1990s to reach 9.5 litres a year in 2004, a rise of 20% on 1980 levels. Since then, consumption has waned and in 2009, the latest year for which figures are available, stood almost 12% lower than its 2004 peak of 9.5 litres (Nicholls 2010). However, total consumption figures form only part of a politically and economically intricate story. Indeed, it is worth noting that in stark contrast to the beer-dominated drinking habits of the early 20th century, the past hundred years have witnessed not only a shift in *how much* the nation drinks, but also *what* it drinks.

In 1900, beer made up over 70% of all alcohol consumed in the UK. By 2007 and defying the 'materialisation of the late 1980s lager lout' through the relentless media uptake of a phrase coined by the media in response to a 1988 Association of Police Chief Officers' inquiry on public disorder (McMurran and Hollin 1989; Measham and Brain 2005, 263), beer composed less than 50% of all alcohol consumed. Since the 1960s, wine consumption has risen rapidly from negligible figures. Family Spending Survey figures show that wine now accounts for 40% of on- and off-trade weekly spending on alcohol and 52% of alcohol spending in supermarkets (Office of National Statistics 2008). This stands in contrast to beer spending, which stood at an average of £7.40 a week per household in 2008, or just under 35% of total alcohol spending of £21.30 a week. Beer sales have been gradually declining in the off-trade, with the average household now spending £2.60 a week in supermarkets and off-licences. Beer therefore remains a drink

Figure 25: Per capita alcohol consumption in the UK, 1990–2008

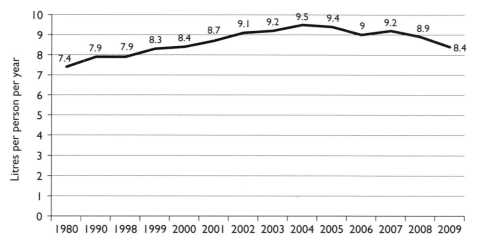

Source: British Beer and Pub Association 2009

of the on–trade and, in particular, the pub. In 2008, beer still accounted for 52% of alcohol spending in licensed premises. By comparison, wine accounted for 17% of on–trade spending, spirits 13% and (despite their extreme vilification) alcopops only 2%.

The coexistence of a decline in *overall* consumption in the UK and a shift in its *composition* is a point worth dwelling on, not least for the manner in which it challenges current alcohol policy discourses, which are disproportionately based on an assertion that,

> while consumption has fallen over recent years in most of the wine-producing countries, British alcohol consumption continues to rise. If present trends continue, the UK will rise to near the top of the consumption league within the next ten years. (Prime Minister's Strategy Unit 2004: 10)

As the most recent figures demonstrate, the suggestion that British consumption is rising and is 'now higher than any European country' according to a 2010 NHS Confederation briefing is empirically unfounded. This is clear when OECD data for 2003 (the latest year for which it is consistently available) is considered, especially as it shows the persistence of higher consumption rates in nine other countries: Ireland, the Czech Republic, Luxembourg, France, Spain, Hungary, Portugal, Austria and Denmark (see Figure 26). Moreover, with mean consumption of 10.7 litres of pure alcohol per person per year across the 21 European countries examined, the UK's consumption of 11.2 litres hardly warrants the hyperbolic cries of consumption league-topping drinking that has become such a pervasive government and media rhetoric.

Figure 26: European alcohol consumption in 2003

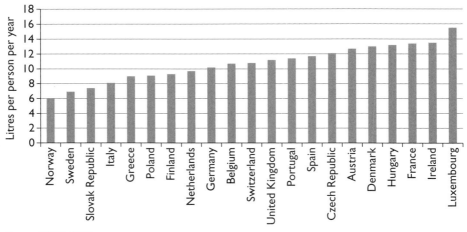

Source: OECD 2009

The argument for intervening in a 'drinking culture' that represents significant economic and social costs to the British state and taxpayers rests on more than an assertion of temporal changes in drinking habits and a definitive European geography of severity. In essence, this interventionist rationale is far more deeply embedded in what Measham and Moore describe as 'the crest of a new wave of criminalisation of contemporary cultures and an increasingly repressive regime of governance' (2008: 284). This logic runs through the governance of lifestyle choices and their varying impacts in the UK. In the case of drinking, such repression rests on a particularly arbitrary distinction between 'the majority [who drink] with no problems the majority of the time' and 'alcohol misuse by a small minority' (Prime Minister's Strategy Unit 2004: 2) that straddles, albeit unevenly, health and crime and disorder agendas. Underpinning the majority/minority distinction that forms the basis of a regulatory regime that a number of authors have painted in various shades of repression (Measham 2004; O'Malley and Valverde 2004; Hadfield 2007; Moore 2008) is a conceptual and pragmatic concern with what 'sensible behaviour' *is* (in technical terms) and *should be* (in moral terms). Therefore, before turning to a wider discussion of the significance and consequences of such thinking, the mechanics of sensible drinking must first be examined.

Constructing the sensible drinker

> The Government's vision is to produce a long-term and sustainable reduction in the harms associated with alcohol and drugs, where . . . there is a safe, sensible and social drinking culture where violent and anti-social behaviour is not tolerated; where young people are prevented from experiencing poor outcomes resulting from alcohol misuse; where those who drink alcohol are aware of the risks involved;

and where those that are drinking too much receive the advice and support they need. (HM Treasury 2009: 3)

Drinking is a distinct regulatory conundrum because of the persistent and gross mismatch between the highly regularised parameters that delineate the risk of alcohol-related harm and individual behavioural choices that expressly disavow these, rendering the 'vision' of a 'safe, sensible and social drinking culture' expressed above evasive (Hackley et al 2008). Even though the lifestyle behaviours discussed in this book highlight the gap between the intention or aspiration of being healthy and the reality of actions that are frequently far from healthy, drinking represents perhaps a far more complex form of what has been elsewhere termed a 'value–action gap' (Barr 2006). Underlying this complexity is a deep-seated 'moral confusion at the heart of policy' (Hackley et al 2008: 72) which requires a far more detailed critical analysis than has yet been carried out in the alcohol literature. Just as with eating and being physically active, drinking in a manner that is officially defined as 'sensible' is often rendered a difficult aspiration by a general and pervasive 'ambivalence' towards the social norms of drinking (Room 1976). Room's neotemperance understanding of ambivalence is of an explanatory model for the 'deviance' that he suggests underpins chronic drinking (Room 1976: 1051). By contrast, the version of ambivalence put forward here eschews moral judgement on individual behaviour and instead focuses on the policy significance of the innate coexistence of contradictory values and emotions by individuals towards drinking. Drinking behaviours in the UK are increasingly at odds with official advice concerning risk thresholds (Banerjee et al 2006; NHS Confederation 2010), and the goal of fostering a populace predisposed to 'sensible drinking' habits remains frustratingly elusive. As a recent National Audit Office report (2008) highlights, 10.5 million adults (or 31% of men and 20% of women) in England drink at levels classified as above sensible limits. If this is the case and eschewing sensible drinking is a regular occurrence for many, what is it about the particular delineations of sensibleness that normalises such persistent rebellion?

Sensible drinking guidelines represent, in the first place, a statement of relative risk – they set a threshold above which the risk of alcohol-related health harms increase significantly. They also serve as an educational, social normalising and 'harm prevention' tool (International Center for Alcohol Policies 2009). Banerjee et al usefully define sensible drinking as:

> Drinking enjoyably, socially and responsibly. It includes not drinking at all when the effects of alcohol will put someone's safety or health at risk. It also means being aware of the risks of young people and special groups drinking alcohol. (Banerjee et al 2006: 24)

Such a definition highlights the entwinement of enjoyment, sociality and moral obligation to oneself and society that accompanies a simple drink – a combination of loaded expectations situated within a tight, quantified framework that serves to delineate risk thresholds. Safe or sensible drinking thus requires an initial, standard measurement of alcohol against which to plot the gradations of such health risks. As Hackley et al instructively note, sensible drinking is a 'more complex construct involving implicit behavioural norms and, by implication, wider issues of class, race and gender with overtones of paternalism' (2008: 69). In the UK, the basis for this construct is known as the unit, whereas in other countries drinking guidelines may be in grams of pure alcohol. In the UK, a unit is 8 grams of pure alcohol. The origins of this measurement remain clouded in mystery; the most frequently-cited source is Susan Dight's 1976 paper on Scottish drinking habits, in which the unit was developed as a means of effectively and simply quantifying imperial drink measures for large-scale, longitudinal survey analysis. However, as a tool of risk communication, the unit is distinctly problematic and contentious, not least due to the well-documented and dramatic changes in drink strengths and the measures in which they have been sold over the past 30 years. In turn, this calls into question the very possibility of a 'standard drink' on which to base risk communication (International Center for Alcohol Policies 2009). Such discrepancies also resulted in the adjustment of units data for the HSE, GHS and ONS in 2007 (Office of National Statistics 2007). The unit is an abstract measure and, even when this is communicated through labelling total units on packaging, the shades of grey that constitute the multiple contexts that shape sensible practices (rather than sensible guidelines) hold clear potential to undermine efforts to communicate risk:

> 'I think that you get simply a unit, if you know what units to look at and if you bother to look at the units, which is usually on a very small picture of a bottle with a very small number, right at the edge of the corner. Then on that very simplistic level it's just giving you information about the number of units in that bottle, what it doesn't tell you is what would be a sensible drinking level. So if you are going to drink the whole bottle of wine in one go, that is binge drinking. And there's really no context attached to it.' (London Primary Care Trust, interview, 2009)

It is also important to note that sensible drinking has a distinct and somewhat well-documented history (Ball 2003; Ball et al 2007). Sensible drinking has its conceptual origins in the belief in 'controlled drinking' as an alternative harm reduction strategy for dependent drinkers in the 1950s and 60s (Banerjee et al 2006). The belief that controlled drinking was possible reflects a profound split among addiction experts between those advocating abstinence as the only route to recovery for alcoholics and those suggesting that alcoholics could return to drinking only in a controlled, tightly supervised manner. By the 1970s and 1980s, epidemiological studies were pointing to the possible protective health effects of 'moderate' alcohol consumption; an idea that would later play a significant role in the aspiration for a café culture characterised by 'moderate drinking'. Ball (2003) suggests that the most recent history of 'sensible drinking' guidelines in the UK can be traced to the 1979 Royal College of Psychiatrists' report *Alcohol and Alcoholism*, which set safe drinking limits at an exceptionally generous 8 units a day (56 units a week). However, by 1981 the then Department of Health and Social Security in its discussion paper 'Prevention and health: drinking sensibly' shied away from giving information about drinking limits, fearing that this might, inadvertently, constitute too permissive a stance towards drinking. Instead, as Ball et al (2007) highlight, the report suggested that Britons should drink in moderation and in a fashion appropriate to circumstances, but that ultimate responsibility for this was firmly in the hands of the individual. In 1984, the Health Education Council published a pamphlet in which it set a recommended limit of 2 or 3 pints, two or three times a week for men and two or three standard drinks two to three times a week for women. This would equate to 8–18 units a week for men and 4–9 units per week for women. Adding to the confusion, the Royal College of Psychiatrists issued advice in 1986 stating that alcohol–related harm increased greatly above 50 units per week for men and 35 for women, but cautioned the need for common sense in the interpretation of these limits. By the time of a 1987 Health Education Authority booklet, the government had agreed to the 21/14 units a week message and in 1992, the *Health of the Nation* report used these limits to set the target to reduce the proportion of men exceeding them from 28% in 1990 to 18% by 2005, and the proportion of women exceeding them from 11% in 1990 to 7% by 2005.

In 1995, as concern with the UK's emergent 'lager lout' culture and the first wave of mass panic over alcopops took hold, the government commissioned a review of its sensible drinking guidelines. The review 'concluded that it was more appropriate to set benchmarks for daily than for weekly consumption of alcohol, partly because of concern about the health and social risks associated with single episodes of intoxication' (Department of Health 1995; Goddard 2007: 4). The report stated that 'regular consumption of between three and four units a day for men and two to three units a day for women does not carry a significant health risk, but that consistently drinking above these levels is not advised' (Office of National Statistics 2007: 4). Such advice about *regular* drinking was also motivated by new research suggesting that 'moderate' levels of alcohol consumption might reduce the risk of coronary heart disease (CHD) through its effect on lipids and homeostatic factors (Rimm et al 1999). Such research stemmed, in large part, from curiosity over what has become popularly known as the 'French Paradox' or the coexistence of low rates of CHD and high levels of red wine, red meat and fat consumption in France (Renaud and de Lorgeril 1992). The suggestion of alcohol's 'protective effect' is still subject to a debate of varying degrees of intensity, for reasons that leap beyond the biomedical and squarely into the realm of political economy, national protectionism and populist policy making. However, research into the relationship between wine consumption and CHD rates in France do reinforce the assertion that there is a fundamental difference between the health effects of 'moderate' wine drinking and more irregular episodes of heavy sessional beer and spirits consumption (Ferrières 2004). These studies also raise the question of the causal role of other confounding lifestyle choices such as stress, physical activity, smoking and diet, as well as the role of the environment and context within which drinking takes place. Yet, it is important to note that research into the French Paradox has also had the effect of conferring a certain legitimacy and prestige to wine drinking, marking it out as potentially good for you and therefore somehow an inherently different category of alcoholic drink within the orbit of sensible behaviour. The distinction of wine drinking will consequently be revisited in Chapter Eight as it illustrates the ways in which class, taste and socioeconomic difference overlap in the creation of the alcohol control debate and its associated judgement of the boundaries of responsibility.

Building from this interest in the relative safety of Southern European drinking styles, shifts in the delineation of both risk and sensible behaviour were underpinned by a fear that maximum *weekly* 'limits' offered up the temptation of consuming them in their entirety on a single drinking occasion, thus sanctioning risky binge-drinking practices. This also dovetailed with a turn in both epidemiological and political thinking to the risks attached to specific drinking patterns and, as Gill and O'May highlight, ways 'to help people avoid drunkenness' (2006: 303). Despite this, it is interesting that the review's claim that there is 'no significant health risk' of drinking up to the daily limit (of 2/3 or 3/4 units for women and men respectively) in effect condones weekly consumption of 28 units a week for men and 21 for women. Furthermore, given that the new advice rested heavily on the shaky and contentious science of the relationship between alcohol and CHD risk in older age (Edwards 1996: 1), additional advice was given to older people (who abstain or rarely drink) that they 'may wish to consider the possibility that light drinking may benefit their health' (*Ibid*). The 1995 report also turned away from the language of safe drinking 'limits', drawing instead on the far more malleable term 'benchmarks'. This subtle semantic shift signalled some degree of flexibility and uncertainty in official advice and, as Ball (2003) asserts, garnered intense opposition in the biomedical and public health community and was quickly condemned by the British Medical Association in its 1995 report *Alcohol: Guidelines on Sensible Drinking*. As a result, the daily and weekly unit recommendations were kept with the caveat that drinkers should ensure at least two drink-free days a week. However, sensible drinking has not been without controversy, and a history of 'conflicting advice on sensible drinking in Britain has left confusion in its wake' (Ball et al 2007: 100). As a result, it has also irrecoverably dented public trust in the reliability of sensible drinking guidelines. This dent still shapes public ambivalence towards drinking and reinforces the complexity of the public health task, especially given the residual belief that there is poor understanding of both alcohol units and how these relate to personal acute and chronic health risks through the drinking limits. As Ball et al contend, 'the sensible drinking message is confused and poorly understood . . . [it] is not an effective approach to reduce excessive alcohol consumption and this needs to be addressed urgently' (2007: 101).

Adding further to the confusion, the drinking guidelines also serve as the basis for a tripartite subdivision of risk categories – hazardous, harmful and binge drinking – that have been taken up as key indicators of alcohol-related harm (both health and crime and disorder). In technical terms, consumption below 21 or 14 units a week is considered 'low risk'. However, given the ongoing 'lack of consensus' (Szmigin et al 2008: 364) over the definition and parameters of 'binge drinking', such high-risk drinking patterns can also plausibly occur within the safe weekly limits – an exceptionally grey definitional sphere in which the problematic status of 'problem' drinking remains fiercely contested. The language of a 'binge' in relation to drinking long pointed to an extended period of intoxication (usually two days or more) associated with dependent or chronic drinkers (Plant and Plant 2006). However, in more recent years, binge drinking has undergone a profound semantic and political shift, leaving persistent inconsistencies between the supposed objectivity of drinking guidelines and the subjective translation of these into health behaviours (Herring et al 2008a).

The General Household Survey (GHS) – one of the key data sources for alcohol consumption in the UK since 1978 – classifies binge drinking as consuming twice the recommended daily limit on the heaviest drinking day in the last week. This equates to 8 units for men and 6 units for women. However, within UK policy documents such as the 'Alcohol Harm Reduction Strategy for England' or AHRSE (Prime Minister's Strategy Unit 2004) and 'Safe, Sensible, Social' (Department of Health 2007), binge drinking is underpinned by the additional motivation of the express purpose of getting drunk. Thus binge drinking can be defined in quantitative terms, in terms of behavioural intentions and, moreover, 'pervades media discourse on contemporary youth alcohol consumption' (Hackley et al 2008: 66). Related to this, 'the definitions are really not that useful because they are too broad and usually describe the drinking habits of the young' (Norris and Williams 2008: 259). As a result and unsurprising, given New Labour's repeated focus on youth agendas (Minton 2009), binge drinking has developed 'a politically loaded character' (ibid) that all too often fails to acknowledge the social contexts and mediations through which drinking practices are undertaken. As one interviewee noted, the normalising role of these mediations and milieus is essential if binge drinking is ever to be *de*normalised:

> 'You're talking about people where particular behaviours are the norm rather than the exception . . . so that sort of cultural milieu that you're in is very important. So drinking would be a classic one where you create your bubble of people who probably have similar drinking patterns to you, and therefore you wouldn't necessarily view say binge drinking or heavy drinking as being abnormal because that's probably what everyone else does with you.' (Central London PCT, interview, 2009)

Such contentions around relative understandings of sensibleness were not helped when, in 2007, *The Times* reported that Richard Smith, former editor of the *British Medical Journal* and a member of the Royal College of Physicians (RCP) working party that had been charged with revising the guidelines, told a journalist that 'those limits were plucked out of the air. They were not based on any firm evidence at all. It was a sort of intelligent guess by the committee.' It was a guess taken under significant pressure to address 'growing evidence of the chronic damage caused by heavy long-term drinking'. Mr Smith further explained how the committee's epidemiologist had stated that 'it is impossible to say what's safe and what isn't', the reason being 'because we really don't have any data whatsoever' (Norfolk 2007). The reaction to *The Times* exposé was instant and searing, and the sensible drinking message has never quite recovered. As one *Guardian* journalist scathingly questions in relation to the risks presented by alcohol:

> How do they know this? Without the aid of an Orwellian two-way telly in every living-room, how did they conclude what constitutes too much? They simply applied their own measures to the 13,000 homes they polled. It was the government that plucked out of thin air a weekly 14 units for women and 21 units for men as the limit for 'sensible and safe' drinking. It was the government that worried over the size of the glasses holding these units. Why do they waste their time and ours on this nonsense? Statistics, advice, guidance, warnings, threats and general interference don't do much more than irritate everyone, since those who choose what they drink don't need to hear it and those who are in denial about booze can't or won't hear a word said against it. (Aitch 2009)

The intersections of scientific uncertainty and public enjoyment of drinking are both deeply politicised and particularly contentious. This is rendered even more so when the international variations in the delineation of sensible drinking guidelines are considered. As Table 6 demonstrates, not only do guidelines vary in their expression between daily or weekly limits, but also between upper limits or 'safe' ranges for both men and women. It might rightly be asked how 'safe' drinking can vary between 165g a week for Finnish men and 252g a week for South African men. Similarly, daily upper limits vary between 20g for Swedish men and 42g a day for men in the US. The international variations are equally great for women, ranging from 20g a day in Sweden to 40g a day in Australia. While there are genetic and racial differences in the effects of alcohol on the body – for example, the increased propensity to flush among East and South-East Asian populations (Chan 1986) – such variations would not account for the dramatic differences in purportedly 'safe' limits between nations with majority Caucasian populations. As such, it is clear that the business of delineating and communicating the risk thresholds of drinking are far from an exact science and, moreover, are influenced by factors that stray far from public health and biomedicine.

When set against its international comparators, the genesis of the current epistemology of sensible drinking suggests a situation where 'moderate consumption of alcohol is condoned, excessive consumption is condemned and drunkenness is increasingly criticised' (Measham and Moore 2008: 274). However, as the AHRSE states:

Table 6: International sensible/safe drinking guidelines

Country	Men	Women
Australia	20–40g/day	20–40g/day
Czech Republic	24g/day	16g/day
Finland	165g/week	110g/week
Italy	24–36g/day	12–24g/day
Japan	19.75–39.5g/day	19.75–39.5g/day
Netherlands	39g/day	39g/day
New Zealand	60g/day or 210g/week	40g/day or 140g/week
South Africa	252g/week	168g/week
Sweden	20g/day	20g/day
UK	32g/day or 168g/week	24g/day or 112g/week
US	42g/day or 196g/week	28g/day or 98g/week

Source: International Center for Alcohol Policies 2009

> it is vital that individuals can make informed and responsible decisions about their own levels of alcohol consumption. Everyone needs to be able to balance their right to enjoy a drink with the potential risks to their own – and others' – health and wellbeing. (Prime Minister's Strategy Unit 2004: 3)

Sensible drinking guidelines are thus a lynchpin in the enactment of responsible behaviour. However, the drive to foster what Hobbs et al somewhat scathingly term 'righteous consumption' (2003: 245) has not been without scrutiny. With knowledge and awareness of both units and the guidelines increasing year on year in the UK, but relatively little change in the propensity to exceed them, there are vital questions to be raised about the tenability of the civilised café culture aspirations of UK licensing and alcohol policy. More than this, there is also a need for sustained critical engagement with the idea that:

> Changing the regulations that govern alcohol consumption in order to change behaviour is a complex task, a task that requires more rigorous and detailed analysis than has been applied hitherto in a British context. How a continental café´ culture might be achieved within the framework of British law is neither obvious nor straightforward. (Roberts et al 2006: 1123)

The faith that behaviour can be changed into something more closely resembling the official aspirations of sensible drinking guidelines rests on bridging the gap between awareness, intention and action that characterises so many of the lifestyle choices underpinning health outcomes. Unlike physical activity and eating, alcohol is, in many ways, 'no ordinary commodity' (Babor et al 2003). This is not only in its physiological and psychological effects, but also because of the complex ways in which the political economy of alcohol actively – and often insidiously – shapes health risks. Moreover, given that the political economy of alcohol has distinct geographical and place-based effects, more attention is needed to the nature of drinking places as sites of risk. This will be further explored in the next chapter.

Knowing and doing?

> A campaign that advocates moderation may be damaged by its internal contradictions, but a movement that insisted that people gave up drinking alcohol altogether would be laughed out of court. (Barr 1995: 323)

> As the great political chipmunk herself, Hazel Blears, put it a couple of years ago, after reflecting on the failure to reduce the bingeing: 'we enjoy getting drunk'. (Whitworth 2010)

While prohibition has yet to gain a foothold in UK alcohol policy, in the eyes of many, even sensible drinking messages are out of synch with the drinking habits and social norms of the British public. Indeed, there is a clear disjuncture between evidence suggesting the public's increasing awareness of units and their seeming apathy towards acting on this awareness. As Measham contends, there is a 'credibility gap between recommended and actual practices for drinkers, alcohol manufacturers and retailers' (2006: 263). In other words, and because of this 'gap', being sensible is usually approached somewhere along a spectrum between religious fervour and abject apathy. Such 'cognitive dissonance' (Roberts 1988; Makela 1997) or the existence of feelings of unease when personal behaviour is at odds with self-perception (in this case of prospective risks) is, however, not generalised across the whole population. Between 2000 and 2008, awareness of units climbed from 80% to 86% and awareness of specific unit benchmarks from 64% to 70% (Figure 27). However, there was no change in the disparity between these two figures, indicating the resilience of the divide between a basic awareness of units and a more advanced understanding of the guidelines.

While it may be predictable that awareness of the specific guidelines would be lower than that of the existence of units alone, it is perhaps less obvious that the knowledge of benchmarks would be roughly equal between men and women (Figure 28). When the numbers are further broken down, they demonstrate, somewhat counterintuitively, that the more likely a person is to have heard of units, the more they are likely to drink. Even more counterintuitively given the vilification of youth drinking framed in New Labour's crime and disorder agenda, such unit awareness is greatest among those aged 16–24 (Figure 29). HSE data from 2008 shows that among those drinking more than 22 units a week ('hazardous' drinkers), 95% had heard of units. By contrast, among those that did not drink at all, only 55% had heard of units. This also corroborates findings that highlight an age gap in awareness with those aged over 65 the least likely to know about units (75%) and those most likely aged 25–44 (88%) or 16–24 (86%). There is also a marked difference in awareness by socioeconomic status, with 93% of men and

Figure 27: Awareness of units and unit benchmarks 2000–08

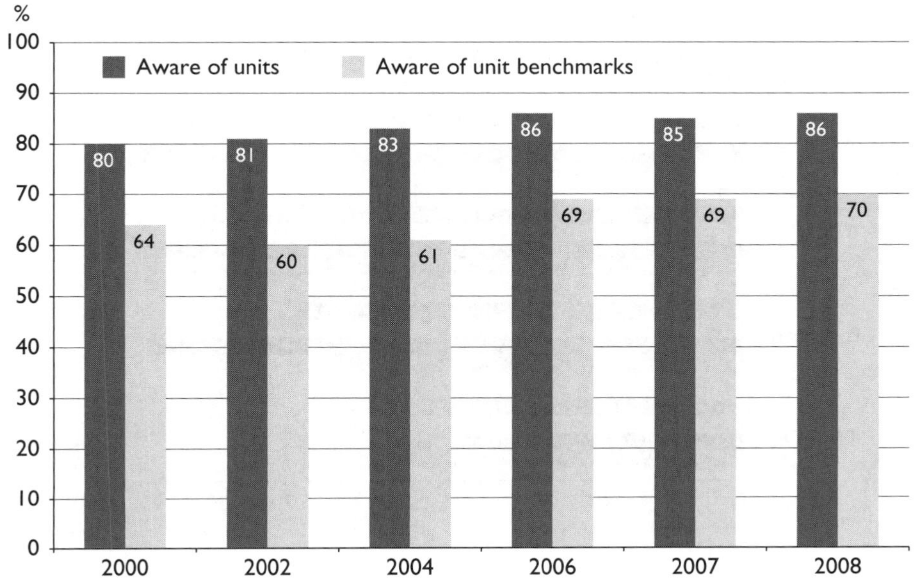

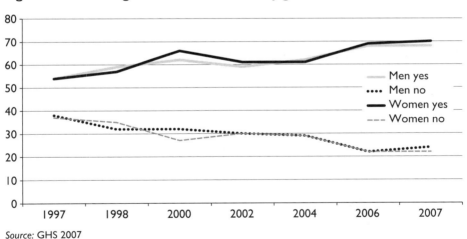

Source: Department of Health (2008)

Figure 28: Knowledge of unit benchmarks by gender 1997–2007

Source: GHS 2007

women in 'managerial/professional' roles in contrast to 79% of women and 76% of men in 'manual' roles stating their awareness of units (Figure 30). However, even while knowing more about units, Figure 31 shows that women identifying as professional/managerial drink markedly more than women in manual roles (more than 12 units a week compared to fewer than 8 units a week). The pattern

Figure 29: Awareness of units by age and average consumption in 2007

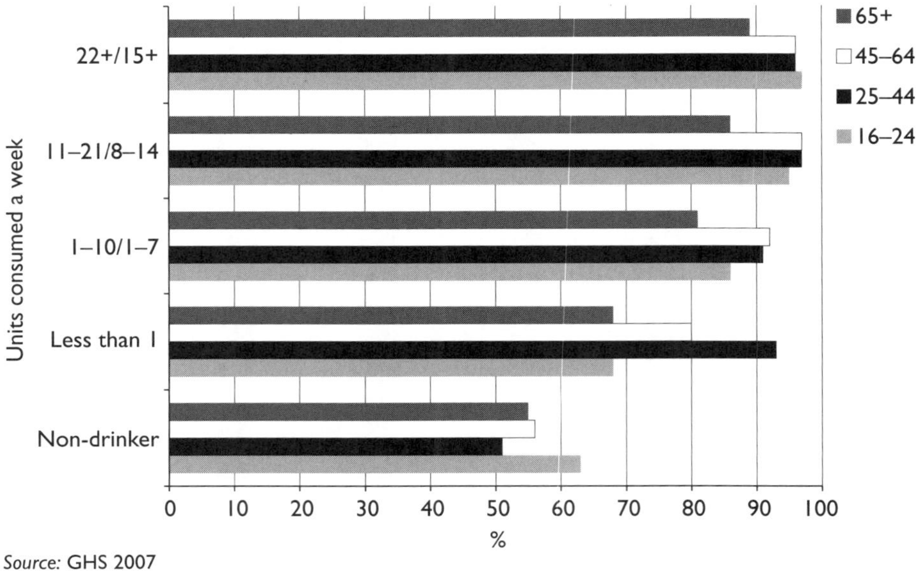

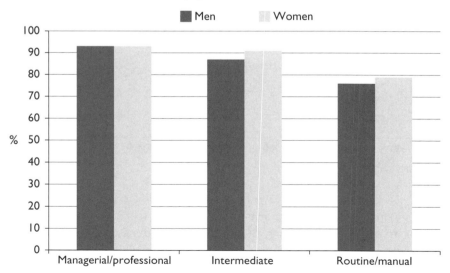

Source: GHS 2007

is slightly different for men as, on average, those in both socioeconomic groups drink roughly the same. It is therefore clear that *knowledge* of units is far from an accurate predictor of propensity to drink; not only is there a high level of public apathy over the system delineating sensible behaviour, but there is also evidence of more complex risk–denial mechanisms that call into question the overriding

Figure 30: Awareness of units by gender and socioeconomic status

Source: GHS 2007

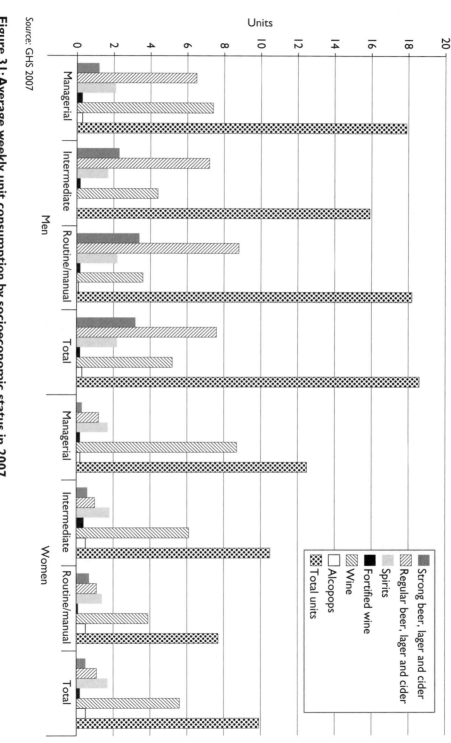

Source: GHS 2007

Figure 31: Average weekly unit consumption by socioeconomic status in 2007

faith being placed on technologies of risk communication and 'cultural change' as a vehicle for managing alcohol-related harm.

This general *awareness* of daily benchmarks does not necessarily translate into specific *knowledge* of their relationship to risk thresholds. Indeed, while only 46% of respondents in the 2007 GHS guessed the correct benchmark for men and 50% guessed the correct benchmark for women, there was no significant change in the level of benchmark knowledge in the period 1997–2007. Knowledge of units remains the object of concern for an education-orientated public health paradigm (Cabinet Office 2004), yet there remains a fundamental gap in the process of translating knowledge into action. As Figure 32 shows, between 1997 and 2007, the proportion of women claiming to be 'keeping an eye' on their alcohol intake rose from 12% to only 14% and from 14% to 16% for men. Curiously, this negligible increase occurred alongside exponential growth in media concern with drinking and its harms. Whether this is an outcome of apathy, ambivalence or a fundamental mismatch between the social norms of drinking and the expectations of sensibleness laid down in unit benchmarks is a key question for public health policy. What is clear is that the message may be raising awareness slightly, but persistently low levels of people self-monitoring their intake indicates an absolute lack of *will* to alter behaviour. Perhaps, as Labour MP Hazel Blears once conceded, it might be fair to say that 'we just like getting drunk'. While this might be the case, there is a far greater case to be made for the failure of the drinking guidelines to resonate with either the contemporary drinking environments discussed in the next chapter or 'myopic' short-termist personal rationalisations of risk (Offer 2007). Moreover, this societal cognitive dissonance seems to be rampant across almost all drinking sectors of the population, even though there is a persistent

Figure 32: Percentage of people monitoring their alcohol consumption by gender, 1997–2007

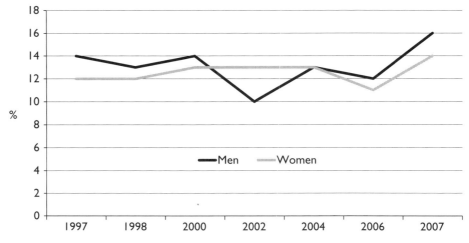

Source: GHS 2007

claim that such deviance is contained among a clearly demarcated group that comprises the young and, more recently, the middle classes (Berry and Fleming 2007; Boseley 2007a; Brown 2007; Beckford 2009).

The NHS Alcohol Statistics 2010 showed clearly that those in professional and managerial roles both drank the most and were most likely to drink on every day of the week, prompting Professor Ian Gilmore, president of the RCP, to highlight:

> those who regularly exceed the recommended limits are more likely to work in office jobs, and range in ages from their mid twenties to early sixties . . . it is vital that government does not lose sight of this group most at risk of developing serious health complications and the pivotal role of cheap supermarket drink and widespread availability. (Devlin 2010)

In reply, Anne Milton, the (then) public health minister reiterated the line that the government should 'prevent the harm that alcohol can cause without penalising those who drink sensibly' (ibid). But, with the very constitution of sensible drinking so contested, the line between permitted and unacceptable risk taking is easily crossed by even the most 'respectable' of middle-class consumers.

The limited allure of sensible behaviour and the persistence of pleasure

There is a curious myopia in approaches to alcohol underscored by a continued faith by government in what Room et al (2005: 525) term the 'popular but ineffective' use of education to convert an 'irresponsible minority' into a responsible majority. However, as the figures discussed above suggest, this minority is a far from an exclusive group and, by extension, 'irresponsibility' is a far from unusual behaviour. This deserves a return to the very notions of responsibility set out in Chapter Two. Unlike obesity, which raises some deep-seated moral complexities in the context of the luck egalitarian argument, drinking alcohol is a lifestyle choice with both foreseeable and unforeseeable consequences. Therefore, it is fair to assert that, with the marked exception of dependent drinkers, those who choose to drink do so in the knowledge that their actions may have negative outcomes. For many, however, the consequence of intoxication (as a liminal state with negative and positive attributes) is appeal enough. Indeed, as Walton suggests:

> intoxication is its own justification . . . Whatever other physiological processes are going on while we drink, our brains are experiencing intoxication symptoms, and the pleasure, satisfaction and relief that affords were the reason we scrabbled through the draw for the corkscrew in the first place . . . This [pleasure] is the most forceful argument it is possible to offer against the unit-counting, binge-policing mentality. (Walton 2001: 204)

The allure of pleasure is undeniable. But, as Hadfield asserts, New Labour's governance of the 'business of pleasure', and the ensuing alcohol control debate, has been 'accompanied by the placing of ever greater responsibilities on the consumer' where 'rational, autonomous and strong-willed individuals have the capacity to make informed decisions about their own repertoire of pleasure-seeking behaviours' (2007: 19). This 'pleasure ethic' (ibid) is both undertheorised and under-elucidated in studies of lifestyle behaviours, including eating and exercising. While this is partly predictable given the residual 'pathology paradigm' (Moore 2008: 353) that frames understandings of health behaviours, the study of pleasure has been marginalised in many academic accounts of practices such as drinking (O'Malley and Valverde 2004). Yet, without taking pleasure into account, the unwavering faith in the possibility of a responsible majority capable of informed choice cannot fully explain the persistent allure of risky drinking, not to mention unhealthy eating and being lazy. Perhaps we need to think more carefully, therefore, about how and why 'intoxication is in itself the opportunity for a temporary escape from the moderation that the rest of life is mortgaged to' (Walton 2001: 205). Here 'moderation' is the antithesis of pleasure, not because moderate behaviour necessarily precludes the possibility of measured pleasure, but because it places moral boundaries on the exercise of personal freedoms. As such, exercising personal responsibility in drinking may well be 'the cost of freedom' that Roemer (1993) suggests.

Pleasure is an embedded sentiment that takes shape in the context of certain social norms, environments and cultural practices. However, pleasure enjoys a particularly tumultuous relationship with responsibility in the context of drinking in the UK, especially given the ways in which being sensible is being written into the very structures that condition drinking. With unit labelling (on drinks packaging) not yet compulsory, but increasingly and voluntarily being taken up by producers as part of their corporate social responsibility portfolios (Portman Group 2007), pleasure and responsibility have been entwined in new ways. As this chapter has explored, the delineation of sensible behaviour has long been translated through the language and logic of units. Unit labelling thus serves as an awareness-raising tool and an educational technique that holds the potential to transmit and concretise sensible drinking admonitions by visually demonstrating risk in product form. While great faith has been placed in this method of risk communication (Webster-Harrison et al 2002), there is evidence to suggest that, among the 'risk group' of young people, such labelling may instead signify the possibility of pleasure. For example, to the savvy teenager, unit labelling spells out the number of units per pound spent, allowing them to put this information to good use by maximising their unit intake for the smallest possible cost through the off-trade. While this might seem like a particularly sceptical stance, it does corroborate Coveney and Bunton's (2003) assertion that we need to pay more attention to 'pleasure-seeking activities', especially in the context of trying to corral pleasure into the strictures of sensibleness.

Given that pleasure is a motive for action, and intoxication is widely agreed to be pleasurable, then perhaps we need to explore further why a belief in 'drunkenness' over 'determined drunkenness' (Measham 2006) has become an ingrained part of the narrative of British drinking. The *determination* or agency inherent within quests for intoxication fully negates the argument that it is a lack of education and awareness that promotes such behaviour. Rather, the question should be: why, despite high levels of awareness, does risk taking persist? The answer to this lies not just in assertions of pleasure as a point of resistance against 'the forces of unwanted "authoritarian" control of individual choice' (Coveney and Bunton 2003: 166), but also in the allure of alcohol as an accessible pleasure in a particularly unequal and often inaccessible society. Pleasure is thus one means by and through which difference can be temporarily suspended and the deep social divisions that perpetually reinforce popular narratives around drinking, intoxication, risk taking and irresponsibility forgotten. Just as with obesity, the alcohol debate is one that is very firmly skewed by class-based elisions of inequality and irresponsibility. Moreover, this occurs in ways that distort the significant health risks of excessive drinking. As Barr suggests, 'the fact that moderate alcohol consumption is (and was) positively beneficial does not mean that excessive alcohol consumption has not been positively harmful' (1995: 287). The delineation between moderation and excess on one hand, and benefit and harm on the other is not biomedically defined. Rather, it is deeply embedded in class, cultural and political discourses, suggesting that being sensible with respect to alcohol-related harms is an enterprise that only the privileged few will be able to attain, regardless of their actual behavioural choices. As O'Malley and Valverde helpfully suggest:

> The moderate middle-class wine lovers, the cocktail set and the quiet toper in the rural pub can all warrantably be aligned with pleasure, in the quiet enjoyment of their property. Pleasure is mobilized by liberal government as a discursive tactic: pleasure is Good and, warrantably, can only be assigned to the Good. (O'Malley and Valverde 2004: 39)

Conclusion

This chapter has critically interrogated the construction, delineation and deployment of what have been termed 'codes of sensibleness' with respect to drinking. In so doing, it has torn apart three of the most common assertions that guide and structure the hesitant logic of the UK's alcohol control debate. In the first place, it has argued that while there remain demonstrable differences between Southern and Northern European drinking cultures, the gap is closing at a far quicker pace than ever considered by the DCMS in its 'extraordinary naivety in believing the Licensing Act 2003 would bring about "civilised cafe culture"' (Health Select Committee 2010: 119). That Southern European drinking practices and places remain the goal of UK policy is curious in both its impracticality and its idealisation of observation-based assumptions. Processes of cultural homogenisation are pushing Northern and Southern European drinking habits ever closer and, in the process, delegitimising the ongoing alcohol control debate's claims of clear geographical disparities.

This feeds directly into the second assertion that 'heavy sessional' or binge drinking is an innately British pastime. While it is not to be doubted that heavy sessional drinking is a characteristic of British consumption patterns, it should not be assumed that this is a practice confined to the UK. There is strong evidence to suggest that, just as total alcohol consumption in France, Italy, Spain and Portugal continues to fall from very high levels, beer drinking is rising and binge drinking (among young people) is becoming an established phenomenon. The discourse of bingeing (in the UK and beyond) is inextricable from far more generalised discourses of youth culpability, whereby young people are seen as the chief culprits in the UK's 'alcohol epidemic'. However, data from the GHS demonstrates that binge-drinking rates are highest among those with the highest incomes (over £1,000 a week), who are highly likely to be older. The GHS data show that the highest drinking rates (total units per week) are found among men aged 45–64 (21 units a week), exceeding that of 16- to 24-year-old men (17.3 units); among women, 16- to 24-year-olds drink the most per week (11.3 units). However, as ages rise, the amount being consumed does not fall to any significant degree, with those aged 25–44 consuming 10.2 units a week and those aged 45–64 putting away an average 9.9 units. Thus, not only is heavy sessional drinking not clearly an innately British trait, but it is also not one that cannot fairly be ascribed solely to young people. Young women may drink more over the course of a week than older groups, but the difference is not sufficiently marked to identify this group as the clearly defined risk-takers that policy and media accounts so often suggest (Day et al 2004).

The third contention questions the degree of novelty of such 'excessive' and 'irresponsible' behaviour; this chapter has argued that not only have historical drinking rates been far higher than they are at present, but that the British relationship with alcohol has been far from a linear progression towards widespread inebriation. Most importantly and running contrary to overly simplistic assertions that Britain has seen a 'decline' into alcohol-fuelled debauchery, historical accounts demonstrate the profound ways in which drinkers, drink and the places where it is consumed have served as touchstones for wider societal hopes and fears. What marks out the contemporary period as distinct is the proliferation of media and communication channels, which have fundamentally altered the nature of a night out. Not only are drinking behaviours immortalised through TV documentaries, reality shows, Facebook and Bebo, but the normalisation of 'unsafe' or non-sensible drinking – in the sense of going beyond the recommended limits – has also been inexorably reinforced through these same pathways. As one interviewee from a central London drug and alcohol action team suggested:

> 'I think that there is evidence that drinking among young people is stabilising. It's not reducing and I think young people use alcohol as

escape. You know even when I was young, alcohol wasn't this massive thing . . . now you don't spend the evening drinking a half and lime with your mates; what you do is you get all your mates to come round to my house and you get plastered because you can't afford the prices of drinks in the pubs and you go out drunk. You're drunk before you have your evening out. I think you throw it down your neck, you know, the end point is to get drunk and off your face. It's not really to, you know, oil the wheels of social intercourse like we used to when we were . . . yeah right! But you know what I mean? You used to, it's much more like drug taking and it's spirits, getting drunk is the thing and getting drunk is funny and showing your knickers and I mean you could run round showing your knickers – it's hilarious! You can put a picture up on Facebook and everybody laughs at it. It's weird!' (interview, 2008)

The notion that we are now witnessing a period of demonstrably excessive drinking is deeply problematic as total consumption has fallen since 2004 and this trend looks likely to continue. Nor is it correct to assert that the current period is novel for being a 'problem' of young people. The data instead demonstrate that the popular image of heavy sessional drinking as solely a problem of young people both underplays the demographic and cultural complexity of the situation and denies the multiple ways in which heavy sessional drinking can take place, including at home. Again, the focus on crime and disorder – rather than health – favoured by policies such as the AHRSE has meant that *public* drinking (and therefore youth drinking) has become the primary cause for concern, a focus that will be more fully explored in the next chapter.

The regulation of alcohol is inherently complex, not least as the delineation of what and who is sensible is fraught with conceptual and pragmatic difficulties; delineating risk thresholds through units is an uncertain and inexact science and communicating certainty in such conditions of contestation is practically challenging. In this vein, this chapter has explored the emergence and expression of sensible drinking and, building from this, the misplaced faith in education as a means of increasing awareness and therefore using this pathway to inculcate sensible behaviour. As this chapter has shown, there is a continued and persistent mismatch between the public's awareness of units and their reported self-monitoring of their alcohol intake. This demonstrates either a high level of apathy or a determination to drink despite sensible drinking messaging. It may also be reflective of the manifold social roles that alcohol plays. Drinking is a very particular battleground, which, like eating and physical activity, is drawn out firmly along class lines. This battle extends not just to judgements of how much people drink, but what they drink and where. To be young and in a town centre on a Friday or Saturday thus comes to stand for deviance, regardless of an individual's actual behaviour. A middle-aged drinker at home may consume more alcohol in total, but the ways in which sensible drinking has been defined as primarily linked to 'violent and anti-social behaviour' and 'young people' means that their 'irresponsibility' as a 'silent majority of heavy drinkers' (Emslie et al 2009: 13) is far too often overlooked. This has clear consequences for the manner in which the regulation of alcohol repeatedly curtails the freedoms of the young, while leaving the middle-class wine drinker and the off-trade largely unscathed. The conundrum of sensible drinking is not, however, merely a story of definitions, it is also a narrative of place. It is for this reason that Chapter Eight turns to discuss the dialectical relationships between drink, drinkers and drinking places. The lived tensions between freedom and regulation can only properly be explored in situ; being sensible is fine in theory, but ultimately meaningless without action.

EIGHT

Spatial governance and the night-time economy

Introduction

This chapter explores the contentious rise and rise of London's night-time economy (NTE) as a means of investigating the increasingly spatialised logic underpinning the techniques and rationales being deployed to foster a sensible drinking culture in the UK. As such, this chapter speaks directly to the third contention of this book as set out in Chapter Three. In this reading, the enterprise of governing alcohol lays bare particular governmental and non-governmental aspirations for urban environments and societies. However, this vision is distinctly ambiguous in that while certain urban agendas are being pursued *through* alcohol (for example through 'drink-led regeneration'), other urban aspirations are being achieved by *regulating* alcohol consumption and its harms. However, both ventures are predicated on a certain vision of the spatial and its impact on behaviour. Governing drinking is consequently inextricable from efforts to govern drink and drinkers. By extension, this also means that governing (and therefore theorising) drinking *places* – despite being an essential element of the alcohol control debate – has been omitted by sociological, anthropological, psychological, biomedical and psychiatric studies and has only recently started to be developed by geographers (Jayne et al 2006: 55, 2008a, 2008b), 2010; Kneale and French 2008).

To address this omission, this chapter will specifically focus on the example of London's NTE. With the nation's largest selection of bars, pubs and nightclubs, drinking has been a key strategic element in the city's broader economic successes (Elvins and Hadfield 2003; Roberts and Turner 2005; Hadfield 2006; Roberts et al 2006). Indeed, over the past two decades, the landscape of London's leisure industry has changed beyond all recognition and, with this, so have the consumption habits of those who frequent the city's diverse range of NTE venues. Above and beyond the critique of the commodification and homogenisation of the branded, commercialised night-time experience so maligned by some urban geographers and sociologists (see for example Chatterton and Hollands 2003; Hollands and Chatterton 2003), shifts in the city's drinking environments have come under attack for fundamentally altering existing codes of sanctioned behaviour and, in the process, creating urban 'no-go areas' (Roberts 2006). In conscious efforts to create the '24 hour city' and foster a European-style café culture through licensing reform; drinking practices and the risks associated with them have been inevitably and irrevocably altered (Bianchini 1995; Montgomery 1995, 1997; Heath 1997).

In turn, these shifts have created complex socio–spatial governance challenges that will be further discussed in this chapter.

Set within this context, London offers a fascinating case study as it acts as both exception and rule, mirroring and disavowing national patterns of work and play. Indeed, it has the lowest rate of binge drinking in the UK (Health and Social Care Information Centre 2010), despite the city's West End having the highest density of licensed premises in the country (Elvins and Hadfield 2003). This complicates the tendency to equate causality for risky drinking practices with the density of licensed premises (Graham and Homel 2008; Roberts 2009). London has not been uniformly transformed by the development and expansion of the NTE over the past two decades. Rather, the effects have been unevenly distributed and are most marked in certain hotspots, including the West End, Clapham, Islington's Upper Street, Clerkenwell, Shoreditch, Brixton and the City of London. While town and cities outside the capital have been transformed through the creation of drinking circuits and zoned drinking quarters (Jayne et al. 2008a), London's NTE

Table 7: Policy agendas at a national and mayoral scale that seek to govern alcohol directly or indirectly

Scale	Policy title
National	Crime and Disorder Act 1998
	Urban Renaissance (Urban Task Force 1999)
	Criminal Justice and Police Act 2001
	Licensing Act 2003
	Anti-Social Behaviour Act 2003
	Choosing Health (DH 2004)
	Alcohol Misuse Interventions: guidance on developing a local programme of improvement (DH 2004)
	Hidden harm (Home Office 2004)
	Alcohol Harm Reduction Strategy for England (Prime Minister's Strategy Unit 2004)
	Planning Policy Statement (PPS) 6, Planning for Town Centres (2005)
	Violent Crime Reduction Act 2006
	Social Responsibility Standards for the Production and Sale of Alcoholic Drinks (2007)
	How to Manage Town Centres (DCLG 2007)
	Safe, Sensible, Social (HM Government 2007)
Mayoral	London Plan (2004, 2008)
	Sounder City: London's Ambient Noise Strategy (2004)
	The London Agenda for Action on Alcohol (2005)
	London Anti-Social Behaviour Strategy (GLA 2005)
	London's Night-time Economy (GLA 2005)
	London Tourism Vision and Action Plan (LDA 2009)
	Economic Development Strategy (LDA 2010)
	Transport Strategy (2010)
	London Cultural Metropolis (2010)

offerings have remained extremely diverse. This cosmopolitan NTE thus acts as an interesting counterpoint to the town centre-based focus that dominates critical accounts of the NTE. Moreover, London's mixed and dense NTE offerings also raise distinctive sets of issues for the management and governance of drinking (Mayor of London 2003, 2006). London is thus a perspicuous site for exploring the conceptual tensions at the heart of efforts to create sensible drinkers through fashioning sensible drinking places. Because London both resembles and is markedly different to other places, it presents valuable opportunities for contrast and comparison, as well as generalisation and specificity in discussions of the governance of the NTE.

Returning to the third contention of this book, this chapter asks in what ways London's NTE not only demonstrates the current spatial turn within social and public policy, but also the consequences of this mode of thought. Governing drinking means acting on the practices of drinkers and the spaces in which they consume alcohol. In turn, this is based on particular readings of risk and responsibility in relation to the urban environment and, by extension, how these are produced and experienced by urban dwellers. The much-maligned 2003 Licensing Act may have been the most high-profile piece of legislation with respect to the spatial governance of alcohol in recent years, but it is important to note that it sits at a vortex of a host of other, interrelated policy, legislative and strategy agendas (of which Table 7 lists only a cross-section). In this policy maelstrom, the UK's response to alcohol has been complex, but underpinned by a series of socio-spatial governance strategies that attempt to shunt responsibility for individual conduct onto licensed premises through a comprehensive system of penalties and sanctions (Talbot 2006; Tierney 2006; Foster 2008). When set within the context of the socio-spatial governance of alcohol, being sensible goes beyond simply sticking to drinking guidelines, but also involves fitting into expectations of civil conduct appropriate to the consumption ethic of the revamped 24-hour city (Hobbs et al 2005). Managing drinking in urban environments has long been, and overwhelmingly remains, a crime and disorder issue. As a result, the health agenda has been largely reduced to the target laid down in PSA 25: to reduce the harm caused by alcohol and drugs by reducing the number of alcohol-related hospital admissions. As such, the sensible drinker is judged by his or her public actions and the risks that these pose. In framing drinking through the strictures of crime and disorder reduction agendas, the urban is often reduced to a criminogenic space of actual and potential risk, a place where fun and menace coexist. This chapter will therefore critically explore the alcohol harm reduction agenda in the UK as exemplifying the tension between the need to manage the risks produced by the 24-hour city and the parallel need to foster drinking-led economic growth by stimulating appropriate and desirable (sensible) consumer demand for leisure and entertainment.

To address these concerns, this chapter proceeds in three parts. The first will briefly explore the UK's 24-hour city agenda, before turning to London's changing nightscapes in order to explore the shifting landscapes of risk attached to drinking and, therefore, the strategies enacted to mitigate these. The second part draws on interview material to discuss the socio-spatial governance strategies currently being developed to encourage sensible behaviour to reduce alcohol-related harm. In so doing, it will also explore the contention that the drive to create sensible places to mitigate the effects of the 24-hour city's focus on alcohol-led growth and regeneration may, in eroding the possibilities for spontaneity and pleasure through spatial management strategies, actually be reinforcing a broader cultural shift away from drinking in pubs and bars and towards drinking at home. In so doing, this chapter further argues, the individual health risks associated with drinking are multiplied even as such actions are repeatedly sanctioned in two ways: by virtue of occurring in a private space and by the fact that drinking at home does not necessarily add to the burden of visceral crime and disorder. In tandem, while this may produce a more sensible civic and public realm as measured through crime, disorder and anti-social behaviour indicators, it does little to foster sensible drinking behaviours for the sake of better public health. Drinking practices and places are therefore increasingly becoming a means by which to judge both risk and those indulging in those risky practices such as binge drinking discussed in the previous chapter. We must not therefore always ask how we can solve the UK's drinking problem, but rather why and how drinking has come to signify a far broader and deeper set of 'problems' within urban environments that act to perpetuate drinking as a societal crisis.

Fashioning an urban renaissance in the 24-hour city

The rapid growth of the UK's NTE has courted both substantial interest and substantial criticism (see for example Lovatt and O'Connor 1995; Roberts 2006; Talbot 2006; Tierney 2006; Tiesdell and Slater 2006; Roberts and Eldridge 2007). Ken Worpole's 1992 book *Towns for People*, based on the Gulbenkian Foundation's 1991 Out of Hours study was among the first to set out an agenda to address a purported 'crisis facing British towns and cities' (Worpole 1992: 1; Roberts 2004, 2006). The study suggested that British town centres had remarkably underdeveloped evening and night-time economies when compared to their European counterparts and in stark contrast to the vibrancy of their own daylight economies. The report lamented the overwhelming dominance of retail-led development in town centres and, as a result, the loss not only of independent retailers but of the potential for the kind of 7 am–11 pm urban space needed to foster greater diversity, vitality and viability. The report noted Britain's 'underdeveloped café and open air culture' and its over-reliance on a weekend youth 'fashion circuit of city-centre pubs' (Worpole 1992: 41) and argued strongly for bringing back city-centre living. Worpole also focused heavily on perceptions of town-centre crime, lambasting inadequate and unsafe public transport, poor lighting, inadequate taxi regulation and a paucity of woman-friendly town-centre spaces. The report further identified the 'hijacking' of town-centre life 'by the young at the expense of all other sections of the population' (ibid: 66). Worpole's assertion of a youth-led 'territorial colonisation underscored by the threat of violence' (ibid: 67) seems a remarkably familiar refrain given the more recent media hysteria over 'an alarming rise in binge drinking' (Waszkiewicz and Szulc 2009) and related patterns of anti-social behaviour assumed to be dominated by the young. The management of the NTE and urban crime reduction agendas have, therefore, long been entwined. However, the hope that this entanglement would be a 'virtuous circle' (Hadfield 2006: 47) into urban renewal now seems a far more problematic aspiration.

The report further identified some now-familiar problems with the UK's NTE: standardised closing times, the conversion of 'traditional' pubs into hybrid 'youth pubs' or 'disco-pubs', the mono-functionality of contemporary drinking spaces, their intimidating appearance to many women, the pub's inability to accommodate children, a lack of outdoor seating and minimal diversity in night-time venues. In order to address this 'crisis', Worpole called for a 'people-centred cultural strategy' that would Europeanise the drinking experience in the UK to 'bring towns and cities back to life' and bring back a 'culture of hope'. Reinforced by similar calls being made by Montgomery (1995, 1997), the 24-hour city concept and vision was born. In this, the role of drinking was an express concern and it was felt that the 24-hour city needed longer opening hours for licensed premises to avoid the creation of crime and disorder flashpoints caused by large numbers of people on the streets after a single closing time. The 1988 Licensing Act and the 1995 (Sunday Hours) Licensing Act theoretically allowed premises to open from 11 am to 11 pm, seven days a week. However, as the Office of the Deputy Prime Ministers's (ODPM) report, *The Evening Economy and the Urban Renaissance* noted, 'there is very little activity in most British town and city centres between 5 and 8 o'clock in the evening' (ODPM 2003: 7). Instead of a vibrant, mixed and inclusive evening economy therefore, British towns and cities suffered a late-night economy dominated by the young, who 'gather in vertical drinking venues . . . standing up . . . where music is played at high volume' (ibid). In this logic, the evening economy was to be sustained and supported and the late-night alcohol-driven economy regulated and managed through a variety of new tools and techniques.

It is worth noting that the 1988 Supply of Beer (Tied Estate) Order (more commonly known as the 'Beer Orders') has had an equally profound effect on the nature of British drinking habits and the direction taken by the urban renaissance. The Beer Orders effectively produced both the managed house and the pub company (or PubCo), paving the way for the current and frequently maligned corporate dominance of the NTE. The Beer Orders resulted from a 1989 Competition Commission report that expressed concern at the monopoly held by breweries over 'tied' pubs (for example, they were required to buy beer from that brewery only) as, at that time, six brewers effectively controlled 75% of tied houses. The new regulation thus placed a limit on the size of brewers' estates at a maximum of '2,000 pubs plus half the highest number of pubs over 2,000 held by the brewer' since 10 July 1989. This provided the impetus for an unparalleled land grab fuelled by venture capitalists, producing behemoth PubCo empires such as Enterprise Inns, Punch and Pub Master. In 2002, the Beer Orders were repealed for, in the words of then-Parliamentary Under-Secretary for Trade and Industry Melanie Johnson, no longer being 'relevant to today's industry'. The repeal actively coincided with the enactment of New Labour's 'market-led' Urban Renaissance agenda, within which the NTE held a central, if underexplored, role (Urban Task Force 1999; Imrie and Raco 2003; ODPM 2003). As an active result of this legislative about-turn, Enterprise Inns now runs an estate of almost 7,200 managed houses and Punch 7,100, according to their latest 2010 annual reports. These companies form just one sector of a lucrative leisure market governed from the 'boardrooms of corporate interests' and 'led by the demands of the marketplace' (Hobbs et al 2005: 174–5).

Intermingled with the dictates of the market also came a drive to emulate the European-style drinking cultures explored in the previous chapter. In a bid to create a more civilised European ambiance (Roberts et al 2006), shifts in planning regulations in the 1990s encouraged the liberalisation of the NTE through profligate granting of licences, irrespective of existing concentrations of licensed premises or 'need' (Roberts 2004, 2009). When this legislative environment was laid over the growth in high-street leisure corporations with their branded and themed night-time venues (Hobbs et al 2005; Hadfield 2006), the result was a spectacular and now well-documented expansion in the number and range of licensed premises in town and city centres across the UK. Moreover and inseparable from this, this growth has also spurred an attendant and trenchant critique of the negative externalities of the newly vibrant NTE. However, amid this, the drive to Europeanise British cities in a bid to foster the sensible drinking cultures perceived to exist south of the English Channel was not lost. In 2000 further strides were made to further deregulate the licensing laws to facilitate a 'continental ambiance' (Roberts et al 2006; Tierney 2006; Jayne et al 2008a) set against the backdrop of a homogenised 'post-industrial leisure economy' (Hadfield 2006: 45).

The ODPM's 'urban renaissance' report was commissioned alongside the development of the 2003 Licensing Act – New Labour's controversial move to liberalise and modernise the UK's archaic licensing laws (Department for Culture Media and Sport 2001). The Licensing Act – thanks in part to a dedicated campaign by *The Daily Mail* newspaper – is instead now synonymous with the goal of permitting '24 hour drinking' through the provision of 24-hour licences. However, it is worth noting that the 7,400 premises with 24-hour licences represent a mere 3.4% of all licensed premises in the UK (Department for Culture Media and Sport 2009). Furthermore, the focus on drinking hours oversimplifies a piece of legislation that was actually part of a far broader strategy for 'modernising and integrating the alcohol, public entertainment, theatre, cinema, night café and late refreshment house licensing systems' (Department for Culture Media and Sport 2001: 7) through simplification and streamlining. The legislation was principally designed to act as a mechanism to address alcohol-related crime and disorder by enabling the emergence of a contemporary NTE within a system that gave greater powers to local residents. While these aspirations are laudable, it was the interlinking of the rationale for the new legislation and arguments for staggered and later closing times with the potential for a Europeanised drinking culture that courted particularly sustained criticism. As the Health Select Committee's report noted, 'the worst fears of the Act's critics were not realised, but neither was the DCMS's naive aspiration of establishing café society: violence and disorder have remained at similar levels, although they have tended to take place later at night' (2010: 92). The Act and the subsequently published AHRSE (Prime Minister's Strategy Unit 2004) were also criticised for ignoring public health goals relating to alcohol. This is a sentiment echoed by Goodacre, who argues that:

> To increase availability of alcohol at a time when the problem is escalating, as the Licensing Act does, appears to lack common sense. Unless the new powers to close problem premises are used effectively the Act will just exacerbate an already serious problem. Meanwhile, emergency clinicians will have to carry on clearing up the mess. (Goodacre 2005: 682)

Thus, instead of widening the field associated with the governance of alcohol, the Act and strategy reinforced drinking as a crime and disorder agenda. This process also served to solidify a distinctly spatialised governance logic. More than this, they instigated a renewed moral panic around the deregulation and liberalisation of the high street, deepening the perceived synonymity of the NTE, and by extension the 24-hour city model, with uncontrolled and uncontrollable drinking spaces. The contemporary town and city centre are thus never far from political, public and popular scrutiny, but ardent criticism does little to foster a deeper understanding of how the NTE is governed and why.

While much has been written boosting the aspirations enshrined in the 24-hour city concept, more has since been written decrying the limitations to what Hobbs et al have called this 'new urban script which promised a café society' in that it, 'delivered only a flow of capital into the development of venues selling alcohol' (2005: 163). The result, they argue, has not been any great social revolution into civility, but rather that alcohol remains 'the core commodity that attracts individuals into the night-time city' (ibid). While the voluminous sociological and criminological work of Dick Hobbs, Phil Hadfield, Simon Winlow and Stuart Lister is exceptionally valuable, it also offers a particularly vehement critique of the government's drive to instigate an urban renaissance reliant on 'a night-time economy that constitutes an imperfectly regulated zone of quasi-liminality awash on a sea of alcohol' (Hobbs et al 2005: 165). They argue that the resultant 'criminogenic growth' of the increasingly privatised and purified 'public' space of the high street (Hadfield 2006: 55) has been the inevitable outcome of a blind faith in the model of a 24-hour city understood, overwhelmingly, as a space of consumption. In this reading, citizens are also to be treated solely as consumers, particularly where their behaviour starts to be marked out as problematic. Hadfield asserts, this 'promotes an individualised mode of governance in which control of consumption, and any harms relating to it, become the responsibility solely of the consumer' (2006: 162). While this individualisation of responsibility is true of a neoliberal ethic more broadly, it seems hollow when set against the burgeoning array of sanctions and regulations laid on the licence holder under the new Licensing Act. Indeed, the NTE may be a discursive domain of individual responsibility, but it is a regulatory domain increasingly defined by the responsibilisation of on-trade licence holders and the clear recognition that a sensible NTE is an entity that cannot evolve organically, but rather must be moulded through processes of active management (Greater London Authority 2002, 2007; Roberts 2004; Tiesdell and Slater 2006).

There is a sense that, as Hobbs et al argue, 'the processes of commercial agglomeration, consumer colonisation and cultural purification that have accompanied the de-regulation of the night-time high street have generated an array of social and environmental harms' (2005: 163). It is therefore fair to argue that the current alcohol harm reduction agenda exemplifies a domain of governance that permeates almost all elements of urban life and liveability. If, as Hobbs and colleagues argue, alcohol defines the night-time city, then urban governance agendas (and even national election agendas) are now also defined by the management of alcohol and its manifold harms (see for example, Mayor of London 2004). Their trenchant critique of the neoliberalisation of a NTE now surrendered to market forces also argues that such a governmentality is characterised by a 'prevailing hypocrisy' in the state's retreat from controlling the negative externalities of its own urban growth strategies (Hobbs et al 2005: 178). Instead, control has been hybridised and privatised, farmed out and devolved to newly created agencies such as the Security Industry Association (SIA) which now licenses door staff. In London, for example, the preference of Westminster police to work with known and respected companies means that control of venue doors is dominated by just one company, TSS, which now employs 2,800 security operatives (aka bouncers). In keeping with the corporatisation of the NTE, assigning responsibility has become structurally more complex through the new powers of the Licensing Act and a new array of bylaws, fixed penalty notices (FPNs) and regulatory tools such as alcohol control zones, Designated Public Place Orders, dispersal zones, alcohol disorder zones, Drinking Banning Orders and curfews attached to the Anti-Social Behaviour Act. These measures are being targeted disproportionately at the on-trade as a part of a broader crack-down of youth presence on the high street, with the off-trade (such as supermarkets) escaping lightly. With the regulatory burden and moral panic precipitated by constant press attention aimed at a criminalised on-trade, it comes as little surprise that the 24-hour city model is not just under attack, but also now under threat. The recession means that the high street is dying a slow death and the model of an urban renaissance predicated on economic growth has ground to a standstill. The British Beer and Pub Association claims that pubs are now closing at a rate of 40 a week and supermarkets' share of the British alcohol spend remains resolutely above that of pubs and restaurants (see Figure 33). Such political economic shifts

Figure 33: Consumer purchasing: off-trade and on-trade 2000–07

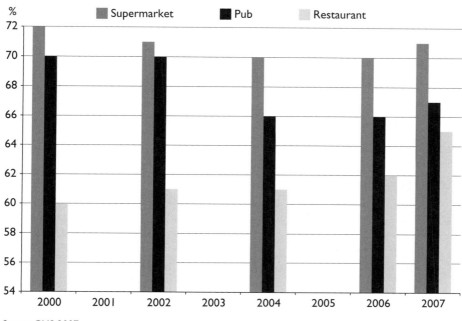

Source: GHS 2007

are altering not just where Britons drink, but what and how, which is crucial when considering the entwined governance of alcohol and urban spaces.

The 2008 Living Costs and Food Survey showed that 56% of consumers' weekly spending on alcohol was bought through the on-trade and 46% through the off-trade (such as supermarkets and off-licences) (Office of National Statistics 2008), but this does not adequately reflect the volume or quantity of alcohol bought. Indeed, with beer regularly retailing in supermarkets at a fifth of what it would cost in a pub (for example 48p a pint versus £2.80 in a pub outside London) (Clark 2010), the current recession seems likely only to further reinforce the turn to cheaper at-home drinking (Measham and Ostergaard 2010). Such an assertion is corroborated when the 35% fall in on-trade beer consumption since 1997 is considered (Figure 34), alongside a corresponding 73% climb in at-home wine consumption since 1992 (Figure 35). The high street might thus be ground zero for the alcohol-related crime and disorder agenda, but the home is increasingly and necessarily becoming the heartland of the health agenda. As such, the governance of alcohol has specific spatial ascriptions according to the nature of the harm under question. The 24-hour city model may well have exacerbated a criminogenic high street, but the regulation of these spaces has ironically produced new private sites of risk sanctioned by recourse to the same discourses of European civility that underscored the original aspirations for an urban renaissance.

Figure 34: Consumption of alcohol outside the home (on-trade) 2000–07

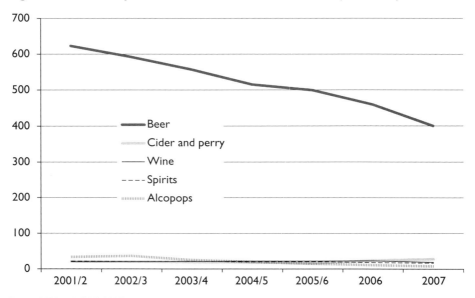

Source: NFS and GHS 2007

Figure 35: Consumption of alcohol in the home (off-trade) 2000–07

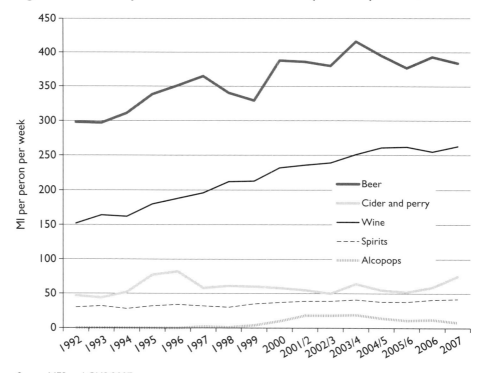

Source: NFS and GHS 2007

Spaces of sense and sensibility: governing London's drinkers

London's NTE is, in the words of the city's Chamber of Commerce (CoC), 'big business'. The CoC's 2006 report on London's NTE identified that the capital's leisure industry had grown by 30% since 1995 and, in 2005, was home to over 9,000 pubs and 522 nightclubs, making up an annual market worth roughly £2.2 billion and employing 60,000 people. In addition to its pubs and clubs, the capital also has 2,426 restaurants in a dining sector worth £4.5 billion a year (London Chamber of Commerce and Industry 2006). Licensed premises in the UK generate 3% of GDP and provide £14 billion in excise and VAT revenue every year. London is at the centre of this leisure spending. Indeed, with per capita incomes far above the national average and an unparalleled choice of licensed venues, it is unsurprising that Londoners account for 25% of the UK's annual leisure spend. Further enhancing the economic potential of London's NTE is a catchment area that extends far beyond the city itself, past the endless miles of its suburban hinterland to the 14.1 million tourists that visited in 2009 (Visit London 2010). With an estimated 500,000 people travelling into the city to go clubbing on a Saturday night alone (London Chamber of Commerce and Industry 2006), London's NTE is clearly 'a significant source of income, employment and civic image building' (Chatterton and Hollands 2003: 2) as well forming part of its essential allure as a place for a 'good night out'. However, what makes a good night for some does not make a good night out (or in) for others. The management of London's NTE is thus riddled with tensions and contentions as a 2005 London Assembly report identifies:

> London's thriving night-time economy is good for London, but does it deliver what Londoners want? Does the upside of living in a vibrant world city offset the downside of living with noise, mess and disruption? How can the needs of Londoners and visitors to London who want to enjoy the city at night be balanced with the need for all Londoners to enjoy a good quality of life? (London Assembly 2005: 5)

The intricacies of managing the city's drinking spaces thus fall to a variety of stakeholders, and all boroughs are required to develop alcohol strategies to tackle alcohol-related harm (interestingly, often farming this task out to the same consultancy group). The result is that managing London's NTE is not just about reducing alcohol-related harm, but also about fashioning a city that better meets both residents' and visitors' needs at a time when the former now have powers to complain about licensees through the new Licensing Act.

Geographers concerned with the study of drinking have argued that 'little attention has been paid to the ways in which drink is represented as a spatial problem' (Kneale and French 2008: 233), despite the fact that alcohol in its popular incarnation as a social problem is inextricably entwined with alcohol as a spatial problem. Due to its varied drinking places and spaces, London perhaps provides a more intricate instance of the spatial logic that explicitly and implicitly underpins hopes for a sensible drinking culture laid down in *Safe, Sensible, Social* (HM Government 2007). As Jayne et al (2006: 460) suggest, 'scratching the surface appearance of urban transformation allows depiction not of a homogenised, purified set of spaces and experiences, but of something more complicated and contested' or what Latham describes as 'a new way of inhabiting the city' (2003: 1710). London is a city of multiple town centres, although many would argue that Westminster's 'multiple stress area' of the West End and Covent Garden, Soho, Queensway and Bayswater and Edgware Road represent the city's closest thing to a centre. While these parts of London are popular with locals and tourists alike, their dominance of the NTE would be hotly debated by Londoners, who more often than not see their city divided between central London and its multiple neighbourhoods, which also often have distinct and vibrant NTEs. It is therefore conceptually and empirically difficult to think of London as a unified whole in the context of drinking and its governance. This is even more so given the devolution of alcohol licensing control to local authorities and the distinct consumption niches that particular areas of the city foster and fulfil. The Sloanes of Parson's Green and the Fulham Road might have just started to brave the journey east to Shoreditch, but the Hackney doyens are fleeing to the emergent scenes of New Cross, Dalston, Bethnal Green and Deptford as fast as their fixed-gear bikes will carry them. Once-edgy Shoreditch is now being mainstreamed, Clerkenwell recently lost nightclub Turnmills after almost two decades of shaping the UK's dance scene and King's Cross lost its iconic venue The Cross to the Eurostar. These are just snapshots of the city's exciting and constantly morphing NTE.

In stark contrast to the often-scathing critique of the homogenised and commercialised nature of the UK's NTE that runs through Hobbs et al and Chatterton and Holland's impressive works, this chapter argues that London exhibits a diversity and vitality that might have pleased even the most disaffected of 24-hour city proponents. London also exhibits the kind of 'evening economy' that was deemed to be lacking in the UK. As many Londoners commute into central London on public transport and work long hours, they have markedly different socialisation patterns to other city residents in the UK (ODPM 2003). Depending on where people live, weekday socialising most commonly starts straight from work, with people returning home only later at night. Pubs and bars may be full to bursting in the hours between 5 pm and 9 pm, but then often get much quieter as people head back to tube and train stations. The weekends offer different temporal and social patterns of activity, with people from a broader age range travelling from further afield to eat, drink and partake in a significant and diverse set of cultural offerings. This is not to say that London is without 'flashpoints' that exhibit the traits of the violent, youth-dominated town centres that have courted such public outcry, but the broader picture allows for tentative optimism in terms of the capacity to produce sensible drinkers and drinking spaces. Importantly, the empirical research detailed here puts the long-standing media hysteria surrounding the UK's drinking culture into sharp relief by offering a far more restrained and regulated vision of spatial governance at work. In so doing, it seeks to work through the third contention set out at in Chapters Two and Three: that the spatialisation tendencies of social policy agendas – of which alcohol and drinking are just one part of a much broader trend – are reworking geographical imaginations of risk, risk taking and risk-takers, with marked consequences for the ways in which individual drinking practices are rationalised.

London's drinking spaces and drinkers

> Londoners and visitors to the city are increasingly keen to make the most of evening entertainment in one of the most cutting-edge cities in the world. The diverse nature of London's night-time economy opens up the city for young people, marginalised groups and counter cultures and in doing so offers greater opportunity for self expression and creativity, which is vital for building and sustaining London's creative edge. (Greater London Authority 2007: 5)

In seeking to explore the governance of drinking in London critically and empirically, the research project from which this discussion is derived sought the opinions of a representative cross-section of 'experts' or what Rose (2000) terms 'control workers' that shape the governance agenda or the 'risk gaze'. However, contrary to Rose's assertion that these control workers are locked into 'circuits of surveillance and communication in a perpetually failing endeavour to minimise the riskiness of the most risky' (2000: 333), the governance of alcohol requires not just the risk management of certain 'monstrous individuals' (ibid), but rather the delineation and definition of 'legitimate consumption' in relation to the general drinking population. From an empirical and spatial perspective, the views of London's control workers were solicited in four inner London local authorities (Westminster, Camden, Lambeth and Islington) and, as a point of contrast, the outer London boroughs of Harrow and Croydon. However, the discussion here proceeds thematically, cutting across borough lines, just as drinking practices in London are also geographically fluid and often veer from locale to locale as the night goes on. This, again, is in contrast to the ideas of a singular, spatially constrained drinking circuit linked into town and city centre 'drinking quarters'. As such, the following three sections will explore the co-creation of 'sensible' places and people through efforts to govern drinking and drinkers in London, before turning to an examination of the threatened NTE. This about-turn in the perception of the NTE deserves further elaboration for the way in which it challenges the current logic and parameters of the alcohol control debate. The final section critically examines the inexorable shift to at-home drinking to explore the shifting spatialised parameters of risk and responsibility in relation to the aspirations of sensible citizen–consumers.

The micro-regulation of reckless abandon

In contrast to the images of Hades promulgated by *The Daily Mail* and colleagues in its interpretation of the Licensing Act's deregulated '24-hour drinking', the legislation's end result instead appears to have been an increased regulatory burden on the on-trade, more control for the control workers and a shift in the nature of alcohol-related risks. The Licensing Act has provided tools to create sensible places and, in the process, more sensible consumers through allowing licensing committees to attach numerous conditions to licenses and review them for an array of transgressions. Related to this, a recurring refrain in the alcohol control debate is the ascription of blame to an 'irresponsible minority', set in contrast to a 'responsible majority' who can generally go out drinking without major incident. Thus, actively carving out sensible drinking spaces using the powers accorded to control workers by the Licensing Act means ensuring that this irresponsible minority is either actively excluded from the venue or the venue is refashioned to appeal to a more 'responsible' (for example richer or older) clientele. As one central London police officer explained:

> A: 'What we did is that we worked with the licensed premises to persuade them to change the people they were inviting to come.'
>
> Q: 'And are they open to such things?'
>
> A: 'Most were. A couple weren't. However, when you then start the review process and you enter into negotiations with these people, most of them . . . come round to sort of our way of thinking really and realise.' (police, interview, 2008)

Changing the consumer type can be undertaken through a variety of measures – the types and cost of drinks that are served, the type and volume of music played, decoration and ambience, promotions, offering food, seating configurations and styles, the size of the dance floor, the venue capacity, door staff screening, staff training etc (see also Hadfield 2006; Green and Plant 2007). These preferences are also reflected in the specific conditions attached to licences such as, for example, food must be served. In so doing, these conditions aim to control not just the manner in which people drink, but also the type of drinks (such as wine, cocktails) and thus the people who are likely to drink them. As one licensing officer explained:

> 'A condition would be agreed that alcohol can only be served with a table meal and ancillary to the meal. So people can't stand at the bar or just go in there for a drink. 'Cos what would happen normally is people might finish at a nightclub and then find somewhere that's got a licence until five o'clock in the morning and then want to stand and continue drinking. And the council is against vertical drinking, it wants people sitting and having meals.' (interview, 2008)

Indeed, the coworking between the police and licence holders in order to come to this shared understanding of how the premises should function and, crucially therefore, *who* might come in can be even more detailed:

> 'I can say first hand it's about changing the environment, you know, changing the layout, the environment in the pub. It was things like removing bar stools, changing the layout of the dance floor. Give you an example of the ladies' toilets, the women had to go across the dance floor to get to the ladies' toilets, so of course what was happening is a few drunken blokes were touching the women up as they're going, course, boyfriend says, "You been touching my . . .?" You know, and we're off. So basically they redesigned it a bit, changed the access to the ladies' toilets, removed the ashtrays, before the smoking ban came in, so that everything was plastic, polycarbonate glass, polycarbonate bottles as well, no groups of blokes allowed in, no readmission, no admission after midnight, quite strong around that. And it worked. I'm not saying it cured the problem completely but in terms of crime and disorder it went right down.' (police, interview 2008)

While there has been some consideration of the relationship between premises design and the risk of alcohol-related harm (either through violence or excessive drinking), there have been fewer analyses of the ways in which such spatial techniques are being used as a direct affront to the aspirations of an inclusive and diverse NTE agenda by regulating out those consumers who lack desirable behavioural aspirations. In short, the spatial logic of alcohol control is about creating spaces that foster and validate 'responsible' (premium) drinkers at the expense of others. However, the line between responsibility and irresponsibility is easily breached, with the City of London providing a good example of this persistent tension between perceptions (or assumptions) of civility and the reality of the NTE.

In recent years, the City has seen an explosion of licensed premises, as the corporation embarked on a strategy of encouraging more residential and commercial development in the Square Mile, with prestigious large developments such as the Heron Tower near the Barbican Centre surging ahead despite the recession. As the Heron's own marketing literature highlights:

> The City of London is the financial capital of the world and is being transformed into a vibrant area full of culture, retail outlets and the very finest restaurants . . . the true secrets of the city reveal themselves when the working day ends. It's an area that's dynamic by day, but compelling by night. (Heron 2010).

While many might argue that the hoards of drinkers desperately seeking night buses outside nearby Liverpool Street Station is far from compelling, the City has nonetheless cultivated an aura of sophisticated drinking that is somehow seen as qualitatively distinct from the mainstream, uncouth spaces of the West End due to the socioeconomic profiles of City workers. As one borough councillor put it when questioned about the correlation between income and drinking:

> Q: 'It doesn't really explain why alcohol consumption is highest among higher earners than lower earners.'
>
> A: 'Well, higher earners drink in a different sort of way.'
>
> Q: 'Yeah. I mean, if you go to the City on a Friday or Saturday night, it's not that much different, I mean it's a different venue for drinking, it's a different amount of money that you're spending but there's still an extraordinary amount of alcohol being consumed and some quite lewd behaviour.'
>
> A: 'Yes. But it's sort of different lewd behaviour, isn't it? And what's more it's happening in a completely non-residential area.' (Central London Licensing Committee, interview, 2008)

Such assertions of fundamental difference are characteristic of the blatant class judgements that underscore many public health debates. Obesity, drinking and physical (in)activity are thus conceptually linked in the frequent elision of deprivation, income, ethnicity (in this case, white) and (wilful) ignorance. Thus, the City is a different type of drinking and a different type of drinker purely because 'high earners drink in a different sort of way', regardless of the reality examined in Chapter Seven that the highest earners drink the most consistently and the highest amount by occasion, therefore presenting significant public health risks of their own. Such logic then undoubtedly has a knock-on effect for the kind of urban spaces that are envisaged and imagined through the enterprise of alcohol governance. The City, long seen as problematic under the 24-hour city paradigm for being deserted after work and at weekends, is now suffering the effects of the profligate granting of licences while also actively seeking to expand its residential population. The result has been a rise in tensions between residents and the on-trade:

> 'The City have got all of these people living there who are seeing the explosion of the City as a business centre, but also as a leisure centre as well, so there is going to be some form of conflict in the City because of all of this.' (PubCo, interview, 2009)

There has also been a conflict over the types of nightlife permitted in the Square Mile and what Pratt (2009) has called its 'City Fringe'. As an example, a campaign to save the Light Bar, an eclectic venue just a few minutes north of Liverpool Street into Hackney, was started in 2008 after plans for a 1 million square feet mixed-use development by Foster and Partners were brought to Hackney Borough Council. This was finally resolved in 2009 after English Heritage threw its weight behind the Light Bar's fight to save Shoreditch's historical buildings from yet another developer's high-rise tower. Hackney Council ruled in favour of extending the

Shoreditch conservation zone and thus the Light Bar escaped a fate by bulldozer. The story of the Light Bar is, on the one hand, a classic gentrifier vs gentrified stand-off, but, on the other hand, when set within the specific context of the changing governance of the NTE, it exemplifies the ways in which alcohol is bound into competing narratives about who and what urban spaces should be for. In the case of 'edgy' Shoreditch, this is precisely *not* its neighbouring city boys. As *Time Out* states in its review of the Light Bar:

> On busy evenings, you can't move for booze-hungry drones, who celebrate the end of the day by invading each other's personal space and shouting loudly. Shame, really, because there are a number of high points, from the large beer garden and lengthy wine list to the loft-style top floor and balcony, which hosts the odd proper rave-up and lots of funky house. Developers have their eye on this place, so get there while you can. (*Time Out London* 2008).

It is worth noting that *Time Out* clearly proffers its preference for 'authentic' drinking experiences in its reviews and, as such, offers up particular aspirations for London's NTE which are often in stark contrast to the vision made reality through the Licensing Act. This is particularly evident when applied to the capability the Licensing Act gives to residents to complain about 'nuisance' premises that might provoke behaviours deemed anti-social (such as noise, public urination and vomiting, littering and violence). Even though this provides residents with greater powers to oppose existing and new licences, it has also meant a shift in the balance of power within the urban NTE:

> 'The Licensing Act gave the ability to people to suddenly say, "Oh, I'm not happy with that pub." It might have been there 300 years but again, the person might say, "I've been disturbed ever since I moved in here." The pub, on the other hand, might turn round and say, "Yeah, well, you chose to move in next to a pub." Which they'll often turn around and say, "Well, we've been here 300 years, we're part of this society."' (PubCo, interview, 2008)

This conflict has been made worse by the tendency of developers to build on urban infill sites often above or directly adjacent to existing or planned licensed premises, often thereby bringing incoming residents into direct conflict with the (often established) socialisation habits of others. Frequently, it is the problems of noise associated with the city's crowded pavements outside pubs and in beer gardens that have caused the most problems. These gatherings have been reinforced by the smoking ban and, as a response, residents' complaints have soared. For example, in Westminster: "One of the biggest problems we have is people drinking outside pubs, and there the most severe penalty we've established so far is to stop people being able to drink outside pubs after six o'clock at night" (Licensing Committee, interview, 2008). While this style of vertical alfresco drinking might be a very British variation on the DCMS's café culture aspirations, it has found itself caught in a legislative trap. In boroughs such as Westminster and Camden, the relationship between residents and the responsibility placed on the on-trade is further complicated by the significant through-flow of drinkers from outside the borough, which as one interviewee from the Licensing Committee argued, meant that their conduct was likely to suffer:

> 'The majority of people that drink in Westminster are not residents, certainly on a Friday and Saturday night within the West End, the number of residents drinking in there is not high, whereas in other areas of London it would be quite significant. So people that come to an area where they don't live, may either socialise frequently or have some connection through work or whatever, I think are prone to perhaps be . . . less inhibited in their behaviour at times, whereas elsewhere in London there's the fear of peer pressure, being recognised by family and friends.' (Licensing Committee, interview, 2008)

With few of the classic high streets of lore, London perhaps presents an even more contested nightscape than other cities. The drive to then create sensible people through the development of regularised, sensible drinking spaces by the conditions and sanctions attached to the Licensing Act is fraught with difficulty due to the problematic delineations of responsibility for transient drinkers. As a Camden Council representative highlighted: "We are, in a way, responsible for them because they are impacting on the residents that live there, but it does make things hard because you haven't got a captive audience, they're not accessing our services" (interview, 2009).

Using licensed premises as spaces of transformation to create the responsible, sensible drinker is thus often a wasted enterprise on highly mobile consumers. Under Section 141 of the Licensing Act, the licensee or their staff may risk a Fixed Penalty Notice of £80 or a fine of up to £1,000 for serving someone who is drunk, but once that person has left the premises, responsibility for their actions is technically passed on. The introduction of 'last drink analysis' in custody and Accident and Emergency settings has attempted to identify the premises to blame for individuals' later actions. But this seems ineffectual against persistent alcohol-related anti-social behaviour and/or harm. The last drink is not technically the one that causes the trouble to self and others, but rather it is the numerous drinks throughout the evening that set the stage for mischief. Thus, last drink analysis in an age of preloading is bound to vilify the on-trade disproportionately, instigating a causal link between premises and individual actions that may often have had their genesis in a much earlier trip to the supermarket. As Moriarty and Gilmore contend, 'we know that much of the alcohol that fuels the social disorder is bought at supermarkets and off licences, often heavily discounted, and drunk before going out, and now we have the prospect of "topping up" in the small hours at cheap prices in the corner shop or petrol station' (2006: 94). Yet, the Licensing Act still reinforces a vilification of the on–trade even while it piles control on control and regulation on regulation. The result, when set against the recession, the smoking ban and changing consumer habits, has been a shift in narratives of the NTE from pubs as culprits to (some) pubs as victims. This offers a new dynamic to designations of risk and responsibility in the alcohol control and sensible drinking debate.

The threatened NTE

The smoking ban, significant alcohol duty rises (2% above the rate of inflation imposed in March 2010), the recession that started in 2008, the beer tie and changing demographic and socioeconomic community profiles have hit the on-trade exceptionally hard, with the BBPA pressing particularly keenly to redirect the public debate away from binge drinking and onto the role and value of 'community' pubs (Muir 2008; Foster et al 2009). To this end, the BBPA has been vociferously transmitting the message that 40 pubs a week (1,973 in 2008) are closing in the UK, thus ensuring that this memorable statistic consistently finds a place in newspaper articles bemoaning the demise of the pub. More specifically, the BBPA's research has highlighted that there is a geographic logic to these closures, with suburban pubs the hardest hit (19 closures a week), followed by rural pubs (14) and then town centre establishments (8). With scarce credit to open new pubs, the total number of pubs in the UK has fallen by 4,271 since 2005 (CGA Strategy 2009). Not only do these statistics sit in stark contrast to assertions of the unfettered growth of the NTE, but they have also, understandably:

> '. . . generated a lot of concern, because pubs are perceived to be a British institution, an element of stability within a community, it's the thing that has probably had the biggest single effect in recent years. There really has been a concern amongst the media and amongst politicians.' (trade association, interview, 2009)

In London, 329 pubs closed between 2005 and 2009 and 30 pubs closed in Westminster alone between 2007 and 2009 (CGA Strategy 2009). This translates into a closure rate of 11 a week or a 5% loss since 2005, demonstrating that although London's NTE may exhibit stark differences to the rest of the country, similar factors are still precipitating pub closures. In order to explore this, interview respondents were asked whether and how drinking in London was different to the rest of the country. From a business and socioeconomic perspective, many saw a clear contrast. The capital's economy has shown to be more buoyant and resilient than many parts of the UK (boosted by tourism and spillovers from the City), as one respondent identified:

> 'London is a different country . . . the economic environment's just so much more robust in London compared to other places, the market here performs better from a bar point of view than probably anywhere else in the country. The use of pubs is very different . . . London's a

very young market. It's younger, it's more female, it's more affluent.'
(PubCo, interview, 2008)

Yet London also has a very transitory population, with a degree of mobility that sits at odds with expectations that a community pub should have a set of grounded and enduringly loyal locals. The threatened NTE thus represents the novel and underresearched elision of two debates – one on the nation's cultural ineptitude and incivility in the face of alcohol and the other on the pub as a cherished element of the nation's cultural identity. Furthermore, discourses about the threatened NTE represent a value judgement about the relative importance of the constitutive elements that compose a night out. At a political level, the importance of the pub was clearly articulated through the appointment of MP John Healey as minster for pubs in early 2010, but at the time of writing, no new minster had been appointed by the coalition government, despite the heartfelt pleas from the Campaign for Real Ale (CAMRA) and trade associations for the government to rethink the disproportionate compliance burdens that alcohol harm reduction legislation places on smaller pubs. Clearly, the momentum behind campaigns such as CAMRA's Save Our Pubs has served as a useful tool to start to think about the NTE in a more nuanced, variegated way, where 'responsible operators' can and do exist alongside irresponsible ones in an increasingly challenging marketplace. This sentiment of victimisation is made clear by the following interviewee: "We're not an industry that can cope with any more, you know, so if the government is intent on destroying us, well it's not going to take very much at the moment" (trade association, interview, 2008).

While for many in the public health lobby the demise of any drinking establishment might seem to mark renewed potential for creating a nation of sensible drinkers, pub closures lay bare a further and deeper level of contestation within the NTE. Pubs are exceptionally emotive places, an element of the drinking debate that is often overlooked in favour of highlighting drinking itself as an emotive and social practice and drinking places as loci of irresponsibility and danger. The fears over the threatened NTE are not, however, universally applied and often pertain only to fears over the loss of community and/or local pubs, rather than larger chain pubs or bars – a designation that is as much a qualitative statement concerning feelings of membership and inclusion as it is an expression of a particular business model operating according to 'impersonal' economies of scale. This value judgement, however, holds the potential to reinforce the current moral panic and widespread denigration of mass volume vertical drinking establishment and its irresponsible youth drinkers. Instead, responsible pub operators are suffering the disproportionate effects of legislative and economic pressures, with significant knock-on effects for the vitality and diversity of urban (and rural) locales. Somewhat problematically for those who enjoy denouncing youth excess, but also wish to keep hold of their local boozers, it is clear that while the two types of premises occupy different places in popular values systems, they both still rely on consumers drinking, whether sensibly or not.

It is clear that the recession has exposed gaping holes in the business and finance models of large PubCos and nightclub chains, but academic work on alcohol has been slow to think through their likely effects. Enterprise Inns hit the headlines in 2009 for its mammoth £3.5 billion debt, sparking a property sale with the company raising £60 million from the sale of 50 pubs in late 2009. Times are also tough for nightclubs. Operator Luminar Leisure, which runs 87 clubs in the UK – and is often maligned as being a core proponent of the youth-centred, binge drinking-fuelled NTE – saw its pretax profit fall from £31.5 million in 2008 to £4.4 million in 2010. Such a downturn in the company's performance has been attributed to a number of factors: spiralling youth unemployment (78% of Luminar's customers are aged 18–24) and the impact of later licences for pubs and bars on the nightclub trade. Luminar's annual report also highlights the competition that nightclubs face from other elements of the leisure industry, such as restaurants and cinemas as evidenced by a fall in sales of almost 20% in 2010 as admissions rates fell by 11% (Luminar Group Holdings plc 2010) across the country. Luminar is now locked into ensuring that its clubs remain 'fashionable, relevant and attractive to [their] core consumer' (ibid) – a difficult task among fickle and flighty young consumers faced with record levels of unemployment. However, those cheering the demise of the youth nightclub trade should also spare a thought for some of London's illustrious venues – Matter at the O$_2$ in North Greenwich has closed its doors after defaulting on a £3.2 million loan in early 2010 and, shortly after, superclub Fabric went into administration. The story of London's threatened NTE thus extends far beyond simple discourses of responsible and irresponsible drinking practices and policies.

The perilous state of the on-trade reveals a central irony: adherence to a neoliberal free market ideology is being blamed for fostering premises that promote binge drinking culture through mechanisms such as drinks promotions at the same time as a *lack* of free market competition in the licensed trade (the higher cost of 'tied' beer contracts forced onto licensees by PubCos) is causing massive pub closures. The difference is that the former venues are cast as 'irresponsible' (despite having to adhere to the multiple minutiae of licensing stipulations as discussed in the previous section), whereas the latter are deemed to be responsibly-run 'locals'. This double standard is captured by one interviewee:

> 'Consumption, for example, is declining, pubs are closing left, right, and centre, so you know, what actually is going on there? I mean, we can all see the BBC and people behaving stupidly, mostly young people behaving stupidly on the streets, but people's inhibitions are lower and society's sanctions on misbehaviour are less stern so they get away with it, and then the television cameras turn up and everybody says, "Oh my God, it didn't happen in my day, it's awful, awful, what you going to do about it, Mr Government?" And the government, who hates being nasty to people, except by taxing them, looks around, as I would describe it, for a stationary target with deep pockets and that

> looks like the pub. So if somebody's been sick in the streets outside the Dog and Duck it's probably the Dog and Duck's fault, isn't it?' (trade association, interview, 2008)

The layers and layers of compliance costs now placed on the on-trade have helped precipitate the current threat to the 'stationary target' of certain elements of the NTE. It is thus unsurprising that the industry representatives interviewed were keen to point out the multitudinous threats to the (well-run) pub, while those working in the public health field were concerned with the effect of pub closures in London only in so far as they might precipitate the prevalence of 'hidden harm' by reinforcing a turn to drinking in the home (Home Office 2003). This is perhaps unsurprising given that the objectives of the Licensing Act contain no reference to health and, as a result, a more holistic vision of drinking as part of a broader set of place-based activities that link into social capital accumulation is absent in public health policy thinking. In turn, this reveals the limits to public health's engagement with ecological or spatial thinking. This is despite the centrality of alcohol to the NTE; the NTE to public health; and the ecological to both the NTE and public health. Thus, health and planning remain pragmatically distanced, even as they grow ever closer in a conceptual sense.

The current threats to London's NTE demonstrate the importance of theorising alcohol not just as a drinking problem, but as a broader spatially conditioned socialisation problem. In turn, the changing face of Briton's socialisation habits and trends demands more nuanced attention from those in public health for they have distinct repercussions for health agendas. However, with a target-driven governance system, the lack of any health-specific targets for PSA 25 on alcohol and drugs severely undermines the possibility of bringing the spatial fully into health agendas, particularly for alcohol. As one interviewee suggested:

> 'I think the difficulty is the things that make a difference for health, those environmental factors, sit outside of health agenda. So there's a whole, this kind of joining up of environment and health means that there's this whole kind of world of people and it's not one holistic, although you're one person and your health is just what happens, what you experience, in professional terms there's a whole range of different professionals that you have to influence to make that happen on the ground.' (planner, interview, 2008)

Hence, while discourses of the threatened NTE are starting to open up much-needed new angles in the alcohol control debate, it does seem to mark the ongoing limit to public health's capacity to engage directly with urban and spatial agendas, a lack reinforced by the continued drive to keep alcohol firmly within the domain of crime and disorder. The quotation earlier also demonstrates that spatial thinking in a policy sense often goes beyond the logic dictated by present governmental structures and roles. Thus, in order for modes of thinking to be challenged and transformed and the division between the crime and public health lobbies in alcohol to be opened up, a far wider host of actors need to be brought together than is currently the case. In essence, the threats to the NTE reveal as much about the unsustainability of the political economy of the NTE as they do about the model of alcohol consumption that this is predicated on. At present, however, the NTE is threatened most of all by the extreme differences in cost between the on- and off-trade, and cheap drinking with home comforts seems now to be the logical endgame for both consumers and any hope of the 24-hour city. Governing public and private drinking are conceptually distinct undertakings and the retreat to the home (with a DVD and a six-pack) represents a definite challenge to alcohol harm reduction efforts that is inextricably linked into both the recession and the associated demise of the NTE.

Governing the public in private

The Licensing Act is underpinned by four objectives: the prevention of crime and disorder; ensuring public safety; the prevention of public nuisance; and the protection of children from harm. However, while disorder and nuisance are the most visceral effects of alcohol, it is the health harms (acute and chronic) that have the most sustained, long-term effects and, therefore, costs. With alcohol bought through the off-trade now sustaining growth in the alcoholic drinks market, at-home drinking has become a 'widely accepted social practice' (Holloway et al 2008: 543). As Foster et al argue, 'the portrayal of alcohol-related harm is concentrated upon binge drinking and the *visible* consequences presented by problematic drinkers. Furthermore, policy responses tend to be a reaction to the *visible* problems presented by binge drinking' (2010: 5, emphasis added). They further contend that 'drinking at home is uncontrolled and unregulated' and that this 'lack of scrutiny' is precisely one of the reasons why the home has become such an attractive, judgement-free place to drink (ibid). The culture of domestic drinking and preloading has, however, only recently caught academic attention (Plant and Plant 2006; Room and Livingston 2009; Wells et al 2009a, 2009b; Measham and Ostergaard 2010). As a result, the alcohol-control debate has only just started to acknowledge the consequences of an at-home drinking culture facilitated by increasing disparities between the on- and off-trade in terms of unit cost, levels of surveillance and regulation (Holloway et al 2008). Since the private realm of the home represents a fundamentally different locus for the genesis of sensible behaviours, this trend demands closer critical inspection for what it lends to debates concerning the spatialisation of urban alcohol governance agendas and, therefore, efforts to co-create sensible people and places.

Home drinking has profound consequences for the alcohol and health agenda. Wells et al argue, 'policies focused upon reducing drinking in licensed premises may have the unintended consequence of displacing drinking to pre-drinking environments, possibly resulting in greater harms' (2009a: 4). This is a form of spatial and social displacement, the effects of which are felt unevenly across age and socioeconomic groups. As Figure 36 clearly shows, the propensity to drink at

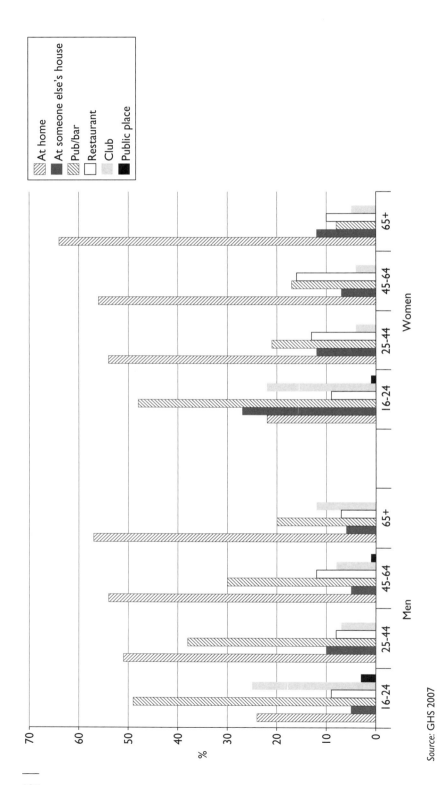

Source: GHS 2007

Figure 36: Location of respondent's heaviest drinking day last week by age

home rises with age, with only 24% of male and 22% of female 16- to 24-year-olds enjoying their heaviest drinking day at home, compared to 57% of male and 64% of female respondents aged over 65. However, when analysed by units consumed on the heaviest drinking session, a slightly different pattern emerges where at-home drinking is associated with lower levels of overall consumption compared to pubs and bars (Figure 37). For example, among men, 63% of drinking occasions within the daily guidelines occurred at home and only 21% in pubs or bars. By contrast, 32% of binge drinking occasions (more than 8 units) among men occurred at home, in contrast to 46% in pubs or bars. The pattern is slightly different among women, where 59% of 'sensible' drinking occurs at home and only 11% in pubs or bars. However, binge drinking among women is almost equally likely to take place at home as in pubs or bars (38% and 40% respectively), which marks out a particularly challenging governance issue.

There is thus a gendered inclination to drinking at home and, moreover, doing so at levels that constitute binge drinking. This has definitive consequences for a policy agenda centred on trying to create a sensible drinking culture through the application of regulations to licensed premises. For, as Wells et al (2009a, 2009b) assert, little consideration has been given to the policy implications of these practices. This is a particular oversight, especially given that domestic drinking is not only 'socially sanctioned', but that the 'ideological power of the home . . . legitimises hazardous/harmful drinking practices and leaves those consuming to unsafe levels in the home feeling unwarrantably insulated from concern' (Holloway et al 2008: 533). In governance terms, it is this dialectic between insulation and legitimation that represents a self-sustaining vortex from which it seems to be increasingly difficult to extricate workable understandings of what sensible behaviour means in both theory and practice. Moreover, although the turn to home drinking means that Britons are now spending less on alcohol than before, as Figure 38 shows, a fall in expenditure does not necessarily indicate a fall in volume – a problem exacerbated still further by the greater likelihood of home drinkers to underestimate their unit intake when compared to those drinking set measures through the on-trade.

The Licensing Act aims for 'the prevention of unreasonable diminution in the living and working amenity and environment of interested parties in the vicinity of premises balancing those matters against the benefits to be derived from leisure' (ODPM 2003: 31). While this is a worthy objective, it is spatially and temporally myopic when set against the increasing propensity of people to drink *away* from licensed premises. Furthermore, it seems insufficient when set against a political economic backdrop in which:

> 'Duty went up by about nine percent in the April 2008 budget and the week after the supermarkets were selling alcohol cheaper than they were selling it before because they're big enough to absorb that increase whereas pubs aren't. So pub prices go up and supermarket prices came down. And that's contributed to this shift in consumption

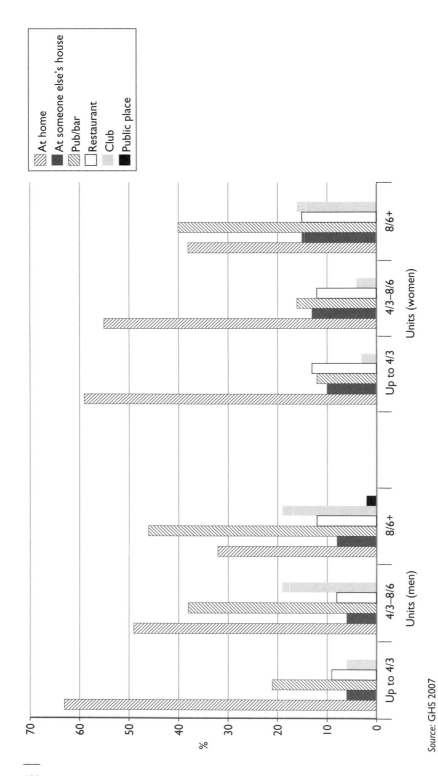

Source: GHS 2007

Figure 37: Location of heaviest drinking session in last week by average units consumed in 2007

Figure 38: Weekly household spend on alcohol

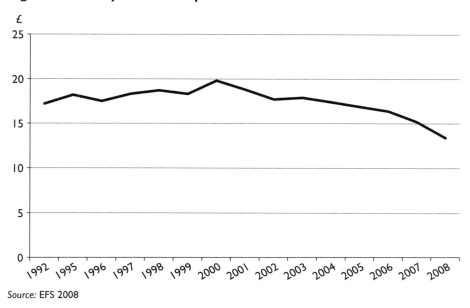

Source: EFS 2008

away from regulated licensed premises to drinking at home, it's just, "Why do I want to go out and spend all that on a pint of beer or a bottle of wine when it's going to cost me this much from Tesco?"' (nightclub, interview, 2008)

Home drinking is thus as much a rational economic choice as it is an emotive social practice that may or may not be viewed as problematic by either individuals or society (Holloway et al 2008). However, when drinking is contained in the home, it does not necessarily trivialise the health risks, even if the risks of being a victim of the crime, disorder or violence popularly associated with the NTE are reduced. Instead, home drinking brings with it new risks and rationalities of risk taking which, in turn, demand revised techniques of governance, given that the spatial logic of risk minimisation through environmental modification discussed earlier in this chapter cannot logically pertain to the home. As one industry respondent suggested:

'Alcohol consumption is increasing and it's going down in the pubs so it must be going up in the home. So if you're trying to affect that, to do so by legislation or tax is very difficult. I think you have to do it by behaviour and culture.' (PubCo, interview, 2008)

Until now, EU competition law has been invoked in order to stave off government regulation of the off-trade through measures to control and restrict supply, leaving education and behavioural change as the residual paradigms. As such, while the price of alcohol in the on-trade can be far more actively influenced through duty rises, this has a smaller effect on the off-trade, which has, as the quotation indicates, been able to absorb these rises and sell alcohol below the price of duty as a loss leader or pass on costs to producers through price promotions. In turn, recent strides towards developing a minimum pricing policy (of 40p a unit) have been cast aside in Scotland and are still under review in the UK. While there is some evidence to suggest that minimum pricing does reduce demand, especially for stronger drinks (spirits and strong lagers and ciders) most associated with alcohol-related harm (Chaloupka et al 2002; Anderson et al 2009; Wagenaar et al 2009), there has been strong political opposition to penalising the 'responsible majority' of drinkers through price rises. This libertarian viewpoint has been pounced on by some elements of the alcohol industry, who have argued that:

> 'If you introduce a measure like minimum pricing what you're actually doing is you're penalising everybody, so the people who enjoy a couple of glasses of wine a week at home face the same penalties as those who do actually abuse alcohol, so we would prefer to see policies and interventions that target those people that misuse.' (industry producer, interview, 2008)

This argument squarely reinforces a perceived divide between 'responsible' at-home drinking (which is rarely cast as excessive) and the abuse of alcohol most often assumed to be done through particular types of on-trade establishments. By extension, therefore, and because minimum pricing would serve to realign on- and off-trade prices (it is worth noting that, at the time of writing, Sainsbury's are selling thirty 440 ml cans of Strongbow for £15, or 50p each, in marked contrast to the average cost of a pint of Strongbow in a London pub at £3.20), it would have the effect of undoing the distancing of the two spatial and social spheres to which they pertain. The increased affordability of off-trade alcohol relative to income has courted considerable media attention and there would seem to be agreement that supermarkets are deeply culpable in fuelling a more complex set of risks in relation to alcohol than is conveyed by simplistic discourses of youth, town centre binge drinking. In short, the reduction of problem drinking to just these instances erases other loci of risk from both popular discourses and policy intervention, thereby reinforcing the difficulty in communicating sensible drinking messages. For, as one DAAT respondent suggested:

> 'It's much more a sense of how do you get a message out there about safe limits? And of course as soon as you get into safe limits people don't necessarily understand what those limits are. So we do work about people's understanding of what units are, and, boy, are they big compared to what you'd expect them to be . . . And but also that people quite often drink at home now, then obviously when people pour their own drinks the evidence indicates that they actually tend to be more liberal rather than less. So it's a complicated message to get out there.' (PCT, interview, 2008)

Indeed, as they further suggest, this complexity is reinforced by persistent, socially sanctioned risk tasking:

> 'So you know, it would be quite easy to think of a dinner party in someone's home where people get through a bottle of wine each. I'm sure that happens quite a lot but that doesn't seem to attract the same sort of set of issues.' (DAAT, interview, 2008)

Drinking at home represents a complex disjuncture. On the one hand, home is a space of safety and sanctity away from the perceived dangers of the NTE. On the other, given the freedoms of home consumption, measures and units are effectively nullified, undermining the quantitative logic of the sensible drinking messages discussed in the previous chapter. As Holloway et al (2008) have also asserted, home drinking involves complex discourses of justification and legitimation that, interestingly, rehearse the very café culture aspirations that characterised the rhetoric accompanying the DCMS's 24-hour city agenda. Moreover, they also have a tendency to mirror the logic found in the management of the on-trade where more expensive, cosmopolitan drinks are presumed to equate a more desirable clientele. Britain's ever-increasing wine consumption is thus valorised through a framework that combines European civility, taste and prestige, regardless of the total volume and frequency of consumption. The largely unknown nature of home-drinking patterns in comparison to the visibility of public drinking means that it can legitimately be argued that home drinking is, *tout court*, responsible drinking:

> 'You go into a bar and there's an offer on you're going to drink the alcohol there and then, so really cheap offers, large quantities of alcohol, tend to create drunkenness, anti-social behaviour and general harm, whereas an offer on a 24-pack of beer in Sainsbury's, supermarkets argue you might take home and drink over the course of one, two and three months.' (industry producer, interview, 2009)

While common sense dictates that it is possible, although deeply unlikely, for a pack of beer to last three months, the off-trade has still argued this line, given the lack of any evidence to the contrary. Yet, since home drinking increases with age and a lack of unit awareness means that home drinkers are less likely to self-identify as binge drinkers (both in terms of units consumed and because they do not exhibit the stereotypical 'determined drunkenness' tendencies associated with the term), there is a clear potential for hazardous and harmful levels of drinking reinforced through such dissociations (Griffin et al 2009). From a public health perspective, the consequences of the 'hidden harms' of domestic drinking are thus of clear concern. However, with drinking as a problem measured through targets such as 'perceptions of drunken and rowdy behaviour' and 'alcohol-related crime', governance structures conceived from a harm reduction standpoint barely impinge on domestic drinking, while the libertarian rhetoric of freedom for the responsible majority ensures that the real and imagined distancing of private and public drinking will continue.

Conclusion

This chapter has explored the limits to the spatial logic underpinning the governance of the contemporary NTE and its aspirations for a sensible drinking culture in the UK. Moving from the vision of the 24-hour city to the broader goals of New Labour's urban renaissance, it has charted the complex entanglements of urban, public health and crime and disorder agendas that have long marked alcohol harm reduction policies and strategies. Within these entanglements, the introduction of the 2003 Licensing Act has rendered drinking spaces strategic locations for the regulation and risk minimisation of drinking practices. In this logic, drinking practices can be used as vehicles to produce the desirable and urbane and to corral those deemed irresponsible, excessive or dangerous. However, such socio-spatial thinking, dedicated to the coproduction of sensible people and places is a logic limited to the public realm. In reality, drinking is increasingly shifting from the public spaces of bars, pubs and clubs to the private spaces of the home. In approaching these tensions between the public and private in responsibilisation strategies, this chapter has also questioned the persistent characterisation of the NTE as underregulated and out of control. In contrast, the discussion presented here argues that it is the overregulation of the NTE with its associated and increasingly complex burdens of regulatory compliance that is fundamentally undermining the NTE's very viability. The town centre thus remains a site of anxiety around particular excesses of youth drinking, but mitigating these anxieties has produced exceptionally comprehensive and often effective spatial management strategies. The research discussed here has demonstrated clear instances where these strategies are working actively to craft the NTE in a more regulated, desirable image, yet still clear tensions remain when trying to instrumentalise and rationalise the NTE to create a sensible drinking culture. As Norris and Williams suggest:

> Policies seeking to control the negative aspects of an alcohol-fuelled night-time economy through a combination of statutory regulation, enforceable penalties and an appeal to citizenship, responsibilisaton and the building/rebuilding of a civic culture are likely to break down at the frontier of the citizen-consumer dichotomy. (Norris and Williams 2008: 261)

This dichotomy is key to understanding the machinations of the NTE: while citizenship calls for responsible restraint, the figure of the good consumer really calls for another drink. It is also a particularly fluid dichotomy that necessitates exploration in situ. Such a geographic framework also reveals further layers of complexity contained in efforts to govern drink, drinking and drinkers. The research findings presented here were gathered during fieldwork in London, but the city's NTE must be understood as being both representative of broader issues in the UK and as being distinct and, in many ways, exceptional. As one respondent suggested:

'I think one of the problems we've got in London is it's so London focused. We've got a whole kind of debate about, oh, wine glasses, they're too big these days, all of our data shows that the only place that really has 250 ml wine glasses is London and the big urban capitals, other than that most places, most country pubs have 125 ml glasses. So we focus a whole kind of thought process on what they see in the bars around Westminster, isn't it dreadful?' (trade association, interview, 2008)

While criticism is often angled at the London-centric focus of the UK, it is important that in discussions of the NTE a focus on the capital does not falsely understate the scale and extent of binge, hazardous and harmful drinking. It is acknowledged that there is ample scope for Londoners to be more sensible with respect to drinking, and that their NTE exhibits many of the traits of diversity and vitality that characterised early calls for the 24-hour city. London's temporal and spatial patterns of socialising and sociability are quite distinct from other cities in the UK due to the effects of longer working hours, commuting, public transport use, a young population, greater affluence (as well as greater income inequalities) and a mobile population, 31% of whom were foreign-born at the time of the 2001 census (Wrendell and Salt 2005). Furthermore, with the greatest concentrations of foreign-born Londoners in the central boroughs – congruent with the city's core NTE – it is clear why diversity and difference are matched by the city's predilection for the maligned chain bars and pubs that throng high streets across the country. However, a discussion of the NTE needs to move beyond the fascination with 'the causes of the current culture in the young and how to change it' (Moriarty and Gilmore 2006: 94) and instead focus on bringing together a workable and systematic governance system that can combine harm reduction in a spatial paradigm that is able to inculcate the multiple pleasures associated with drinking. This seems increasingly unlikely within the tight regulatory confines ironically resulting from the liberalising intentions of the Licensing Act. The control of drinking establishments has not necessarily produced more controlled drinking, but it has produced more regularised environments in which pleasure is often sublimated to the micro- and macro-management of risk. Freedom and coercion thus meet in the spaces of the NTE and together shape not only risk and risk taking, but also a 'good night out'.

NINE

What life is this? Some concluding thoughts

As I write this conclusion, the UK and US are undergoing major governance upheavals. In the UK, the arrival of the coalition government in May 2010 instigated great debate about the future of public services and, therefore, the kinds of behavioural expectations, rights and responsibilities being placed on citizens. This renewed debate is notable principally because it demonstrates the temporal and spatial pervasiveness of the arguments about the role of sensible behaviour in urban governance regimes put forward in this book, as well as the entrenched and intractable nature of the risks associated with diet, sedentarism and drinking. In the US, Barack Obama has toiled to push health up the agenda, passing the landmark health care reform bill through the Senate in early 2010 and has since faced constant threats from the Right to repeal these advances. His wife, Michelle, has championed the cause of childhood obesity prevention through the Let's Move! programme and the transformation of a part of the White House lawn into a community garden. Yet, despite these efforts, preventing obesity, encouraging greater physical activity and moderating alcohol intake remain what Hunter (2009: 202) has pertinently described as 'wicked issues', or those which have 'complex causes and require complex solutions'. The discussions that have unfolded in this book have spanned the Atlantic and a five-year time period. They have also clearly illustrated this complexity as well as the intractability of the 'wicked' and the clear need to interrogate the variegated politicisations and problematisations of health. However, and as Hunter further identifies, the persistence of these wicked issues remains a facet of government 'preferring to regard such problems as being ones of individual lifestyle rather than being socially and structurally determined' (2009: 203). The inevitable result of this way of thinking is 'always to direct interventions to changing individual lifestyle rather than to reducing the health gap between social groups' (ibid). It is clear that as long as this oversight remains, then wicked issues will remain just so.

On both sides of the Atlantic, therefore, the debate over where the lines of responsibility should be drawn for health and ensuring the uptake of healthy lifestyles continues with little sign of resolution. The fact that this debate is so enduring gives an indication of the disjuncture between the outward simplicity of healthy lifestyle messaging (eat more fruit and vegetables, move more, drink less alcohol) and the pervasive complexity of defining, delineating and communicating what it is to be sensible and, moreover, encouraging the uptake of such behaviours. In large part, it is possible that this disjuncture is so entrenched because being sensible in contemporary neoliberal societies has come to symbolise far more than just health. Indeed, as this book has argued, sensible behaviour exists as both a spatial and a social strategic tool or 'fix' for some of the core tensions in neoliberalism, while also ensuring that its negative externalities can be transmogrified from risks to innovative market opportunities. Thus, in placing great expectation on the possibility and plausibility of being sensible and the host of commercial opportunities that these generate (such as advances in the leisure and fitness industry, new bar designs and formats and 'healthier' food choices), there is a danger that addressing the structural *causes* of poor health becomes overlooked in favour of providing new consumption solutions couched in the justificatory language of choice. For example, while MPREs offer a motivational route to increased participation in exercise, they do nothing to address the environmental barriers to activity at a city or local level. Moreover, their 12-week 'communication plan' offers little more than a temporary fix and is not tied in any way to the promotion of local sports facilities or clubs. This represents a real missed opportunity for the health promotion agenda. In this brief conclusion, the three core contentions of this book will be revisited, before we dwell in greater detail on the key findings and significance of this work through a critical reflection on the comparisons and contrasts between the empirical examples discussed.

Revisiting the three contentions

This book has centred on three core contentions that, in turn, have been critically examined through a series of empirical examples and case studies. In the first instance, it has argued that there needs to be far greater attention paid to the relative influence of 'luck' on responsibility and informed choice and, therefore, the plausibility of adopting sensible behaviour. In turn, the influence and significance of individual and geographical luck also demands further exploration. The operationalisation of informed choice and personal responsibility in neoliberal rhetoric, policy and practice is frequently communicated through the language, categorisation and expectation of sensible behaviour. Yet, despite semantic suggestions to the contrary, sensibleness is a dynamic and thoroughly malleable category, the definition of which has long mirrored social and political aspirations and fears. However, sensible behaviour does not exist extraneous to individual and collective luck and its expectation runs the risk of over-emphasising personal capacity for exercising the appropriate and necessary degree of responsibility and persistently underplaying the individual circumstances that may impede its realisation. The resultant culture of blame does nothing to improve health outcomes or the places that condition them.

In order to explore this contention, Chapter Two examined the centrality of informed choice and personal responsibility in neoliberal ideology, with a particular focus on the ascent of New Labour's public service reform Choice Agenda (Jordan 2006) and mounting political concern with individual lifestyle as risk. The neoliberal ideology of 'personalisation' (of state services) and 'responsibilisation' (of the self in relation to such services and fellow citizens), cast at an individual level, does not, however, sit easily with a perspective of social determinants of health that views health as patterned at broader, structural levels (Marmot 2005). The focus on personal responsibility assumes the existence of choice and yet, when such choices are patterned in ways that evade individual control there needs to be greater appreciation of the role of individual circumstance or luck in determining health outcomes. Under the present financial circumstances and particularly as medical services begin to be rationed in the NHS, moral ascriptions of responsibility and choice are only likely to increase in significance. Thus, attention to personal and geographical luck (or the fate of birthplace) is of central importance when arguing for behaviour change and the adoption of healthy lifestyles. Some places, as this book has shown, do not always enable true choice. Sometimes choices do exist, but rather the problem remains the assumption by those governing that the 'wrong' choices will be made by a culturally stereotyped population. This conflation of the spatial and the cultural was certainly the case in East Austin in attempts to prevent and manage obesity, but also has a strong presence in discourses of youth drinking in London. Risk, responsibility, choice and luck are complex moral and practical terrains, but often these categories become elided in the minds of those 'control workers' interviewed for this book. As a result, stereotyping of health behaviours is rampant and was often found to guide policy practice to a far greater degree than the use of baseline data.

The second contention for which this book argues concerns ways in which sensible behaviour has emerged as a strategic tool for the reconciliation of tensions inherent in neoliberal societies and economies. In effect, being sensible or the 'ordered obedience of the desired subjects of civic culture' (Miller 1993: xi) enables the consumption of self-control. Consumption is absolutely essential to the growth of the neoliberal economy, while self-control acts as a form of risk mitigation in a landscape across which risks are pervasive and can be pernicious. In order to manage these risks, the neoliberal subject must constantly balance three sets of elements: the urge for self-indulgence with the need for self-restraint; the promise of freedom with the persistence and necessity of coercion; and the realms of supply and demand. The examples discussed here demonstrate the dialectical relationships at work between these categories and, in the acts of their governance, in bringing them to some kind of resolution. Being prudent and, in the case of diet, exercise and alcohol, pursuing moderation (although *more* exercise is preferable for the majority of people) is, somewhat ironically, now also a huge market opportunity. This is less surprising when it is considered how poor health is routinely figured as a problem of incorrect supply (as well as irresponsible demand). To thus commodify sensible behaviour in the shape of new 'healthier' food products, the constantly evolving gym and leisure industry (Smith Maguire 2008) or through new bar and pub formats seems a logical market response to accusations of supply-side irresponsibility on the part of industry. However, simply ensuring supply does not guarantee demand, even when choice is touted as the rhetorical backbone of lifestyle.

The third contention that underpins this book argues that encouraging sensible behaviours with respect to healthy lifestyles exhibits a spatial logic and spatialising tendencies that extend far beyond public health and into, for example, the realms of urban planning, crime and disorder reduction, social inclusion agendas and urban regeneration. Indeed, such policies are indicative of a far wider turn to the spatial in both explaining and seeking solutions to public policy conundrums. However, the examples discussed here clearly demonstrate the limitations to the uptake and realisation of this spatial logic, despite its clear conceptual value and ethical significance when considered alongside the role of individual and geographical luck in health outcomes. Eliding the language and epistemology of behavioural and cultural change with framework of environmental determinants of health fundamentally reorientates the ways in which individuals and communities are called to task for their own health. This is primarily because of the limitations to divining causal influences on health at a variety of scales (for example individual, family, neighbourhood, city) and, therefore, delineating the most appropriate policy orientations and productive distribution of resources. Thus, with the built environment increasingly being cast in instrumental terms as a 'tool' for the realisation of this broad range of social policy objectives, exploring the problematics of public health therefore also comes to stand as a metonym for a host of broader urban issues and reflective of concerns and fears over the contemporary urban condition.

Chapter Three explores this re-spatialised public health, arguing that this mode of thinking engages health in complex dialectical interactions with environments (understood as an interlacing of built form, culture and political economy). In other words, in examining the intricacies of contemporary debates in public health on the ground, this book also explores how urban liveability (in its broadest sense) is now also being governed 'in the name of health'. Thus Gesler and Kearns (2002) assert, health is both a powerful metaphor and one that 'can steer place-making activities' (Geores 1998: 52). As such, and in recognition of Petersen and Lupton's (1996) call for greater attention to the political strategies deployed in the name of advancing the 'healthy city', Chapter Three also makes a case for the series of city-focused case studies that form the empirical core of this book. Yet, the interactions between urban spaces and public health exigencies exhibit marked variations depending on the lifestyle behaviour in question. For example, the urban politics of sensible drinking are far more politically entrenched in the UK than are those of obesity risk reduction, principally due to the ways in which drinking is repeatedly framed as an issue of crime and disorder rather than health (Herrick 2010). Problematisations of drinking among those interviewed thus exhibited strong geographical imaginations of cause and consequence. While those engaged in preventing obesity and encouraging sport also had a certain awareness of the salience of the spatial, the construction of policy priorities (targets) allowed little room to think through ways in which geographical risks might be managed or mitigated. As such, all three 'diseases of comfort' discussed in this book shed light on an array of conceptual and pragmatic limits to managing city environments in the name of health (Peterson and Lupton 1996: 136), where certain 'ecologies' (or ecological niches) are inherently more pathogenic or risky than others.

The governmental enterprise of encouraging and eliciting sensible behaviour among its citizenry has the hypothetical triple goal of creating better health, better places and better people. However, in reality and as the research discussed throughout this book shows, those engaged in developing and deploying policies or shaping the parameters of health debates often have a very limited appreciation of the spatial, despite the geographical referents and imaginaries included in an increasing array of government policy documents (see for example Department of Communities and Local Government 2007; Sport England 2008; Department for Communities and Local Government 2009; National Institute for Health and Clinical Excellence 2009; Lee et al 2010). This pervasive disjuncture between policy and practice represents a consistent impediment to heath improvement in all the cities discussed in this book. Crucially, this book is novel for exploring these limitations, inconsistencies and consequences of risk mitigation logic and strategies in situ and, in so doing, critically interrogating the lines of similarity and different between eating, exercising and drinking as risky behaviours. Such questions are exceptionally important for two reasons. First, eating habits, sedentarism and drinking in aggregate make up lifestyle and, therefore, risk. As such, disentangling causality and the relative effects of certain behaviours is virtually impossible (for example, might type 2 diabetes be primarily caused by elevated body mass as a result of excess calories or insufficient exercise?) However, the interlocked nature of these risks does not quash attempts to quantify and separate their causal influence on mortality and morbidity and, therefore, economic costs of all three behaviours, even as the methodologies used to do so (for example risk attributable or aetiologic fractions in the case of obesity) have been subject to huge criticism (Mokdad et al 2004; Couzin 2005; Mark 2005; Herrick 2007).

Second, there is limited evidence of best practice for preventing obesity, encouraging physical activity uptake and moderating drinking. Thus, with evidence-based policy the gold standard but with evidence scarce, there have been concerted efforts to learn from and draw parallels with other risky health behaviours and the tactics and techniques of their associated industries. For example, there have been concerted efforts to think through the commonalities between the history of effective tobacco control and the relative inertia of efforts to prevent obesity (Chopra and Darnton-Hill 2004) and to encourage moderate drinking (Bond and Daube 2009; Bond et al 2010). Of particular concern have been the tactics of Big Tobacco, Big Food and Big Booze respectively, and tracing the history of tobacco companies' promotional and regulation-evading strategies as a potential predictor for the future tactics of the food and alcohol industries. This insight is especially important given the political currency such companies hold as major contributors to national duty and tax income, and as large-scale employers as well as sitting on government advisory boards (the coalition's Responsibility Deals being a clear case in point here). Moreover, such comparisons are also useful for what they show about the relative efficacy of demand-side versus supply-side strategies for encouraging sensible behaviour and for the ways in which demand-side explanations of behaviour are often used as a convenient foil for protecting against increased regulation of supply such as the minimum pricing of alcohol or fat taxes, despite ardent calls to regulate supply by the public health lobby.

Eating, exercising and drinking: overlapping and discrete lifestyle risks

The discourse of 'healthy lifestyles' often elides quantitatively and qualitatively different behaviours. As a counter to this tendency, this book has brought together those behavioural realms that are too often considered as conceptually distinct issues or, famously in the case of alcohol, as 'no ordinary commodity' (Babor et al 2003). This assertion is immediately problematic as the risks discussed here are so potent *because* and not *in spite of* their ordinariness. As part of everyday, ordinary life, eating, exercising and drinking test the boundaries of choice and responsibility in markedly different ways. For example, individuals can, realistically, rarely exercise too much (although there are clear instances where this can happen in conjunction with eating disorders), and even gentle exercise is better than no exercise at all. However, the messaging for eating and drinking is more complex as it involves asking people to 'moderate' (usually reduce) their consumption and therefore remains open to wilful and self-serving interpretation. As Chapter Seven argues, the long-standing debate over units and risk thresholds for alcohol in the UK demonstrates very clearly the difficulties in deciding not just the levels at which risks lie, but also the degree to which such advice is likely to be socially and politically sanctioned. Despite their centrality to the direction taken by health policy, there has been far too little attention paid to the importance and dynamics of these sanctioning processes in urban environments. In response to this deficit, the research that underpins this book has uncovered some particularly interesting findings concerning the social and political negotiations over meanings that go into health promotion activities. In short, how a problem is framed will guide its likely solution. In this case, eating, drinking and exercise are framed in quite different ways for different risk groups in different locales.

This research has further revealed the dynamic and fleeting nature of health concerns. To clarify: a number of historical works have clearly shown the ebbs and flows of social and political concern with corporeal fatness (Schwartz 1986; Stearns 1997) over the last century. National fitness levels have been of episodic concern since John F. Kennedy's Cold War call to arms in the 'The soft American' (1960). In this he evocatively stated that 'the physical vigor of our citizens is one of America's most precious resources' and if this was to 'dwindle and grow soft' then America would be 'unable to realize [its] full potential as a nation'. Interestingly, this nationalistic concern with sports participation also mirrors the kind of language now being used to describe popular fears over the UK's levels of alcohol consumption vis-à-vis other (supposedly more disciplined) countries. While there is also a long history of concern with drinking (Kneale 1999;

Berridge 2005, 2006; Herring et al 2008a), it is only in recent years that data on consumption levels and trends has allowed for international comparisons. As Chapter Seven discussed, the assertion that the UK has the 'worst' drinking habits in Europe (NHS Confederation 2010) has realigned the alcohol-control debate in more geographically comparative terms. However, over the shorter time scales explored in this research, interest in such risk behaviours often shifts according to the funding and ideological priorities of government. These shifts, while often temporary, are rarely innocuous.

In the case of obesity, for example, such a situation was found in both London and Austin. Even in the time between my two visits to Austin in 2005 to 2006, there was a palpable sense of disappointment that the energy and enthusiasm so clear in 2005 had not been harnessed into any concrete and concerted city-wide action to prevent further rises in obesity. One interviewee aptly summed up this sentiment when he said "it feels a little like fatigue, fat fatigue . . . The interest in it is there, but not as fanatical as it was" (TDHHS, interview, 2006). Another interviewee also corroborated this malaise with the suggestion that, "the media spotlight has waned, the attention, the obsession, has gone onto other things" (PR and media, interview, 2006). While those in public health and the voluntary and community sector in both Austin and London were exceptionally keen to exploit political momentum around obesity prevention, it was often the case that short-term funding streams (that is, the money from Choosing Health) would often only pay for someone to be in post for a couple of years to oversee, for example, a PCT's obesity strategy. This was also the case for funding posts around alcohol harm reduction and in sports promotion. Thus, while the historical accounts discussed here suggest some degree of continuity in social attitudes towards health risks, the empirical research demonstrates a temporal mismatch in governmental commitment. In spite of the tone of David Cameron's Big Society thesis, coordinated heath action needs money. When this is short lived, or the conditions attached to it have a propensity to change suddenly (as in the sudden shift from a concern with women's health to men as a more significant health risk group in the UK), then health promotion and risk reduction work suffers.

As this book has shown, there are clear practical and financial constraints to shaping individual and population health behaviours in more sensible ways. However, the arguments made to justify differing resource allocations also highlight the varying ways in which each of the behaviours discussed here contributes to or risks the diminution of 'the good life' or 'wellbeing'. This is particularly the case as 'individualized freedom of choice can undermine social attempts to consider appropriate levels of consumption' (Hanlon et al 2010: 310). It is this tension between individual wants and social needs that so often undermines the pursuit of the good life. The split between the desire to grant and take advantage of freedom and the need to set boundaries based on risk calculations is evident in all the case studies. However, the risk calculations are constantly contested, often contradictory, subject to international variations and often communicated in ways that leave the consumer either bemused or determined to reinterpret risk thresholds in a manner that gels more neatly with prevailing social norms. This is particularly the case with regards to the self-denial and short-term risk calculations that so often accompany drinking, but is also plainly evident in the mismatch between high *awareness* levels of guidelines such as 'five a day' and relatively low consumption rates of fruit and vegetables. The exceptionally slow rises in sports participation despite financial investment, clear government interest and continual advances in the political economy of leisure is also testament to the creative and self-legitimising inertia of many consumers. To be sensible is thus to be torn between the consumption habits that are the right of freedom and the constraint that is needed to skirt the threat of coercion that so often hangs heavily and uneasily over neoliberal societies.

Is there a way forward?

It is not the goal of this book to offer a list of definitive policy recommendations. Instead, it would seem fitting to ask what lessons can be learned from bringing together this set of health risks across a number of case study sites. These, it is argued, are fivefold. First, while eating, drinking and exercise are considered separately in this book, they also need to be theorised in tandem. Such thinking is antithetical to governmental agenda and priority setting (which most often proceeds in strategies defined by health risk), but it is only in seeing these risks as mutually reinforcing that these practices might start to incorporate broader conceptions of wellbeing that might also expand discussions to include environmental modifications, rather than simply focusing on narrowly measured indicators of individual health (such as BMI).

Second, any examination of health, as Wilkinson (2005) reminds us, sheds light on the problems with place. In so doing, it also offers up some idea about the ways in which places might be improved in order to influence health outcomes positively. While the research found a keen awareness of the influence of place on health among some interviewees, it was more often the case that targets (for example NI8 for sports participation) tended to focus on individual outcomes rather than on removing the structural barriers to behaviour change and thereby addressing certain social determinants of health. What was so often missing was a genuine desire to redesign quality environments and places, despite such spatial aspirations being of core importance to the original aspirations of public health (MacKian et al 2003) and an increasing prevalence of design guidelines for more active communities. Poor health demands a geographical resolution. The current concern with healthy lifestyles represents a huge opportunity to mobilise resources and momentum behind creating better places. So far, these efforts have been far too limited.

Third, the actions of a few influential individuals can often have more impact than the actions of many. This was clear in both Austin and Newcastle, where the business interests of Paul Carrozza and Brendan Foster respectively have been productively and profitably interwoven with public health concerns. While the impact of MPREs on longer-term sports participation is clearly dubious and in need of far more research, the influence of their champions is marked. This 'go-getting' spirit is something to be harnessed rather than dismissed. Those in Austin were able to do this through Paul Carrozza's role on the Governor's Council. However, the inability of those in Newcastle to harness the resources and influence of Foster's company remained a profound source of frustration, especially given the clear value that would be derived from any collaborative effort.

Fourth, private and public sector roles in health are becoming increasingly blurred, especially as corporate social responsibility agendas allow industry to enter the realm of health promotion. This is not necessarily of concern in itself, but rather for the ways in which it problematises the contractual relationship between the state and individuals that forms the bedrock of admonitions to be sensible. This blurring is symptomatic of the changing nature of health information and advice which is now overwhelmingly to be found online rather than in medical settings, but it is also indicative of the changing direction of public trust as well as the permeation of health agendas into a host of other political policy arenas. In short, while individuals might once have looked to the state to ensure their right to good health, this orientation is increasingly taking in the private and voluntary and community sectors. While the irony of companies such as Nestlé or Kraft promoting healthy lifestyles may seem ironic, the resources that they bring and their capacity to fund research present perhaps the greatest threat to the public sector's hold on health promotion. There thus needs to be greater critical exploration of these shifts rather than their dismissal if health promotion is to avoid being hijacked and commodified.

This leads to the fifth and final point; more research is needed that critically interrogates the relationships between political economy and health behaviours. For many in public health, 'industry' is a dirty word, and the bitter taste left by the business practices and legacies of Big Tobacco has understandably lingered. Moreover, in seeking to second guess the future tactics of the food and drink industries, some sight has been lost of the role played by consumer demand in creating health risks. While supply is a significant element of the genesis of risk, it is only one part of the political economic contract. It is clear that demand is infinitely malleable. However, consumer demands are also symptomatic of the kind of discordant interactions between self and environment that this book has discussed. In other words, consumer demands often express a profound individual or group need; they also clearly exemplify specific sites of societal anxiety where self-efficacy is persistently absent. One clear example is the socially normative assumption that an alcoholic drink will bolster confidence and sexual attractiveness on a night out. The UK government has tried to discredit this with its 'Know your Limits' campaign, in which the consequences of a drunken night out are replayed in reverse to the viewer from finish to start with the strapline, 'You wouldn't start a night like this, so why end it this way?' However, we still have insufficient knowledge of the contextualising processes that make definition of risk thresholds socially resonant. This is a crucial knowledge deficit, especially given the ongoing work of industry to reframe biomedical research, shape the ensuing debates and, therefore, fundamentally alter the processes of contextualisation that serve to legitimise certain risk-taking behaviours. For these reasons, future research needs to be attuned to the politicisations of the political economic and the significance of these processes for the dynamic interactions of supply and demand.

Osborne suggests that the concept of health possesses both an 'essential elasticity' and 'indeterminacy' and that, for this reason, 'health cannot be associated with normality, but only with normativity, with the capacity to impose new norms' (1997: 180). As he further asserts, when political attempts are made to 'absolutise' or 'make determinate' the concept of health, then health itself is transformed from a *right* to a *duty* of citizenship. In all the examples discussed in this book, health sits – albeit in various ways and to varying degrees – at the fulcrum of right and duty. This is especially the case given that the health risks under consideration often arise through legitimate and socially sanctioned consumption norms. Yet, when health becomes a necessary duty in order to qualify for treatment, as is increasingly becoming the case in the resource-starved NHS, then these risky consumption practices may need not just to be questioned but also restricted. To do so would require the brave and exceptionally unpopular move of regulating choice and, as a result, diminishing certain freedoms. A clear example would be addressing the supply of alcohol through minimum pricing in the UK. This would seem to offer a way to work with consumers' immediate cost aversions in order to reorientate the popular view of alcohol from disposable, cheap commodity to one with greater social value. That this would penalise the 'responsible majority' then depends on how the term 'penalty' is defined and understood. If moderation is the goal, then there is no financial penalty to be had from consuming less alcohol at a higher price. However, if pleasure through freedom is the goal, then any restriction can rightly be construed as penalty. But, with affluent societies irrecoverably divided along socioeconomic and ethnic lines, freedom of consumption is already a misnomer. Consumption habits are fickle and liable to rapid change, yet the geographies of threat and opportunity that so often pattern health behaviours are deeply rooted. It is these roots that need prompt excavation if we are to forge not just healthier people, but also better places.

Bibliography

Abbas, A. (2004). 'The embodiment of class, gender and age through leisure: a realist analysis of long distance running'. *Leisure Studies* **23**(2): 159–75.

Airey, L. (2003). '"Nae as nice a scheme as it used to be": lay accounts of neighbourhood incivilities and well-being'. *Health and Place* **9**(2): 129–37.

Aitch, J. (2009). 'The great alcohol myth'. *The Guardian*, 26 January.

Allum, N. and D. Boyd (2002). 'European regions and the knowledge deficit model'. *Biotechnology: The Making of a Global Controversy*. M. Bauer and G. Gaskell. Cambridge, Cambridge University Press: 224–44.

Anderson, P., D. Chisholm, et al. (2009). 'Effectiveness and cost-effectiveness of policies and programmes to reduce the harm caused by alcohol'. *The Lancet* **373**(9682): 2234–46.

Andranovich, G., M. J. Burbank, et al. (2001). 'Olympic cities: lessons learned from mega-event politics'. *Journal of Urban Affairs* **23**(2): 113–31.

Atkinson, G., S. Mourato, et al. (2008). 'Are we willing to pay enough to "back the bid"?: valuing the intangible impacts of London's bid to host the 2012 Summer Olympic Games'. *Urban Studies* **45**(2): 419–44.

Austin/Travis County Health and Human Services Department (2005). *Steps to a Healthier Austin: Behavioral Risk Factor Surveillance System 2005 Report*. Austin: TDHHS.

Babor, T. F. (2008). 'Tackling alcohol misuse in the UK'. *British Medical Journal* **336**(7642): 455.

Babor, T., R. Caetano, et al. (2003). *Alcohol: No Ordinary Commodity. Research and Public Policy*. Oxford:, Oxford University Press.

Bale, J. (2004). *Running Cultures: Racing in Time and Space*. London, Routledge.

Ball, D. (2003). 'Guest editorial: the limits of sensible drinking'. *Drugs and Alcohol Today* **3**(3): 2–3.

Ball, D., R. Williamson, et al. (2007). 'In celebration of sensible drinking'. *Drugs: Education, Prevention, and Policy* **14**(2): 97–102.

Bandura, A. (1982). 'Self-efficacy mechanism in human agency'. *American Psychologist* **37**(2): 122–47.

Bandura, A. (1995). *Self-efficacy in Changing Societies*. Cambridge, Cambridge University Press.

Bandura, A. (2004). 'Health promotion by social cognitive means'. *Health Education and Behaviour* **31**(2): 143–64.

Banerjee, A., D. Basu, et al. (2006). 'How responsible is responsible drinking: an evidence based review'. *Journal of Mental Health and Human Behavior* **11**(1): 23–33.

Barr, A. (1995). *Drink: An Informal Social History*. London, Bantam.

Barr, S. (2006). 'Environmental action in the home: investigating the "value-action" gap'. *Geography* **91**(1): 43–54.

Bassett, D., J. Puchner, et al. (2008). 'Walking, cycling, and obesity rates in Europe, North America, and Australia'. *Journal of Physical Activity and Health* **5**: 795–814.

Bassler, T. and J. Scaff (1975). 'Letter to the editor'. *New England Journal of Medicine* **292**: 1302.

Bauman, Z. (2005). *Liquid Life*. London, Polity.

Beccaria, F. and F. Prina (2009). 'Young people and alcohol in Italy: an evolving relationship'. *Drugs: Education, Prevention and Policy. 17(2): 99-122*

Beckford, M. (2009). 'Millions of middle-class drinkers putting health at risk with evening tipple'. *The Telegraph*. 22 January.

Bell, D. (2008). 'Destination drinking: toward a research agenda on alcotourism'. *Drugs: Education, Prevention, and Policy* **15**(3): 291–304.

Bell, D. W. and V. M. Esses (2002). 'Ambivalence and response amplification: a motivational perspective'. *Personality and Social Psychology Bulletin* **28**(8): 1143–52.

Berking, H. and S. Neckel (1993). 'Urban marathon: the staging of individuality as an urban event'. *Theory, Culture and Society* **10**(4): 63–78.

Bernays, E. L. (1947). 'The engineering of consent'. *Annals of the American Academy of Political and Social Science* **250**: 113–20.

Berridge, V. (2005). *Temperance: Its History and Impact on Current and Future Alcohol Policy*. London, Joseph Rowntree Foundation.

Berridge, V. (2006). 'New strategies for alcohol policy: lessons from history?' *Drugs: Education, Prevention, and Policy* **13**(2): 105–8.

Berry, A. and N. Fleming (2007). 'Scale of harmful middle class drinking revealed'. *The Telegraph*, 16 October.

Berry, W. (1999). 'The pleasures of food'. *Cooking, Eating, Thinking: Transformative Philosophies of Food*. D. Curtin and L. Heldkee. Bloomington, University of Indiana Press: 374–80.

Bianchini, F. (1995). 'Night cultures, night economies'. *Planning Practice and Research* **10**(2): 121–6.

Black, J. L. and J. Macinko (2008). 'Neighborhoods and obesity'. *Nutrition Reviews* **66**(1): 2–20.

Blair, T. (2005). 'Tony Blair's speech on compensation culture'. London, IPPR. Full text available at www.guardian.co.uk/politics/2005/may/26/speeches.media

Blakely, E. and M. Snyder (1999). *Fortress America: Gated Communities in the United States*. New York, Brookings Institute.

Blythman, J. (2004). *Shopped: The Shocking Power of British Supermarkets*. London, Fourth Estate.

Bond, L. and M. Daube (2009). 'Access to confidential alcohol industry documents: from "Big Tobacco" to "Big Booze"'. *Australasian Medical Journal* **1**(3): 1–26.

Bond, L., M. Daube, et al. (2010). 'Selling addictions: similarities in approaches between big tobacco and big booze'. *Australasian Medical Journal* **3**(6): 325–32.

Booth, D. (2003). 'Hitting apartheid for six? the politics of the South African sports boycott'. *Journal of Contemporary History* **38**(3): 477–93.

Booth, K. M., M. M. Pinkston, et al. (2005). 'Obesity and the built environment'. *Journal of the American Dietetic Association* **105**(5): S110–17.

Boseley (2007a). 'Scale of harmful middle class drinking revealed'. *The Guardian*, 16 October.

Boseley, S. (2007b). 'Date for halting childhood obesity slips back 10 years'. *The Guardian*, 17 October.

Boutayeb, A. (2006). 'The double burden of communicable and non-communicable diseases in developing countries'. *Transactions of the Royal Society of Tropical Medicine and Hygiene* **100**(3): 191–9.

Brenner, H. (1995). 'Political economy and health'. *Society and Health*. H. Amick, S. Levine, A. Tarlov and D. Chapman Walsh. Oxford, Oxford University Press: 211–46.

Brenner, N. and N. Theodore (2005). 'Neoliberalism and the urban condition'. *City: Analysis of Urban Trends, Culture, Theory, Policy, Action* **9**(1): 101–7.

British Beer and Pub Association (2007). *Statistical Handbook 2007*. London. BBPA

British Beer and Pub Association (2009). *Statistical Handbook 2009*. London. BBPA

British Medical Association (1995) *Alcohol: Guidelines on Sensible Drinking*. London: BMA

British Medical Association (2008). *Alcohol Misuse: Tackling the UK Epidemic*. London, BMA.

British Transport Police data (2009). http://data.london.gov.uk/datastore/package/pedal-cycle-theft-incidents-recorded-british-transport-police

Brown, A. L., A. J. Khattak, et al. (2008). 'Neighbourhood types, travel and body mass: a study of new urbanist and suburban neighbourhoods in the US'. *Urban Studies* **45**(4): 963–88.

Brown, D. (2007). 'Hazardous drinking, the middle-class vice'. *The Times*, 16 October.

Brown, T. and M. Bell (2008). 'Imperial or postcolonial governance? Dissecting the genealogy of a global public health strategy'. *Social Science and Medicine* **67**(10): 1571–9.

Brown, T. and C. Duncan (2002). 'Placing geographies of public health'. *Area* **34**(4): 361–9.

Brownall, K. and K. Battel Horgen (2003). *Food Fight*. Boston, McGraw Hill.

Burbank, M. J., G. Andranovich, et al. (2002). 'Mega-events, urban development and public policy'. *Review of Policy Research* **19**(3): 179–202.

Cabinet Office (2004). *Personal Responsibility and Changing Behaviour: The State of Knowledge and its Implications for Public Policy*. London, PM's Strategy Unit.

Cabinet Office (2008). *Achieving Culture Change: A Policy Franework*. London, PM's Strategy Unit.

Cabinet Office (2010). *Mindspace: Influencing Behaviour through Public Policy*. London, Institute for Government.

Campbell, D. (2010a). 'How can we balance personal freedoms with public health?' *The Guardian*, 7 July.

Campbell, D. (2010a). 'Leading doctors call for urgent crackdown on junk food'. *The Guardian*. London, 11 July.

Campos, P. (2004). *The Obesity Myth. Why America's Obsession with Weight is Hazardous to your Health*. New York, Gotham Books.

Campos, P., A. Saguy, et al. (2006). 'The epidemiology of overweight and obesity: public health crisis or moral panic?' *International Journal of Epidemiology* **35**(1): 55–60.

Cappelen, A. W. and O. F. Norheim (2005) 'Responsibility in health care: a liberal egalitarian approach'. *Journal of Medical Ethics* 31(8): 476-480.

Carlsen, J. and A. Taylor (2003). 'Mega-events and urban renewal: the case of the Manchester 2002 Commonwealth Games'. *Event Management* **8**: 15–22.

Carmona, R. (2003). 'The obesity crisis in America: testimony before the Committee on Education Reform, Committee on Education in the Workforce and the United States House of Representatives'. www.surgeongeneral.gov/news/testimony/obesity07162003.htm.

Centers for Disease Control (2005). 'Social marketing'. www.cdc.gov/communication/practice/socialmarketing.htm.

Centers for Disease Control (2007). 'National diabetes fact sheet'. Atlanta, CDC.

Centers for Disease Control (2009) *Behavioral Risk Factor Surveillance System*. Atlanta, CDC.

Centers for Disease Control (2010). 'Healthy weight'. www.cdc.gov/healthyweight/.

Central Office of Information (2009). *Communications and Behaviour Change*. London, COI.

CGA Strategy (2009). *Analysis of Pubs by Constituency (England, Scotland, Wales Only)*. Stockport, CGA.

Chaloupka, F., M. Grossman, et al. (2002). 'The effects of price on alcohol consumption and alcohol-related problems'. *Alcohol Research and Health* **26**: 22–34.

Chan, A. (1986). 'Racial differences in alcohol sensitivity'. *Alcohol Alcohol* **21**(1): 93–104.

Chatterton, P. and R. Hollands (2003). *Urban Nightscapes: Youth Cultures, Pleasure Spaces and Corporate Power*. London, Routledge.

Chief Medical Officer (2004). *On the State of Public Health: Annual Report of the Chief Medical Officer 2004*. London, DH.

Chiolero, A. and F. Paccaud (2009). 'An obesity epidemic booga booga?' *European Journal of Public Health* **19**(6): 568–9.

Choi, B. C. K., D. J. Hunter, et al. (2005). 'Diseases of comfort: primary cause of death in the 22nd century'. *Journal of Epidemiology and Community Health* **59**(12): 1030–4.

Chopra, M. and I. Darnton-Hill (2004). 'Tobacco and obesity epidemics: not so different after all?' *British Medical Journal* **328**(7455): 1558–60.

City of Austin Police Department (2009). *Indexed and Non-Indexed Offenses by Zip Code*. Austin, CAPD.

City of Copenhagen (2002). *Cycle Policy 2002–2012*. Copenhagen, City of Copenhagen.

Clark, J. (2010). 'Supermarkets slash beer prices'. *The Independent*, 5 May.

Clarke, J. (2005). 'New Labour's citizens: activated, empowered, responsibilized, abandoned?' *Critical Social Policy* **25**(4): 447–63.

Clarke, J. (2007). 'Unsettled connections: citizens, consumers and the reform of public services'. *Journal of Consumer Culture* **7**(2): 159–78.

Clarke, J., N. Smith, et al. (2006). 'The indeterminacy of choice: political, policy and organisational implications'. *Social Policy and Society* **5**(3): 327–36.

Clough, P., J. Shepherd, et al. (1989). 'Marathon finishers and pre-race drop-outs'. *British Journal of Sports Medicine* **23**(2): 97–102.

Cobb, N. (2007). 'Governance through publicity: Anti-Social Behaviour Orders, young people, and the problematization of the right to anonymity'. *Journal of Law and Society* **34**(3): 342–73.

Cohen-Cole, E. and J. M. Fletcher (2008). 'Is obesity contagious? social networks vs. environmental factors in the obesity epidemic'. *Journal of Health Economics* **27**(5): 1382–7.

Colls, R. and B. Evans (2009). 'Introduction: questioning obesity politics'. *Antipode* **41**(5): 1011–20.

COMEDIA and the Gulbenkian Foundation (1991). *Out of Hours: A Study of Economic, Social and Cultural Life in Twelve Town Centres across the UK*. London: Coluste Gulbenkian Foundation .

Commission on Social Determinants of Health (2008). *Closing the Gap in a Generation: Health Equity through Action on the Social Determinants of Health*. Geneva, WHO.

Conrad, P. (1994). 'Wellness as virtue: morality and the pursuit of health'. *Culture, Medicine and Psychiatry* **18**(3): 385–401.

Corburn, J. (2004). 'Confronting the challenges in reconnecting urban planning and public health'. *American Journal of Public Health* **94**(4): 541–6.

Cornelissen, S. (2004a). '"It's Africa's turn!" The narratives and legitimations surrounding the Moroccan and South African bids for the 2006 and 2010 FIFA finals'. *Third World Quarterly* **25**(7): 1293–309.

Cornelissen, S. (2004b). 'Sport mega-events in Africa: processes, impacts and prospects'. *Tourism and Hospitality, Planning and Development* **1**(1): 39–55.

Cornelissen, S. (2008). 'Scripting the nation: sport, mega-events, foreign policy and state-building in post-apartheid South Africa'. *Sport in Society: Cultures, Commerce, Media, Politics* **11**(4): 481–93.

Cornelissen, S. (2010). 'Football's tsars: proprietorship, corporatism and politics in the 2010 FIFA World Cup'. *Soccer and Society* **11**(1): 131–43.

Cornelissen, S. and K. Swart (2006). 'The 2010 Football World Cup as a political construct: the challenge of making good on an African promise'. *Sociological Review* **54**(s2): 108–23.

Council of Europe (1992). *European Sports Charter*. Strasbourg, Council of Europe.

Couzin, J. (2005). 'Public health: a heavyweight battle over CDC's obesity forecasts'. *Science* **308**(5723): 770–1.

Coveney, J. (1999). *Food, Morals, and Meaning: The Pleasure and Anxiety of Eating*. London, Routledge.

Coveney, J. and R. Bunton (2003). 'In pursuit of the study of pleasure: implications for health research and practice'. *Health (London)* **7**(2): 161–79.

Coyle, N. and J. Fitzpatrick (2009). *Health and Lifestyle in London: Initial Findings from the London Boost of the Health Survey for England*. London, London Health Observatory.

Coyle, N., J. Fitzpatrick, et al. (2009). *Health Survey for England 2006 London Boost: Health and Lifestyle in London Main Report*. London, London Health Observatory.

Crampton, J. and S. Elden, eds (2007). *Space, Knowledge and Power: Foucault and Geography*. London, Ashgate.

Critser, G. (2004). *Fat Land: How Americans Became the Fattest People in the World*. Denver, CO, Houghton.

Crumley, B. (2008). 'French combat youth binge-drinking'. *Time Magazine*. 17 July.

Cummins, S. (2003). 'From observation to experimentation: one prescription for a geography of public policy'. *Area* **35**(2): 220–2.

Cummins, S. (2007). 'Commentary: investigating neighbourhood effects on health – avoiding the "local trap"'. *International Journal of Epidemiology*: 36(2): 355-357.

Cummins, S., A. Diez Roux, et al. (2007). 'Understanding and representing place in health research: a relational approach'. *Social Science and Medicine* **65**: 1825–38.

Cummins, S. and S. Macintyre (1999). 'The location of food stores in urban areas: a case study in Glasgow'. *British Food Journal* **101**: 545–53.

Cummins, S. and S. Macintyre (2002). '"Food deserts": evidence and assumption in health policy making' *British Medical Journal* **325**(7361): 436–8.

Cummins, S. and S. Macintyre (2002). 'A systematic study of an urban foodscape: the price and availability of food in Greater Glasgow'. *Urban Studies* **39**: 2115–30.

Cummins, S. and S. Macintyre (2006). 'Food environments and obesity: neighbourhood or nation?' *International Journal of Epidemiology* **35**(1): 100–4.

Curtis, J. (2004). 'Should the private sector "sell" health?' *Marketing*, 24 November.

Curtis, S., B. Cave, et al. (2002). 'Is urban regeneration good for health? perceptions and theories of the health impacts of urban change'. *Environment and Planning C-Government and Policy* **20**(4): 517–34.

Davey Smith, G., D. Dorling, et al. (2002). 'Health inequalities in Britain: continuing increases up to the end of the 20th century'. *Journal of Epidemiology and Community Health* **56**(6): 434–5.

Davey Smith, G., C. Steer, et al. (2007). 'Is there an intrauterine influence on obesity? Evidence from parent–child associations in the Avon Longitudinal Study of Parents and Children (ALSPAC)'. *Archives of Disease in Childhood* **92**(10): 876–80.

Davis, M. (1990). *City of Quartz: Excavating the Future in Los Angeles*. New York, Verso.

Davis, M. (2000). *Magical Urbanism: Latinos Reinvent the US City*. London, Verso.

Day, K., B. Gough, et al. (2004). 'Warning! alcohol can seriously damage your feminine health'. *Feminist Media Studies* **4**(2): 165–83.

Dean, M. (1995). 'Governing the unemployed self in an active society'. *Economy and Society* **24**(4): 559–83.

Dean, M. (2007). *Governing Societies: Political Perspectives on Domestic and International Rule*. London, Blackwell.

Dean, M. (2010). *Governmentality: Power and Rule in Modern Society*. London, Sage.

Department for Communities and Local Government (2007). *Place Matters*. London, DCLG.

Department for Communities and Local Government (2009). *World Class Places: The Government's Strategy for Improving Quality of Place*. London, DCLG.

Department for Culture Media and Sport (2001). *Time for Reform: Proposals for the Modernisation of our Licensing Laws*. London, DCMS.

Department for Culture Media and Sport (2005). *Drinking Responsibly: The Government's Proposals*. London, DCMS.

Department for Culture Media and Sport (2009). *Alcohol, Entertainment and Late Night Refreshment Licensing, England and Wales: April 2008–March 2009*. London, DCMS.

Department for Transport (2008). www.dft.gov.uk/pgr/statistics/datatables publications/nts/

Department for Transport (2009). *National Travel Survey 2008*. London: DfT.

Department of Health (1995). *Sensible Drinking: The Report of an Inter-disciplinary Working Group*. London, DH.

Department of Health (2001). *Securing our Future Health: Taking a Long-term View*. London: DH.

Department of Health (2003). *On the State of the Public Health: Annual Report of the Chief Medical Officer 2002*. London, DH.

Department of Health (2004a). *Choosing Health: Making Healthier Choices Easier*. London, DH.

Department of Health (2004b). *On the State of the Public Health: Annual Report of the Chief Medical Officer 2003*. London.

Department of Health (2004c). *At Least Five a Week: Evidence on the Impact of Physical Activity and its Relationship to Health*. London, DH.

Department of Health (2005a). *Choosing a Better Diet: A Food and Health Action Plan*. London, DH.

Department of Health (2005b). *Choosing Activity: A Physical Activity Action Plan*. London, DH.

Department of Health (2007). *Safe, Sensible, Social: The Next Stages in the National Alcohol Strategy*. London, DH.

Department of Health (2008). *Healthy Weight, Healthy Lives*. London, DH.

Department of Health (2009). *Be Active, Be Healthy: A Plan for Getting the Nation Moving*. London, DH.

Department of Health (2010). *Healthy Lives, Healthy People: Our Strategy for Public Health in England*. London, DH.

Devlin, K. (2010). 'Professionals "more likely to drink than those in working class jobs"'. *The Telegraph*, 27 May.

Di Loreto, C., A. Ranchelli, et al. (2005). 'Make your diabetic patients walk: long-term impact of different amounts of physical activity on type 2 diabetes'. *Diabetes Care* **28**(6): 1295–302.

Downs, J., G. Loewenstein, et al. (2009). 'The psychology of food consumption: strategies for promoting healthier food choices'. *American Economic Review: Papers and Proceedings* **99**(2): 1–10.

Duany, A., E. Plater-Zyberk, et al. (2001). *Suburban Nation: The Rise of Sprawl and the Decline of the American Dream*. New York, North Point Press.

Dutta-Bergman, M. (2005a). 'Psychographic profiling of fruit and vegetable consumption: the role of health orientation'. *Social Marketing Quarterly* **9**(1): 19–35.

Dutta-Bergman, M. (2005b). 'The relation between health-orientation, provider–patient communication, and satisfaction: an individual-difference approach'. *Health Communication* **18**(3): 291–303.

Dyreson, M. (2008). 'Epilogue: athletic clashes of civilizations or bridges over cultural divisions? the Olympic Games as legacies and the legacies of the Olympic Games'. *International Journal of the History of Sport* **25**(14): 2117–29.

Ebbeling, C. B., D. B. Pawlak, et al. (2002). 'Childhood obesity: public-health crisis, common sense cure'. *Lancet* **360**(9331): 473–82.

Ecologist, The (2010). 'Industry lobbying sees EU reject "traffic light" food labelling'. www.theecologist.org/News/news_round_up/511976/industry_lobbying_sees_eu_reject_traffic_light_food_labelling.html.

Edgar, T., V. S. Freimuth, et al. (1988). 'Communicating the AIDS risk to college students: the problem of motivating change'. *Health Education Research* **3**(1): 59–65.

Edwards, G. (1996). 'Sensible drinking'. *British Medical Journal* **312**(7022): 1.

Egger, G. and B. Swinburn (1997). 'An "ecological" approach to the obesity pandemic'. *British Medical Journal* **315**(7106): 477–80.

Ehrenhalt, A. (1995). *The Lost City: The Forgotten Virtues of Community in America*. New York, Basic Books.

Elvins, M. and P. Hadfield (2003). 'West End "stress area" night-time economy profiling: a demonstration project'. London: Westminster Council.

Emslie, C., H. Lewars, et al. (2009). 'Are there gender differences in levels of heavy, binge and problem drinking? Evidence from three generations in the west of Scotland'. *Public Health* **123**(1): 12–14.

Etzioni, A. (1968). *The Active Society*. New York, Free Press.

Evans, B. (2006). '"Gluttony or sloth": critical geographies of bodies and morality in (anti)obesity policy'. *Area* **38**(3): 259–67.

Evans, B. and R. Colls (2009). 'Measuring fatness, governing bodies: the spatialities of the body mass index (BMI) in anti-obesity politics'. *Antipode* **41**(5): 1051–83.

Farmer, P. (1993). *AIDS and Accusation: Haiti and the Geography of Blame*. Berkeley, University of California Press

Farmer, P. (1997). 'Social scientists and the new tuberculosis'. *Social Science and Medicine* **44**(3): 347–58.

Farmer, P. (1999). *Infections and Inequalities: The Modern Plagues.* Berkeley, University of California Press.

Feiring, E. (2008). 'Lifestyle, responsibility and justice'. *Journal of Medical Ethics* **34**(1): 33–6.

Feng, J., T. A. Glass, et al. (2010). 'The built environment and obesity: a systematic review of the epidemiologic evidence'. *Health and Place* **16**(2): 175–90.

Ferrières, J. (2004). 'The French paradox: lessons for other countries'. *Heart* **90**(1): 107–11.

Finkelstein, E. A., J. G. Trogdon, et al. (2009). 'Annual medical spending attributable to obesity: payer-and service-specific estimates'. *Health Affairs* **28**(5): 822–31.

Flegal, K. M. (2006). 'Commentary: the epidemic of obesity – what's in a name?' *International Journal of Epidemiology* **35**(1): 72–4.

Flegal, K. M., M. D. Carroll, et al. (2010). 'Prevalence and trends in obesity among US adults, 1999–2008'. *Journal of the American Medical Association* **303**(3): 235–41.

Flegal, K. M., B. I. Graubard, et al. (2005). 'Excess deaths associated with underweight, overweight, and obesity'. *Journal of the American Medical Association* **293**(15): 1861–7.

Foster, C. and M. Hillsdon (2004). 'Changing the environment to promote health-enhancing physical activity'. *Journal of Sports Sciences* **22**(8): 755–69.

Foster, J. H. (2008). 'The Licensing Act 2003: eighteen months down the road'. *Drugs: Education, Prevention, and Policy* **15**(1): 1–6.

Foster, J. H., R. Herring, et al. (2009). 'The Licensing Act 2003: a step in the right direction?' *Journal of Substance Use* **14**(2): 113–23.

Foster, J. H., D. Read, et al. (2010). 'Why do people drink at home?' *Journal of Public Health*: fdq008 32(4): 512-518.

Foucault, M. (1982). 'The subject and power'. *Critical Inquiry* **8**(4): 777–95.

Frank, L. D., B. E. Saelens, et al. (2007). 'Stepping towards causation: do built environments or neighborhood and travel preferences explain physical activity, driving, and obesity?' *Social Science and Medicine* **65**(9): 1898–914.

Freudenberg, N. (2010). 'The biology and politics of obesity'. *The Lancet* **375**(9712): 365–6.

Friedman, M. and R. Friedman (1980). *Free to Choose.* London, Pelican.

Gabriel, Y. and T. Lang (1995). *The Unmanageable Consumer: Contemporary Consumption and its Fragmentations.* London, Sage.

Gaesser, G. (2002). *Big Fat Lies: The Truth about Your Weight and Your Health.* Carlsbad, CA, Gurze Books.

Gard, M. (2009). 'Friends, enemies and the cultural politics of critical obesity research'. *Biopolitics and the 'Obesity Epidemic'.* J. Wright and V. Harwood. London, Routledge: 31–45.

Gard, M. and J. Wright (2005). *The Obesity Epidemic: Science, Morality and Ideology.* London, Routledge.

Gass, J. (1988). 'Towards an "active society"'. *OECD Observer* **152**: 4–8.

Geores, M. (1998). 'Surviving on metaphor: how "health = hot springs" created and sustained a town'. *Putting Health into Place: Landscape, Identity and Well-being*. G. Kearns and W. Gesler. Syracuse, NY, Syracuse University Press: 36–53.

Gesler, W. and R. Kearns (2002). *Culture, Place and Health*. London, Routledge.

Giddens, A. (1992). *The Transformation of Intimacy*. Cambridge, Polity Press.

Giles-Corti, B. and R. J. Donovan (2002). 'The relative influence of individual, social and physical environment determinants of physical activity'. *Social Science and Medicine* **54**(12): 1793–812.

Giles-Corti, B. and R. J. Donovan (2003). 'Relative influences of individual, social environmental, and physical environmental correlates of walking'. *American Journal of Public Health* **93**(9): 1583–9.

Gill, J. and F. O'May (2006). 'People seem confused about sensible drinking messages'. *British Medical Journal* **332**: 302–3.

Gillick, M. R. (1984). 'Health promotion, jogging, and the pursuit of the moral life'. *Journal of Health Politics Policy and Law* **9**(3): 369–87.

Gilman, S. (2004). *Fat Boys: A Slim Book*. Lincoln, University of Nebraska Press.

Girginov, V. and L. Hills (2008). 'A sustainable sports legacy: creating a link between the London Olympics and sports participation'. *International Journal of the History of Sport* **25**(14): 2091–116.

Glassner, B. (1989). 'Fitness and the postmodern self'. *Journal of Health and Social Behavior* **30**(2): 180–91.

Goddard, E. (2007). *Estimating Alcohol Consumption from Survey Data: Updated Method of Converting Volumes to Units*. London, Office for National Statistics.

Gold, J. and M. Gold (2008). 'Future indefinite? London 2012, the spectre of retrenchment and the challenge of Olympic sports legacy'. *The London Journal* **34**: 179–96.

Goodacre, S. (2005). 'The 2003 Licensing Act: an act of stupidity?' *Emergency Medicine Journal* **22**(10): 682–2.

Government Office for Science (2007). *Tackling Obesities: Future Choices: Project Report*. London, Foresight/Government Office for Science.

Graham, K. and R. Homel (2008). *Raising the Bar: Understanding and Preventing Violence in Bars, Clubs and Pubs*. Portland, OR, Willan Publishing.

Gratton, C. and I. Henry, eds (2001). *Sport in the City: The Role of Sport in Economic and Social Regeneration*. London, Routledge.

Greater London Authority (2002). *Late-Night London: Planning and Managing the Late-Night Economy*. London, GLA.

Greater London Authority (2007). *Managing the Night-time Economy: Best Practice Guidance*. London, GLA.

Green, J. and M. A. Plant (2007). 'Bad bars: a review of risk factors'. *Journal of Substance Use* **12**(3): 157–89.

Greener, I. (2009). 'Towards a history of choice in UK health policy'. *Sociology of Health and Illness* **31**(3): 309–24.

Griffin, C., A. Bengry-Howell, et al. (2009). '"Every time I do it I absolutely annihilate myself": loss of (self-)consciousness and loss of memory in young people's drinking narratives'. *Sociology* **43**(3): 457–76.

Grigg, D. (1998). 'Convergence in European diets: the case of alcoholic beverages' *GeoJournal* **44**: 9–18.

Gual, A. and J. Colom (1997). 'Why has alcohol consumption declined in countries of southern Europe?' *Addiction* **92**: 21–32.

Guardian, The (2010). 'The price we pay for our drinking culture'. The *Guardian*, 3 January.

Guthman, J. (2009). 'Teaching the politics of obesity: insights into neoliberal embodiment and contemporary biopolitics'. *Antipode* **41**(5): 1110–33.

Guthman, J. and M. DuPuis (2006). 'Embodying neoliberalism: economy, culture, and the politics of fat'. *Environment and Planning D: Society and Space* **24**(3): 427–48.

Guttman, N. and W. Ressler (2001). 'On being responsible: ethical issues in appeals to personal responsibility in health campaigns'. *Journal of Health Communication* **6**: 117–36.

Hackley, C., A. Bengry-Howell, et al. (2008). 'The discursive constitution of the UK alcohol problem in Safe, Sensible, Social: a discussion of policy implications'. *Drugs: Education, Prevention, and Policy* **15**(s1): 61–74.

Hadfield, P. (2006). *Bar Wars: Contesting the Night in Contemporary British Cities.* Oxford, Oxford University Press.

Hadfield, P. (2007). 'Party invitations: New Labour and the (de)regulation of pleasure'. *Criminal Justice Matters* **67**(1): 18–47.

Hajer, M. (1995). *The Politics of Environmental Discourse: Ecological Modernization and the Policy Process.* Oxford, Oxford University Press.

Hajer, M. and W. Versteeg (2005). 'A decade of discourse analysis of environmental politics: achievements, challenges, perspectives'. *Journal of Environmental Policy and Planning* **7**(3): 175–84.

Hall, C. M. (2006). 'Urban entrepreneurship, corporate interests and sports mega-events: the thin policies of competitiveness within the hard outcomes of neoliberalism'. *Sociological Review* **54**(s2): 59–70.

Hall, C. M. and J. Hodges (1996). 'The party's great, but what about the hangover? the housing and social impacts of mega-events with special reference to the 2000 Sydney Olympics'. *Festival Management and Event Tourism* **4**: 13–20.

Hall, S. and S. Winlow (2006). *Violent Night: Urban Leisure and Contemporary Culture.* London, Berg.

Hamlin, C. and S. Sheard (1998). 'Revolutions in public health: 1848, and 1998?' *British Medical Journal* **317**(7158): 587–91.

Hanlon, P., S. Carlisle, et al. (2010). 'Enabling well-being in a time of radical change: integrative public health for the 21st century'. *Public Health* **124**(6): 305–12.

Hansen, J., L. Holm, et al. (2003). 'Beyond the knowledge deficit: recent research into lay and expert attitudes to food risks'. *Appetite* **41**(2): 111–21.

Hargreaves, S. (2009). 'Hunger hits Detroit's middle class'. *CNNMoney.* Atlanta http://money.cnn.com/2009/08/06/news/economy/detroit_food/

Harris, J. L., J. L. Pomeranz, et al. (2009). 'A crisis in the marketplace: how food marketing contributes to childhood obesity and what can be done'. *Annual Review of Public Health* **30**(1): 211–25.

Harris, P. (2010). 'Detroit gets growing'. *The Guardian*, 11 July.

Harvey, D. (2007). *A Brief History of Neoliberalism*. Oxford, Oxford University Press.

Haskell, W., I. Lee, et al. (2007). 'Physical activity and public health updated recommendation for adults from the American College of Sports Medicine and the American Heart Association'. *Circulation* **116**: 1081–93.

Hastings, G. (2002). 'Marketing diet and exercise: lessons from Mammon'. *Social Marketing Quarterly* **8**(4): 31–9

Hayward, K. and D. Hobbs (2007). 'Beyond the binge in "booze Britain": market-led liminalization and the spectacle of binge drinking'. *British Journal of Sociology* **58**(3): 437–56.

Health Improvement Analytical Team (2008). *The Cost of Alcohol Harm to the NHS in England*. London, DH.

Health Select Committee (2010). *Final Report of Session 2009-2010 on Alcohol*. London, House of Commons.

Heasman, M. and J. Mellentin (2001). *The Functional Foods Revolution: Healthy People, Healthy Profits*. London, Earthscan.

Heath, T. (1997). 'The twenty-four hour city concept: a review of initiatives in British cities'. *Journal of Urban Design* **2**(2): 193–204.

Health and Social Care Information Centre (2010). *Statistics on Alcohol 2010*. London, DH.

Heron, The (2010). 'The Heron'. www.theheron.co.uk.

Herrick, C. (2005). '"Cultures of GM": discourses of risk and labelling of GMOs in the UK and EU'. *Area* **37**(3): 286–94.

Herrick, C. (2007). 'Risky bodies: public health, social marketing and the governance of obesity'. *Geoforum* **38**(1): 90–102.

Herrick, C. (2008). 'To the west and east of Interstate-35: obesity, philanthropic entrepreneurialism, and the delineation of risk in Austin, Texas'. *Environment and Planning A* **40**(11): 2715–33.

Herrick, C. (2009a). 'Designing the fit city: public health, active lives, and the (re)instrumentalization of urban space'. *Environment and Planning A* **41**(10): 2437–54.

Herrick, C. (2009b). 'Shifting blame/selling health: corporate social responsibility in the age of obesity'. *Sociology of Health and Illness* **31**(1): 51–65.

Herrick, C. (2010). 'Why we need to think beyond the "industry" in alcohol research and policy studies'. *Drugs: Education, Prevention, and Policy* **18**(1): 10-15.

Herring, R., V. Berridge, et al. (2008a). 'Binge drinking today: learning lessons from the past'. *Drugs: Education, Prevention, and Policy* **15**(5): 475–86.

Herring, R., V. Berridge, et al. (2008b). 'Binge drinking: an exploration of a confused concept'. *Journal of Epidemiology and Community Health* **62**(6): 476–9.

Heynen, N. and P. Robbins (2005). 'The neoliberalization of nature: governance, privatization, valuation and enclosure'. *Capitalism Nature Socialism* **16**(1): 5–8.

Hiller, H. H. (2000). 'Mega-events, urban boosterism and growth strategies: an analysis of the objectives and legitimations of the Cape Town 2004 Olympic bid'. *International Journal of Urban and Regional Research* **24**(2): 449–58.

Hingson, R., T. Heeren, et al. (2005). 'Magnitude of alcohol-related mortality and morbidity among US college students ages 18–24: changes from 1998 to 2001'. *Annual Review of Public Health* **26**(1): 259–79.

HM Government (2007). *Safe, Sensible, Social: The Next Stages in the National Alcohol Strategy*. London, The Stationery Office.

HM Treasury (2009). *PSA Delivery Agreement 25: Reduce the Harm Caused by Alcohol and Drugs*. London, HM Government.

Hobbs, D., P. Hadfield, et al. (2003). *Bouncers: Violence and Governance in the Night-time Economy*. Oxford, Oxford University Press.

Hobbs, D., S. Winlow, et al. (2005). 'Violent hypocrisy: governance and the night-time economy'. *European Journal of Criminology* **2**(2): 161–83.

Hollands, R. and P. Chatterton (2003). 'Producing nightlife in the new urban entertainment economy: corporatization, branding and market segmentation'. *International Journal of Urban and Regional Research* **27**(2): 361–85.

Holloway, S. L., M. Jayne, et al. (2008). '"Sainsbury's is my local": English alcohol policy, domestic drinking practices and the meaning of home'. *Transactions of the Institute of British Geographers* **33**(4): 532–47.

Holt, M., ed. (2006). *Alcohol: A Social and Cultural History*. London, Berg.

Home Office (2003). *Hidden Harm*. London, Home Office.

Horne, J. and W. Manzenreiter (2006a). 'An introduction to the sociology of sports mega-events' *Sociological Review* **54**: 1–24.

Horne, J. and W. Manzenreiter, eds (2006b). *Sports Mega-events: Social Scientific Analyses of a Global Phenomenon*. London, Blackwell.

House of Commons Committee of Public Accounts (2007). *Tackling Childhood Obesity: First Steps*. London, HM Government.

Hubbard, V. S. (2000). 'Defining overweight and obesity: what are the issues?' *American Journal of Clinical Nutrition* **72**(5): 1067–8.

Hunter, D. (2005). 'Choosing or losing health?' *Journal of Epidemiology and Community Health* **59**: 1010–13.

Hunter, D. J. (2009). 'Leading for health and wellbeing: the need for a new paradigm'., *Journal of Public Health* **31**(2): 202–4.

Imrie, R. and M. Raco, eds (2003). *Urban Renaissance? New Labour, Community and Urban Policy*. Bristol, The Policy Press.

International Center for Alcohol Policies (2009) *ICAP Blue Book*. Washington DC: ICAP.

Isaac, L. and A. Domok (2010). 'Rapid respose: alcohol and public health – potential pitfalls'. *British Medical Journal* **340**: 394.

Jackson, R (2005) 'Commentary on Active Living research'. *American Journal of Preventative Medicine* **28**: 218–19.

Jayne, M., S. L. Holloway, et al. (2006). 'Drunk and disorderly: alcohol, urban life and public space'. *Progress in Human Geography* **30**(4): 451–68.

Jayne, M., G. Valentine, et al. (2008a). 'Fluid boundaries: British binge drinking and european civility – alcohol and the production and consumption of public space'. *Space and Polity* **12**(1): 81–100.

Jayne, M., G. Valentine, et al. (2008b). 'Geographies of alcohol, drinking and drunkenness: a review of progress'. *Progress in Human Geography* **32**(2): 247–63.

Jayne, M., G. Valentine, et al. (2008c). 'The place of drink: geographical contributions to alcohol studies'. *Drugs: Education, Prevention, and Policy* **15**(3): 219–32.

Jayne, M., G. Valentine, et al. (2010). *Alcohol, Drinking, Drunkenness: (Dis)Orderly Spaces*. London, Ashgate.

Jebb, S. A. (1997). 'Aetiology of obesity'. *British Medical Bulletin* **53**(2): 264–85.

Jebb, S. A. (1999). 'Obesity: from molecules to man'. *Proceedings of the Nutrition Society* **58**(1): 1–14.

Jebb, S., T. Steer, et al. (2008). *The 'Healthy Living' Social Marketing Initiative: A Review of the Evidence*. Cambridge, MRC Human Nutrition Research/DH.

Jones, A., G. Bentham, et al. (2007). *Obesogenic Environments: Evidence Review*. London, Foresight Programme of the Office of Science and Innovation, Department of Trade and Industry.

Jones, C. (2001). 'Mega-events and host-region impacts: determining the true worth of the 1999 Rugby World Cup'. *International Journal of Tourism Research* **3**(3): 241–51.

Jordan, B. (2005). 'New Labour: choice and values'. *Critical Social Policy* **25**(4): 427–46.

Jordan, B. (2006). 'Public services and the service economy: individualism and the choice agenda'. *Journal of Social Policy* **35**(01): 143–62.

Joyce, P. (2003). *The Rule of Freedom: Liberalism and the Modern City*. London, Verso.

Kantrowitz, B. and L. Kalb (2006). 'Food news blues'. *Newsweek*, 13 March.

Katan, M. B. (2004). 'Health claims for functional foods'. *British Medical Journal* **328**(7433): 180–1.

Kearns, G. and S. Reid-Henry (2009). 'Vital geographies: life, luck, and the human condition'. *Annals of the Association of American Geographers* **99**(3): 554–74.

Kearns, R. (1991). 'The place of health in the health of place: the case of the Hokianga Special Medical Area'. *Social Science and Medicine* **33**(4): 519–30.

Kearns, R. (1993). 'Place and health: towards a reformed medical geography'. *Professional Geographer* **45**(2): 139–47.

Kearns, R. (1997). 'Narrative and metaphor in health geographies'. *Progress in Human Geography* **21**(2): 269–77.

Kearns, R. and W. Gesler (1998). *Putting Health into Place*. Syracuse, NY, Syracuse University Press.

Kearns, R. and G. Moon (2002). 'From medical to health geography: novelty, place and theory after a decade of change'. *Progress in Human Geography* **26**(5): 605–25.

Keeley, G. and F. Bagenal (2010). 'Young Spaniards turn to "big bottle" binge drinking'. *The Times*, 1 January.

Kennedy, J. F. (1960). 'The soft American'. *Sports Illustrated*, December 26.

Kidd, B. (2008). 'A new social movement: sport for development and peace'. *Sport in Society: Cultures, Commerce, Media, Politics* **11**(4): 370–80.

Klein, R. (1997). *Eat Fat*. London, Picador.

Kmietowicz, Z. (2007). 'MPs deplore poor progress in combating childhood obesity'. *British Medical Journal* **334**(7586): 173.

Kneale, J. (1999). '"A problem of supervision": moral geographies of the nineteenth-century British public house'. *Journal of Historical Geography* **25**(3): 333–48.

Kneale, J. and S. French (2008). 'Mapping alcohol: health, policy and the geographies of problem drinking in Britain'. *Drugs: Education, Prevention, and Policy* **15**(3): 233–49.

Kraak, V. and D. Pelletier (1998a). 'How marketers reach young consumers: Implications for nutrition education and health promotion campaigns'. *Family Economics and Nutrition Review* **11**: 31–41.

Kraak, V. and D. Pelletier (1998b). 'The influence of commercialism on the food purchasing behavior of children and teenage youth'. *Family Economics and Nutrition Review* **11**: 15–24.

Kraak, V. I., S. K. Kumanyika, et al. (2009). 'The commercial marketing of healthy lifestyles to address the global child and adolescent obesity pandemic: prospects, pitfalls and priorities'. *Public Health Nutrition* **12**(11): 2027–36.

Kuczmarski, R. J. and K. M. Flegal (2000). 'Criteria for definition of overweight in transition: background and recommendations for the United States'. *American Journal of Clinical Nutrition* **72**(5): 1074–81.

Kunstler, J. (1993). *The Geography of Nowhere: The Rise and Fall of America's Man-made Landscape*. New York, Touchstone.

Kunstler, J. (1998). *Home from Nowhere: Remaking our Everyday World for the Twenty-first Century*. New York, Free Press.

Kwan, S. (2009). 'Framing the fat body: contested meanings between government, activists, and industry'. *Sociological Inquiry* **79**(1): 25–50.

Lake, A. and T. Townshend (2006). 'Obesogenic environments: exploring the built and food environments.' *Journal of the Royal Society for the Promotion of Health* **126**(6): 262–7.

Lalonde, M. (1974). *A New Perspective on the Health of Canadians*. Ottowa, Department of Health.

Lang, T. (1999). 'The complexities of globalization: the UK as a case study of tensions within the food system and the challenge to food policy'. *Agriculture and Human Values* **16**: 169–85.

Lang, T. (2003). 'Food Industrialisation and Food Power: Implications for Food Governance'. *Development Policy Review* **21**(5–6): 555–68.

Lang, T. (2007). 'Functional foods'. *British Medical Journal* **334**(7602): 1015–16.

Lang, T. and M. Heasman (2004). *Food Wars*. London, Earthscan.

Lang, T. and G. Rayner (2005). 'Obesity: a growing issue for European policy'. *Journal of European Social Policy* **15**(4): 301–27.

Lang, T. and G. Rayner (2007). 'Overcoming policy cacophony on obesity: an ecological public health framework for policymakers'. *Obesity Reviews* **8**(s1): 165–81.

Lansley, A. (2010). 'A new approach to public health'. speech made at London, Faculty of Public Health. 7 July. www..dh.gov.uk/en/MediaCentre/Speeches/DH_117280

Latham, A. (2003). 'Urbanity, lifestyle and making sense of the new urban cultural economy: notes from Auckland, New Zealand'. *Urban Studies* **40**(9): 1699–724.

Lawlor, D. Ness, A. Cope, A. Davis, A. Insall, P. and Riddoch, C. (2003) 'The challenges of evaluating environmental interventions to increase population levels of physical activity: the case of the UK National Cycle Network'. *Journal of Epidemiology and Community Health* **57**: 96–101.

Lawrence, F. (2004). *Not On the Label: What Really Goes into the Food on Your Plate.* London, Penguin.

Lawrence, F. (2010). 'Nanny does know best, Andrew Lansley'. *The Guardian*, 8 July.

Lawrence, R. G. (2004). 'Framing obesity: the evolution of news discourse on a public health issue'. *Harvard International Journal of Press/Politics* **9**(3): 56–75.

Lee, I. M., R. Ewing, et al. (2009). 'The built environment and physical activity levels: the Harvard Alumni Health Study'. *American Journal of Preventive Medicine* **37**(4): 293–8.

Lee, K., D. Burney, et al. (2010). *Active Design Guidelines: Promoting Physical Activity and Health in Design.* New York: New York City Economic Development Corporation.

Lefebvre, R. (1992). 'Social marketing and health promotion'. *Health Promotion: Disciplines, Diversity and Developments.* R. Bunton and G. Macdonald. London, Routledge: 219–46.

Levi, R. and M. Valverde (2001). 'Knowledge on tap: police science and common knowledge in the legal regulation of drunkenness'. *Law and Social Inquiry* **26**(4): 819–46.

Linn, S. (2000). 'Marketing to children harmful: experts urge candidates to lead nation in setting limits'. *Center for Media Education* **2003**: n.p.

Lobstein, T. (2006). 'Commentary: obesity – public health crisis, moral panic or a human rights issue?' *International Journal of Epidemiology* **35**(1): 74–6.

Loewenstein, G., T. Brennan, et al. (2007). 'Asymmetric paternalism to improve health behaviors'. *Journal of the American Medical Association* **298**(20): 2415–17.

London Assembly (2005). *London's Night-time Economy.* London, London Assembly: Economic Development, Culture, Sport and Tourism Committee.

London Chamber of Commerce and Industry (2006). *London After Dark: Licensing and Central London's Late Night Economy.* London, London Chamber of Commerce and Industry.

Longhurst, R. (2005). 'Fat bodies: developing geographical research agendas'. *Progress in Human Geography* **29**(3): 247–59.

Loughren, E. (2009). 'Motivation of first time marathoners to adherence to marathoning'. PhD thesis, College of Health Professions, Temple, PA.

Lovatt, A. and J. O'Connor (1995). 'Cities and the night-time economy'. *Planning Practice and Research* **10**(2): 127–34.

Loveday, B. (2005). 'The 2003 Licensing Act: alcohol use and anti-social behaviour in England and Wales'. *Police Journal* **78**(3): 178–91.

Luminar Group Holdings Plc (2010). *Annual Report 2010.* Milton Keynes, Luminar Group Holdings.

Lupton, D. and A. Peterson (1996). *The New Public Health: Discourses, Knowledges, Strategies.* London, Sage.

McDonald, S. D., Z. Han, et al. (2010). 'Overweight and obesity in mothers and risk of preterm birth and low birth weight infants: systematic review and meta-analyses'. *British Medical Journal* **341**: c3428.

McDougall, C. (2004). *Born to Run: The Hidden Tribe, the Ultra-Runners, and the Greatest Race the World Has Never Seen.* London, Profile Books.

McGuire, M. and S. Hallsworth (2010). *The Criminology of Pleasure.* London, Routledge.

Macintyre, J., A. Ellway, et al. (2002). 'Place effects on health: how can we conceptualise, operationalise and measure them?' *Social Science and Medicine* **12**(3): 125–39.

Macintyre, S. (2003). 'Evidence based policy making' *British Medical Journal* **326**(7379): 5–6.

Macintyre, S. (2007). 'Deprivation amplification revisited; or, is it always true that poorer places have poorer access to resources for healthy diets and physical activity?' *International Journal of Behavioral Nutrition and Physical Activity* **4**(1): 32.

Macintyre, S., S. Maciver, et al. (1993). 'Area, class and health: should we be focussing on places or people?' *Journal of Social Policy* **22**: 213–34.

MacKian, S., H. Elliot, et al. (2003). 'Everywhere and nowhere: locating and understanding the "new" public health'. *Health and Place* **9**: 219–29.

McMurran, M. and C. Hollin (1989). 'Drinking and delinquency: another look at young offenders and alcohol'. *British Journal of Criminology* **29**(4): 386–96.

Maibach, E. (2002). 'Explicating social marketing: what is it and what isn't it?' *Social Marketing Quarterly* **13**(4): 7–13.

Majumdar, B. (2006). 'Tom Brown goes global: the "Brown" ethic in colonial and post-colonial India'. *International Journal of the History of Sport* **23**(5): 805–20.

Makela, K. (1997). 'Drinking, the majority fallacy, cognitive dissonance and social pressure'. *Addiction* **92**(6): 729–36.

Mark, D. H. (2005). 'Deaths attributable to obesity'. *Journal of the American Medical Association* **293**(15): 1918–19.

Marmot, M. (1998). 'Improvement of social environment to improve health'. *The Lancet* **351**(9095): 57–60.

Marmot, M. (2001). 'Inequalities in health'. *New England Journal of Medicine* **345**(2): 134–6.

Marmot, M. (2005). 'Social determinants of health inequalities'. *The Lancet* **365**(9464): 1099–104.

Marshall, A. (2000). *How Cities Work: Suburbs, Sprawl and the Roads not Taken.* Austin, University of Texas Press.

Marvin, S. and W. Medd (2006). 'Metabolisms of obecity: flows of fat through bodies, cities, and sewers'. *Environment and Planning A* **38**(2): 313–24.

Matheson, V. A. and R. A. Baade (2004). 'Mega sporting events in developing countries: playing the way to prosperity?' *South African Journal of Economics* **72**(5): 1085–96.

Matthews, S. (2008). 'The salience of neighbourhood: some lessons from sociology'. *American Journal of Preventative Medicine* **34**(3): 257–9.

Mayor of London (2003). *The London Agenda for Action on Alcohol.* London, Greater London Authority.

Mayor of London (2004). *The London Plan.* London, Greater London Authority.

Mayor of London (2006). *London Agenda for Action on Alcohol: Update Report.* London, Greater London Authority.

Mayor of London (2010). *The London Health Inequalities Strategy.* London, Mayor of London.

Measham, F. (1996). 'The "big bang" approach to sessional drinking: changing patterns of alcohol consumption amongst young people in North West England'. *Addiction Research and Theory* **4**(3): 283–99.

Measham, F. (2004). 'The decline of ecstasy, the rise of "binge" drinking and the persistence of pleasure'. *Probation Journal* **51**(4): 309–26.

Measham, F. (2006). 'The new policy mix: alcohol, harm minimisation, and determined drunkenness in contemporary society'. *International Journal of Drug Policy* **17**(4): 258–68.

Measham, F. and K. Brain (2005). '"Binge" drinking, British alcohol policy and the new culture of intoxication'. *Crime Media Culture* **1**(3): 262–83.

Measham, F. and K. Moore (2008). 'The criminalisation of intoxication'. *ASBO Nation: The Criminalisation of Nuisance.* P. Squires. Bristol, The Policy Press: 273–89.

Measham, F. and J. Ostergaard (2010). 'The public face of binge drinking: British and Danish young women, recent trends in alcohol consumption and the European binge drinking debate'. *Probation Journal* **56**: 415–34.

Miller, P. and N. Rose (2008). *Governing the Present: Administering Economic, Social and Personal Life.* Cambridge, Polity.

Miller, T. (1993). *The Well-Tempered Self: Citizenship, Culture and the Postmodern Subject.* Baltimore, MD, Johns Hopkins University Press.

Minkler, M. (1999). 'Personal responsibility for health? a review of the arguments and the evidence at century's end'. *Heath Education and Behaviour* **26**(1): 121–44.

Minton, A. (2009). *Ground Control: Fear and Happiness in the Twenty-first Century.* London, Penguin.

Mitchell, G. and K. McTigue (2007). 'The US obesity "epidemic": metaphor, method, or madness?' *Social Epistemology: A Journal of Knowledge, Culture and Policy* **21**(4): 391–23.

Mitka, M. (2005). 'Government unveils new food pyramid: critics say nutrition tool is flawed'. *Journal of the American Medical Association* **293**(21): 2581–2.

Mokdad, A. H., J. S. Marks, et al. (2004). 'Actual causes of death in the United States, 2000'. *Journal of the American Medical Association* **291**(10): 1238–45.

Monaghan, L. (2005). 'Discussion piece: a critical take on the obesity debate'. *Social Theory and Health* **3**: 302–14.

Montgomery, J. (1995). 'Editorial: urban vitality and the culture of cities'. *Planning Practice and Research* **10**(2): 101–10.

Montgomery, J. (1997). 'Café culture and the city: the role of pavement cafés in urban public social life'. *Journal of Urban Design* **2**(1): 83–102.

Moon, G. (2009). 'Residential environments and obesity – estimating causal effects'. *Geographies of Obesity*. J. Pearce and K. Witten. London, Ashgate: 251–77.

Moon, G., G. Quarendon, et al. (2007). 'Fat nation: deciphering the distinctive geographies of obesity in England'. *Social Science and Medicine* **65**(1): 20–31.

Moore, D. (2008). 'Erasing pleasure from public discourse on illicit drugs: on the creation and reproduction of an absence'. *International Journal of Drug Policy* **19**(5): 353–8.

Moriarty, K. J. and I. T. Gilmore (2006). 'Licensing Britain's alcohol epidemic'. *Journal of Epidemiology and Community Health* **60**(2): 94–4.

Morland, K., S. Wing, et al. (2002). 'Neighbourhood characteristics associated with the location of food stores and food service places'. *American Journal of Preventive Medicine* **22**: 23–9.

Morris, J. (1994). 'Exercise in the prevention of coronary heart disease: today's best buy in public health'. *Medicine and Science in Sports and Exercise* **26**(7): 807–14.

Morris, J. N., D. G. Clayton, et al. (1990). 'Exercise in leisure time: coronary attack and death rates'. *British Heart Journal* **63**(6): 325–34.

Moss, A., K. Dyer, et al. (2009). 'Knowledge of drinking guidelines does not equal sensible drinking'. *British Medical Journal* **374**: 1242.

Mozaffarian, D. and M. J. Stampfer (2010). 'Removing industrial trans fat from foods'. *British Medical Journal* **340**: 1826.

Muir, R. (2008). *Pubs and Places: The Social Value of Community Pubs*. London, Institute for Public Policy Research.

Murakami, H. (2008). *What I Talk About When I Talk About Running*. London, Vintage.

Murdock, S., S. White, et al. (2002). *Texas Challenge Report*. Austin, Office of the State Demographer.

National Audit Office (2008). *Reducing Alcohol Harm: Health Services in England for Alcohol Misuse*. London, DH.

National Consumer Council. (2005). 'National social marketing strategy for health: realising the potential of effective social marketing.' www.ncc.org.uk/health/NSMS%20LEAFLET%20-%20Realising%20the%20potential%20of%20effective%20social%20marketing.pdf.

National Institute for Health and Clinical Excellence (2009). *Promoting and Creating Built or Natural Environments that Encourage and Support Physical Activity*. London, NICE.

NHS (National Health Service) (2009) *NHS constitution for England*. London: DH

National Institute for Clinical Excellence (2010). *Prevention of Cardiovascular Disease at Population Level*. London, NICE.

Nauright, J. (2004). 'Global games: culture, political economy and sport in the globalised world of the 21st century'. *Third World Quarterly* **25**(7): 1325–36.

Navarro, V. (2004). *The Political and Social Contexts of Health*. Amityville, CA, Baywood.

Navarro, V., ed. (2007). *Neoliberalism, Globalization, and Inequalities: Consequences for Health and Quality of Life*. Amityville, CA, Baywood.

Navarro, V., C. Muntaner, et al. (2006). 'Politics and health outcomes'. *The Lancet* **368**(9540): 1033–7.

Nestle, M. (2000). 'Soft drink "pouring rights": marketing empty calories to children'. *Public Health Reports* **115**: 308–19.

Nestle, M. (2002). *Food Politics: How the Food Industry Influences Nutrition and Health*. Berkeley, University of California Press.

Nestle, M. and L. Dixon (2004). *Taking Sides: Clashing Views on Controversial Issues in Food and Nutrition*. Guildford, McGraw-Hill/Dushkin.

Nettleton, S. (1997). 'Governing the risky self: how to become healthy, wealthy and wise'. *Foucault, Health and Medicine*. R. Bunton and A. Petersen. London, Routledg: 207–22.

Nettleton, S. and M. Hardey (2006). 'Running away with health: the urban marathon and the construction of "charitable bodies"'. *Health:* **10**(4): 441–60.

Newman, P. (2007). '"Back the bid": the 2012 Summer Olympics and the governance of London'. *Journal of Urban Affairs* **29**(3): 255–67.

NHS (2006). *Your Weight, Your Health: How to Take Control of Your Weight*. London, NHS.

NHS Confederation (2010). *Briefing: Too Much of the Hard Stuff. What Alcohol Costs the NHS*. London, NHS.

NHS Information Centre (2009). *Health Survey for England 2008*, Leeds: NHS Information Centre (www.ic.nhs.uk/statistics-and-data-collections/health-and-lifestyles-related-surveys/health-survey-for-england).

NHS London (2009). *Go London! An Active and Healthy London for 2012 and Beyond*. London, NHS.

Nicholls, J. Q. (2006). 'Liberties and licences: Alcohol in liberal thought'. *International Journal of Cultural Studies* **9**(2): 131–51.

Nicholls, J. Q. (2010). 'Drink: the British disease?' *History Today* **60**(1): 10–17.

Norfolk, A. (2007). 'Drink limits "useless"'. *The Times*, 20 October.

Norris, P. and D. Williams (2008). '"Binge drinking", anti-social behaviour and alcohol-related disorder: examining the 2003 Licensing Act'. *ASBO Nation: The Criminalisation of Nuisance* P. Squires. Bristol, The Policy Press: 257–73.

Nova International (2008). Personal communication.

Nova International (2010). 'About us: marketing'. www..greatrun.org/Corporate/Marketing.aspx

Nuffield Council on Bioethics (2007). *Public Health: Ethical Issues*. London, Nuffield Council.

O'Malley, P. and M. Valverde (2004). 'Pleasure, freedom and drugs: the uses of "pleasure" in liberal governance of drug and alcohol consumption'. *Sociology* **38**(1): 25–42.

ODPM (2003). *The Evening Economy and the Urban Renaissance*. London, ODPM.

Oduku, O. and S. Bageen, eds (2009). *Gated Communities*. London, Earthscan.

OECD (Organisation for Economic Co-operation and Development) (2009) *Health Data*. www.oecd.org

Offer, A. (2007). *The Challenge of Affluence: Self-Control and Well-Being in the United States and Britain since 1950*. Oxford, Oxford University Press.

Office of National Statistics (2007). *Estimating Alcohol Consumption from Survey Data: Updated Method of Converting Volumes to Units*. London, Office of National Statistics.

Office of National Statistics (2008). *Family Spending: A report on the 2008 Living Costs and Food Survey*. London, Office of National Statistics.

Office of the Governor: Texas (2004). 'Gov. Rick Perry's remarks at Texas Round-Up launch'. Austin, Office of the Governor. http://governor.state.tx.us/priorities/families/healthier_citizens/texas_round_up_1/

Ogden, C. L., S. Z. Yanovski, et al. (2007). 'The epidemiology of obesity'. *Gastroenterology* **132**(6): 2087–102.

Ogilvie, D., M. Egan, et al. (2004). 'Promoting walking and cycling as an alternative to using cars: systematic review'. *British Medical Journal* **329**(7469): 763–68.

Olberding, D. and J. Jisha (2005). '"The flying pig": building brand equity in a major urban marathon'. *Sport Marketing Quarterly* **14**: 191–6.

Oliver, J. (2006). *Fat Politics: The Real Story Behind America's Obesity Epidemic*. Oxford, Oxford University Press.

Omran, A. (1971). 'The epidemiologic transition: a theory of the epidemiology of population change'. *Milbank Memorial Fund Quarterly* **49**(4): 509–38.

Orbach, S. (1978). *Fat is a Feminist Issue*. New York, Arrow.

Orbach, S. (2006). 'Commentary: there is a public health crisis – it's not fat on the body but fat in the mind and the fat of profits'. *International Journal of Epidemiology* **35**(1): 67–9.

Osborne, T. (1997). 'Of health and statecraft'. *Foucault, Health and Medicine*. A. Peterson and R. Bunton. London, Routledge: 173-188.

Osborne, T. and N. Rose (1999). 'Governing cities: notes on the spatialisation of virtue'. *Environment and Planning D – Society and Space* **17**(6): 737–60.

Painter, J., R. Jee-Hyun, et al. (2002). 'Comparison of international food guide pictoral representations'. *Journal of the American Dietetic Association* **102**(4): 483–9.

Pan, L., D. Galuska, et al. (2009). 'Differences in prevalence of obesity among black, white, and Hispanic adults – United States, 2006–2008'. *Morbidity and Mortality Weekly Report* **58**(27): 740–4.

Parliamentary Office of Science and Technology (2005). *Binge Drinking and Public Health*. London, Parliamentary Office of Science and Technology.

Parr, H. (2004). 'Medical geography: critical medical and health geography?' *Progress in Human Geography* **28**(2): 246–57.

Pearce, J., K. Witten, et al. (2007). 'Are socially disadvantaged neighbourhoods deprived of health-related community resources?' *International Journal of Epidemiology* **36**(2): 348–55.

Peck, J., N. Theodore, et al. (2010). 'Postneoliberalism and its malcontents'. *Antipode* **41**(s1): 94–116.

Peck, J. and A. Tickell (2002). 'Neoliberalizing space'. *Antipode* **34**(3): 380–404.

Pepin, V., S. McMahan, et al. (2004). 'A social ecological approach to the obesity epidemic'. *American Journal of Health Studies* **19**(2): 122–6.

Peterson, A. and D. Lupton (1996). *The New Public Health: Health and Self in the Age of Risk*. London, Sage.

Petrini, C. (2003). *Slow Food: The Case for Taste*. New York, Columbia University Press.

Pickett, K., S. Kelly, et al. (2005). 'Wider income gaps, wider waistbands? an ecological study of obesity and income inequality'. *Journal of Epidemiology and Community Health* **59**: 670–4.

Pillay, U. and O. Bass (2008). 'Mega-events as a response to poverty reduction: the 2010 FIFA World Cup and its urban development implications'. *Urban Forum* **19**(3): 329–46.

Plant, M. and M. Plant (2006). *Binge Britain: Alcohol and the National Response*. Oxford, Oxford University Press.

Pollan, M. (2006). *The Omnivore's Dilemma*. London, Bloomsbury.

Popkin, B. M. (1999). 'Urbanization, lifestyle changes and the nutrition transition'. *World Development* **27**(11): 1905–16.

Popkin, B. M. (2003). 'The nutrition transition in the developing world'. *Development Policy Review* **21**(5–6): 581–97.

Portman Group (2007). *Guidelines on Unit Labelling*. London, Portman Group.

Pratt, A. C. (2009). 'Urban regeneration: from the arts "feel good" factor to the cultural economy – a case study of Hoxton, London'. *Urban Studies* **46**(5–6): 1041–61.

Prentice, A. M. (2001). 'Obesity and its potential mechanistic basis'. *British Medical Bulletin* **60**: 51–67.

Prentice, A. M. (2006). 'The emerging epidemic of obesity in developing countries'. *International Journal of Epidemiology* **35**(1): 93–9.

Prentice, A. M. and S. A. Jebb (1995). 'Obesity in Britain: gluttony or sloth'. *British Medical Journal* **311**(7002): 437–9.

Prentice, A. M. and S. A. Jebb (2003). 'Fast foods, energy density and obesity: a possible mechanistic link'. *Obesity Reviews* **4**: 187–94.

Price, K. (2006). 'Health promotion and some implications of consumer choice'. *Journal of Nursing Management* **14**(6): 494–501.

Prime Minister's Strategy Unit (2004). *Alcohol Harm Reduction Strategy for England*. London, Cabinet Office.

Prochaska, J. and C. DiClemente (1986). 'Toward a comprehensive model of change'. *Treating Addictive Behaviors: Processes of Change*. W. Miller and N. Heather. New York, Plenum Press: 3–27.

Prochaska, J. O., C. C. DiClemente, et al. (1993). 'In search of how people change: applications to addictive behaviors'. *Journal of Addictions Nursing* **5**(1): 2–16.

Provencher, V., C. Begin, et al. (2007). 'Short-term effects of a health-at-every-size approach on eating behaviors and appetite ratings'. *Obesity* **15**(4): 957–66.

Public Health Commission (2010). *Responsibility Deal 2: Working with Businesses to Improve Public Health*. London, Public Health Commission.

Putnam, R. (2000). *Bowling Alone: The Collapse and Revival of American Community*. New York, Simon and Schuster.

Putnam, R. (2002). *Democracies in Flux: The Evolution of Social Capital in Contemporary Society*. Oxford, Oxford University Press.

Putnam, R. and L. Feldstein (2003). *Better Together: Restoring the American Community*. New York, Simon and Schuster.

Raco, M. (2009). 'From expectations to aspirations: state modernisation, urban policy, and the existential politics of welfare in the UK'. *Political Geography* **28**(7): 436–44.

Reidpath, D., C. Burns, et al. (2002). 'An ecological study of the relationship between social and environmental determinants of obesity.' *Health and Place* **8**: 141–5.

Reischer, E. L. (2001). 'Running to the moon: the articulation and construction of self in marathon runners'. *Anthropology of Consciousness* **12**(2): 19–34.

Renaud, S. and M. de Lorgeril (1992). 'Wine, alcohol, platelets, and the French paradox for coronary heart disease'. *The Lancet* **339**(8808): 1523–6.

Rennie, K. L. and S. A. Jebb (2005). 'Prevalence of obesity in Great Britain'. *Obesity Reviews* **6**(1): 11–12.

Rimm, E. B., P. Williams, et al. (1999). 'Moderate alcohol intake and lower risk of coronary heart disease: meta-analysis of effects on lipids and haemostatic factors.' *British Medical Journal* **319**(7224): 1523–8.

Riordan, J. (1999). 'The impact of communism on sport'. *The International Politics of Sport in the Twentieth Century*. J. Riordan and A. Kruger. London, Taylor and Francis: 48–67.

Riordan, J. (2001). *Sport, Politics, and Communism*. London, Blackwell.

Roberts, M. (2004). *Good Practice in Managing the Evening and Late Night Economy: A Literarure Review from an Environmental Perspective*. London, ODPM.

Roberts, M. (2006). 'From "creative city" to "no-go areas": the expansion of the night-time economy in British town and city centres'. *Cities* **23**(5): 331–8.

Roberts, M. (2009). 'Planning, urban design and the night-time city: still at the margins?' *Journal of Criminology and Criminal Justice* **9**(4): 487–506.

Roberts, M. and A. Eldridge (2007). 'Quieter, safer, cheaper: planning for a more inclusive evening and night-time economy'. *Planning Practice and Research* **22**(2): 253–66.

Roberts, M. and C. Turner (2005). 'Conflicts of liveability in the 24-hour city: learning from 48 hours in the life of London's Soho'. *Journal of Urban Design* **10**(2): 171–93.

Roberts, M., C. Turner, et al. (2006). 'A continental ambience? lessons in managing alcohol-related evening and night-time entertainment from four European capitals'. *Urban Studies* **43**(7): 1105–25.

Roberts, R. (1988). 'Hiccups in alcohol education'. *Health Education Journal* **47**(2-3): 73–6.

Robinson, M. and S. Robertson (2010). 'The application of social marketing to promoting men's health: a brief critique'. *International Journal of Men's Health* **9**(1): 50–61.

Robinson, T. and J. Sicard (2005). 'Preventing childhood obesity: a solution-orientated research paradigm'. *American Journal Preventative Medicine* **28**: 194–201.

Roche, M. (1992). 'Mega-events and micro-modernization: on the sociology of the new urban tourism'. *British Journal of Sociology* **43**(4): 563–600.

Roche, M. (1994). 'Mega-events and urban policy'. *Annals of Tourism Research* **21**(1): 1–19.

Rodger, J. J. (2008). 'The criminalisation of social policy'. *Criminal Justice Matters* **74**(1): 18–19.

Roemer, J. (1993). 'A pragmatic theory of responsibility for the egalitarian planner'. *Philosophy and Public Affairs* **22**(2): 146–66.

Room, R. (1976). 'Ambivalence as a sociological explanation: the case of cultural explanations of alcohol problems'. *American Sociological Review* **41**(6): 1047–65.

Room, R. (1984). 'Alcohol control and public health'. *Annual Review of Public Health* **5**(1): 293–317.

Room, R., T. Babor, et al. (2005). 'Alcohol and public health'. *The Lancet* **365**(9458): 519–30.

Room, R. and M. Livingston (2009). '[Commentary] Does it matter where the drinking is, when the object is getting drunk?' *Addiction* **104**(1): 10–11.

Rose, N. (1991). *Governing the Soul: Shaping of the Private Self*. London, Taylor and Francis.

Rose, N. (1996). 'The death of the social? re-figuring the territory of government'. *Economy and Society* **25**(3): 327–56.

Rose, N. (1999). *Powers of Freedom: Reframing Political Thought*. Cambridge, Cambridge University Press.

Rose, N. (2000). 'Government and control'. *British Journal of Criminology* **40**: 321–39.

Rose, N. and P. Miller (1992). 'Political power beyond the state: problematics of government'. *British Journal of Sociology* **43**(2): 173–205.

Rose, N., P. O'Malley, et al. (2006). 'Governmentality'. *Annual Review of Law and Social Science* **2**(1): 83–104.

Rosenberg, G. (2010). 'France cracks down on pop-up drinking parties'. *Time*, 1 June.

Ross, B. (2005). 'Fat or fiction: weighing the "obesity epidemic"'. *The Obesity Epidemic: Science, Morality, Ideology*. M. Gard and J. Wright. London, Routledge: 86–106.

Rovio, S., I. Kareholt, et al. (2005). 'Leisure-time physical activity at midlife and the risk of dementia and Alzheimer's disease'. *Lancet Neurology* **4**(11): 705–11.

Ruppel Shell, E. (2003). *War: The Inside Story of the Obesity Epidemic*. London, Atlantic Books.

Saelens, B. E., J. F. Sallis, et al. (2003). 'Neighborhood-based differences in physical activity: an environment scale evaluation'. *American Journal of Public Health* **93**(9): 1552–8.

Saguy, A. and R. Almeling (2008). 'Fat in the fire? science, the news media, and the "obesity epidemic"'. *Sociological Forum* **23**(1): 53–83.

Salecl, R. (2010). *Choice*. London, Profile Books.

Sallis, J. F., R. B. Cervero, et al. (2006). 'An ecological approach to creating active living communities'. *Annual Review of Public Health* **27**(1): 297–322.

Sallis, J. F. and K. Glanz (2009). 'Physical activity and food environments: solutions to the obesity epidemic'. *Milbank Quarterly* **87**(1): 123–54.

Schlosser, E. (2001). *Fast Food Nation: What the All-American Meal is Doing to the World*. New York, Penguin Press.

Schmidt, H. (2009a). 'Personal responsibility in the NHS constitution and the social determinants of health approach: competitive or complementary?' *Health Economics, Policy and Law* **4**(02): 129–38.

Schmidt, H. (2009b). 'Just health responsibility'. *Journal of Medical Ethics* **35**(1): 21–6.

Schwartz, B. (2004). *The Paradox of Choice: Why Less is More*. London, HarperCollins.

Schwartz, H. (1986). *Never Satisfied: A Cultural History of Diets, Fantasies and Fat*. New York, Macmillan.

Schwarzer, R. (2008). 'Modeling health behavior change: how to predict and modify the adoption and maintenance of health behaviors'. *Applied Psychology* **57**(1): 1–29.

Seiders, K. and R. D. Petty (2004). 'Obesity and the role of food marketing: a policy analysis of issues and remedies'. *Journal of Public Policy and Marketing* **23**(2): 153–69.

Select Committee on Economic Affairs (2006). *Government Policy on the Management of Risk*. London, House of Lords.

Shaper, A. G., G. Wannamethee, et al. (1991). 'Physical activity and ischaemic heart disease in middle-aged British men'. *British Heart Journal* **66**(5): 384–94.

Shaw, M., G. Davey Smith, et al. (2005). 'Health inequalities and New Labour: how the promises compare with real progress'. *British Medical Journal* **330**(7498): 1016–21.

Sheeran, P. (2002). 'Intention–behavior relations: a conceptual and empirical review'. *European Review of Social Psychology* **12**: 1–36.

Singh, G. K. and M. Siahpush (2006). 'Widening socioeconomic inequalities in US life expectancy, 1980–2000'. *International Journal of Epidemiololgy* **35**(4): 969–79.

Smith, A. and T. Fox (2007). 'From "event-led" to "event-themed" regeneration: the 2002 Commonwealth Games legacy programme'. *Urban Studies* **44**(5-6): 1125–43.

Smith, D. M. and S. Cummins (2009). 'Obese cities: how our environment shapes overweight'. *Geography Compass* **3**(1): 518–35.

Smith, R. (2010). 'Andrew Lansley: occasional Mars bar is fine if overall diet is good'. *The Telegraph*, 8 July.

Smith Maguire, J. (2008). *Fit for Consumption: Sociology and the Business of Fitness*. London, Routledge.

Smithson, C. (2009). 'Extreme makeover: gentrification transforms East Austin'. *ABC News*, 27 April.

Sontag, S. (1979). *Illness as Metaphor*. London, Penguin.

Sport England (2004). *Driving Up Participation: The Challenge for Sport*. London, Sport England.

Sport England (2007). *Building Safe, Strong and Sustainable Communities*. London, Sport England.

Sport England (2008a). *Active Design*. London, Sport England.

Sport England (2008b). *Shaping Places through Sport*. London, Sport England.

Sport England (2008c). *Sport England Strategy 2008–2011*. London, Sport England.

Sport England (2010a). 'The value of sport monitor'. www.sportengland.org/research/value_of_sport_monitor.aspx.

Sport England (2010b) 'Active people survey'. www.sportengland.org/research/active_people_survey/active_people_survey_4.aspx

Spurlock, M. (2005a). *Don't Eat this Book*. London, Penguin.

Spurlock, M. (2005b). 'Don't go the American way'. *The Guardian*, 8 June.

Srinivasan, S., L. R. O'Fallon, et al. (2003). 'Creating healthy communities, healthy homes, healthy people: initiating a research agenda on the built environment and public health'. *American Journal of Public Health* **93**(9): 1446–50.

Stamatakis, E. and M. Chaudhury (2008). 'Temporal trends in adults' sports participation patterns in England between 1997 and 2006: the Health Survey for England'. *British Journal of Sports Medicine* **42**(11): 901–8.

Stamatakis, E., U. Ekelund, et al. (2007). 'Temporal trends in physical activity in England: the Health Survey for England 1991–2004'. *Preventative medicine* **45**: 416–23.

Stearns, P. (1997). *Fat History: Bodies and Beauty in the Modern West*. London, New York University Press.

Steps to a Healthier US (2005). 'Steps to a healthier Austin'. www.healthierus.gov/steps/grantees/austin.html.

Stoddart, B. (1988). 'Sport, Cultural Imperialism, and Colonial Response in the British Empire'. *Comparative Studies in Society and History* **30**(04): 649–73.

Story, M. and S. French (2004). 'Food advertising and marketing directed at children and adolescents in the US'. *International Journal of Behavioral Nutrition and Physical Activity* **1**(1): 3.

Sturgis, P. and N. Allum (2004). 'Science in society: re-evaluating the deficit model of public attitudes'. *Public Understanding of Science* **13**(1): 55–74.

Suarez-Orozco, M. and M. Paez (2002). *Latinos Remaking America*. Berkeley, University of California Press.

Sui, D. Z. (2003). 'Musings on the fat city: are obesity and urban forms linked?' *Urban Geography* **24**(1): 75–84.

Sunstein, C. R. and R. H. Thaler (2003). 'Libertarian paternalism Is not an oxymoron'. *University of Chicago Law Review* **70**(4): 1159–202.

Surgeon General (2001). *Surgeon General's Call to Action to Prevent and Decrease Overweight and Obesity.* Washington DC, US Surgeon General.

Swain, D. P. and B. A. Franklin (2006). 'Comparison of cardioprotective benefits of vigorous versus moderate intensity aerobic exercise'. *American Journal of Cardiology* **97**(1): 141–7.

Swinburn, B. and G. Eggar (2004). 'The runaway weight gain train: too many accelerators, not enough brakes'. *British Medical Journal* **329**: 736–9.

Swinburn, B., G. Egger, et al. (1999). 'Dissecting obesogenic environments: the development and application of a framework for identifying and prioritizing environmental interventions for obesity'. *Preventive Medicine* **29**(6): 563–70.

Szmigin, I., C. Griffin, et al. (2008). 'Re-framing "binge drinking" as calculated hedonism: empirical evidence from the UK'. *International Journal of Drug Policy* **19**(5): 359–66.

Take to the Streets (2010). 'Home page'. www.taketothestreets.org/default.aspx.

Talbot, D. (2006). 'The Licensing Act 2003 and the problematization of the night-time economy: planning, licensing and subcultural closure in the UK'. *International Journal of Urban and Regional Research* **30**(1): 159–71.

Tanasescu, M., M. F. Leitzmann, et al. (2002). 'Exercise type and intensity in relation to coronary heart disease in men'. *Journal of the American Medical Association* **288**(16): 1994–2000.

Thaler, R. and C. R. Sunstein (2008). *Nudge: Improving Decisions About Health, Wealth and Happiness.* New Haven, CT, Yale University Press.

Thaler, R. H. and C. R. Sunstein (2003). 'Libertarian paternalism'. *American Economic Review* **93**(2): 175–9.

Thomson, A., R. Sylvester and M. Leroux (2010). 'Raise drink prices and defy "immoral" supermarkets, Tory strategist demands'. *The Times*, 23 January.

Thorburn, A. W. (2005). 'Prevalence of obesity in Australia'. *Obesity Reviews* **6**(3): 187–9.

Tierney, J. (2006). '"We want to be more European": the 2003 Licensing Act and Britain's night-time economy'. *Social Policy and Society* **5**(4): 453–60.

Tiesdell, S. and A.-M. Slater (2006). 'Calling time: managing activities in space and time in the evening/night-time economy'. *Planning Theory and Practice* **7**(2): 137–57.

Time Out London. (2008). 'The Light Bar'. www.timeout.com/london/bars/reviews/13152.html.

Townshend, T. and A. A. Lake (2009). 'Obesogenic urban form: Theory, policy and practice'. *Health and Place* **15**(4): 909–16.

Transport for London (2005). *Transport for London's Five Year Investment Programme 2005/06–09/10.* London, TfL.

Transport for London (2007). *London Travel Report.* London, TfL.

Transport for London (2010). *Cyling Revolution London.* London, TfL.

Treichler, P. (1988). 'AIDS, homophobia and biomedical discourse: an epidemic of signification'. *AIDS: Cultural Analysis, Cultural Activism*. D. Crimp. Boston, MIT Press: 31–70.

Tudge, C. (2004) *So Shall We Reap: The Concept of Enlightened Agriculture*. London: Penguin

Turner, B. (1984). *The Body and Society: Explorations in Social Theory*. Oxford, Blackwell.

Turner, B. (1995). *Medical Power and Social Knowledge*. London, Sage.

Turner, B. (2004). *The New Medical Sociology. Social Forms of Health and Illness*. New York, WW Norton and Co.

United States Department of Health and Human Services (2000). *Healthy People 2010: The Cornerstone of Prevention*. Washington DC: US HHS.

United States Department of Health and Human Services (2008). *2008 Phyiscal Activity Guidelines for Americans*. Washington, DC, US DHHS.

United States Surgeon General (2001). *Surgeon General's Call to action to Prevent and Decrease Overweight and Obesity*. Washington, DC: US Surgeon General.

United States Surgeon General (2010). *The Surgeon General's Vision for a Healthy and Fit Nation*. Rockville, US Department of Health and Human Services.

UNOSDP (2008). *Harnessing the Power of Sport for Development and Peace: Recommendations to Governments*. Geneva, United Nations Sport for Development and Peace International Working Group.

Urban Task Force (1999). *Towards an Urban Renaissance: The Report of the Urban Task Force*. London, Urban Task Force.

Valentine, G., S. Holloway, et al. (2007). *Drinking Places: Where People Drink and Why*. London Joseph Rowntree Foundation.

Valverde, M. (1998). *Diseases of the Will: Alcohol and the Dilemmas of Freedom*. Cambridge, Cambridge University Press.

Van Der Merwe, J. (2007). 'Political analysis of South Africa's hosting of the rugby and cricket World Cups: lessons for the 2010 Football World Cup and beyond?' *Politikon: South African Journal of Political Studies* **34**(1): 67–81.

Vincent, N. (2009). 'What do you mean I should take responsibility for my own ill health?' *Journal of Applied Ethics and Philosophy* **1**: 39–51.

Visit London (2010). *Key Visitor Statistics 2009*. London, Visit London.

Wagenaar, A., M. Salois, et al. (2009). 'Effects of beverage alcohol price and tax levels on drinking: a meta-analysis of 1003 estimates from 112 studies'. *Addiction* **104**: 179–90.

Waitt, G. (2008). 'Urban festivals: geographies of hype, helplessness and hope'. *Geography Compass* **2**(2): 513–37.

Walton, H., A. Longo, et al. (2008). 'A contingent valuation of the 2012 London Olympic Games'. *Journal of Sports Economics* **9**(3): 304–17.

Walton, S. (2001). *Out of It*. London, Penguin.

Wann, M. (1999). *Fat? So?* New York, Ten Speed Press.

Wannamethee, G. and A. G. Shaper (1992). 'Physical activity and stroke in British middle aged men'. *British Medical Journal* **304**(6827): 597–601.

Wannamethee, S. G., A. G. Shaper, et al. (2000). 'Physical activity and mortality in older men with diagnosed coronary heart disease'. *Circulation* **102**(12): 1358–63.

Wardle, J., S. Sanderson, et al. (2002). 'Parental feeding style and the inter-generational transmission of obesity risk'. *Obesity* **10**(6): 453–62.

Wareham, N. J., E. M. F. van Sluijs, et al. (2005). 'Physical activity and obesity prevention: a review of the current evidence'. *Proceedings of the Nutrition Society* **64**(02): 229–47.

Waszkiewicz, N. and A. Szulc (2009). 'Can we better prevent binge drinking?' *Journal of Epidemiology and Community Health* **63**(7): 589.

Waters, E. and L. Baur (2003). 'Childhood obesity: modernity's scourge'. *Medical Journal of Australia* **178**(9): 422–3.

Webb, F. and A. Prentice (2006). 'Obesity amidst poverty'. *International Journal of Epidemiololgy* **35**(1): 24–30.

Webster-Harrison, P., A. Barton, et al. (2002). 'Alcohol awareness and unit labelling'. *Journal of Public Health Medicine* **24**(4): 332–3.

Wechsler, H., A. Davenport, et al. (1994). 'Health and behavioral consequences of binge drinking in college: a national survey of students at 140 campuses'. *Journal of the American Medical Association* **272**(21): 1672–7.

Weitzman, E. R., A. Folkman, et al. (2003). 'The relationship of alcohol outlet density to heavy and frequent drinking and drinking-related problems among college students at eight universities'. *Health and Place* **9**(1): 1–6.

Wells, S., K. Graham, et al. (2009a). '[Commentary] When the object is to get drunk, pre-drinking matters'. *Addiction* **104**(1): 11–12.

Wells, S., K. Graham, et al. (2009b). 'Policy implications of the widespread practice of "pre-drinking" or "pre-gaming" before going to public drinking establishments: are current prevention strategies backfiring?' *Addiction* **104**(1): 4–9.

Whelan, A., N. Wrigley, et al. (2002). 'Life in a "food desert"'. *Urban Studies* **39**(11): 2083–100.

Whitaker, R., J. Wright, et al. (1997). 'Predicting obesity in young adulthood from childhood and parental obesity'. *New England Journal of Medicine* **337**(13): 869–73.

White, M., E. Williams, et al. (2004). 'Do food deserts exist? a multi-level geographical analysis of the relationship between retail food access, socio-economic position and dietary intake. Final report to Food Standards Agency'. Newcastle: Newcastle University.

Whitworth, D. (2010). 'Why we are still binge drinking'. *The Times*, 20 January.

Wikler, D. (2002). 'Personal and social responsibility for health'. *Ethics and International Affairs* **16**(2): 47–55.

Wilkinson, J. (1996). *Unhealthy Societies*. London, Routledge.

Wilkinson, J. (2005). *The Impact of Inequality: How to Make Sick Societies Healthier*. London, New Press.

Wilkinson, R. and K. Pickett (2009). *The Spirit Level: Why More Equal Societies Almost Always Do Better*. London, Allen Lane.

Williams, J. and S. Kumanyika (2002). 'Is social marketing an effective tool to reduce health disparities?' *Social Marketing Quarterly* **13**(4): 14–32.

World Health Organization (2002) *The World Health Report: Reducing Risks, Promoting Healthy Life*. Geneva: World Health Organization.

World Health Organization (2003). *Diet, Nutrition and the Prevention of Chronic Diseases. Report of a Joint WHO/FAO Expert Consultation*. Geneva, World Health Organization.

World Health Organization (2003). 'Obesity and overweight: fact sheet'. www.who.int/hpr/NPH/docs/gs_obesity.pdf.

World Health Organization (2004). *Global Strategy on Diet, Physical Activity and Health*. Geneva, World Health Organization.

World Health Organization (2005). 'Preventing chronic diseases: a vital investment'. www.who.int/chp/chronic_disease_report/contents/en/index.html.

World Health Organisation (2010). *Global Strategy to Reduce the Harmful Use of Alcohol*. Geneva: World Health Organization.

World Health Organisation (2010). Global Information System on Alcohol and Health. www.who.int/gho/alcohol/en/index.html

Worpole, K. (1992). *Towns for People*. Milton Keynes, Open University Press.

Wrendell, M. and J. Salt (2005). *The Foreign-born Population*. London, ONS.

Wright, J. and V. Harwood, eds (2009). *Biopolitics and the 'Obesity Epidemic': Governing Bodies*. London, Routledge.

Wrigley, N., D. Warm, et al. (2003). 'Deprivation, diet, and food-retail access: findings from the Leeds "food deserts" study'. *Environment and Planning A* **35**(1): 151–88.

Yach, D. and R. Beaglehole (2004). 'Globalization of risks for chronic diseases demands global solutions'. *Perspectives on Global Development and Technology* **3**(1-2): 1–21.

Yach, D., M. Kellogg, et al. (2005a). 'Chronic diseases: an increasing challenge in developing countries'. *Transactions of the Royal Society of Tropical Medicine and Hygiene* **99**(5): 321–4.

Yach, D., S. R. Leeder, et al. (2005b). 'Global chronic diseases'. *Science* **307**(5708): 317

Yach, D., D. Stuckler, et al. (2006). 'Epidemiologic and economic consequences of the global epidemics of obesity and diabetes'. *Nature Medicine* **12**(1): 62–6.

Yajnik, C. (2004). 'Obesity epidemic in India: intrauterine origins?' *Proceedings of the Nutrition Society* **63**: 387–96.

Young, L. R. and M. Nestle (2002). 'The contribution of expanding portion sizes to the US obesity epidemic'. *American Journal of Public Health* **92**(2): 246–9.

Yu, S., J. W. G. Yarnell, et al. (2003). 'What level of physical activity protects against premature cardiovascular death? The Caerphilly study'. *Heart* **89**(5): 502–6.

Zaninotto, P., H. Wardle, et al. (2006). *Forecasting Obesity to 2010*. London, DH.

Index

Note: the following abbreviations have been used: *f* = figure; *n* = note; *t* = table

S